Traumatic Scar Tissue Management

Massage therapy principles, practice and protocols

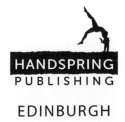

HANDSPRING
PUBLISHING

EDINBURGH

This book is dedicated to our noble colleagues and all the courageous people who grace our treatment tables

> Dear, massage therapist
> that was the best massage
> I ever had. thank you for
> letting me do your nails the
> massag felt so soft,
> On day I will ~~massa~~
> massage you back
> Some day you are the
> best massage therapist
> Thank you

Letter to NKS - from Camp Amigo camper

Traumatic Scar Tissue Management

Massage therapy principles, practice and protocols

Nancy Keeney Smith and Catherine Ryan

Forewords by Pamela Fitch BA RMT • Sandy Fritz BS MS BCTMB

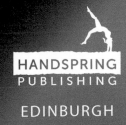

HANDSPRING
PUBLISHING

EDINBURGH

HANDSPRING PUBLISHING LIMITED
The Old Manse, Fountainhall,
Pencaitland, East Lothian
EH34 5EY, United Kingdom
Tel: +44 1875 341 859
Website: www.handspringpublishing.com

First published 2016 in the United Kingdom by Handspring Publishing

Reprinted 2018

ISBN 978-1-909141-223

British Library Cataloguing in Publication Data
A catalogue record for this book is available from the British Library

Important notice
Neither the publishers nor the authors will be liable for any loss or damage of any nature occasioned to or suffered by any person or property in regard to product liability, negligence or otherwise, or through acting or refraining from acting as a result of adherence to the material contained in this book.

Commissioning Editor Mary Law, Handspring Publishing Limited
Design direction by Bruce Hogarth, KinesisCreative
Cover design by Bruce Hogarth, KinesisCreative
Artwork by Bruce Hogarth, KinesisCreative
Copy editing by Lynn Watt
Index by Laurence Errington
Typeset by DiTech Process Solutions
Printed in Malaysia by Tien Wah Press

The
Publisher's
policy is to use
paper manufactured
from sustainable forests

CONTENTS

FOREWORD

Everyone has scars: visible and invisible. Every scar contains stories or secrets about a person's life. They may even represent specific emotions associated with the event that caused the wound. When someone shares the story of their scar or allows the scar to be touched, he or she must recall the story, feel the emotions and relive the secrets.

Applying massage therapy to manage scars reveals an ancient history. 'Rubbing', as the technique was described in antiquity, is mentioned by Hippocrates. First World War nursing sisters massaged patients with complex wounds and burns in order to help them gain function and mobility, long before antibiotics or advanced orthopedic surgical techniques. And yet scar massage therapy principles and evidence have, at times, been forgotten within standard massage therapy training. The reasons for this avoidance seem unclear considering how apt the treatment can be for certain scar conditions.

Once a therapist has acknowledged a scar, questions immediately surface and the therapist must connect with the individual's history and personality. By asking about a scar, a therapist must engage interpersonally and behave compassionately. It is possible that the client may feel pride regarding a scar. Or the individual may feel embarrassed or even ashamed of the scar. It is impossible to simply touch a scar without considering the story or asking questions: what does this scar represent? How did it happen? Did it hurt? Does it hurt now? How does this scar affect the client's capacity to move or function? Does this scar affect the client's self-image negatively or positively?

Massage therapists commonly encounter client scars when they effleurage over the body. Many therapists may feel curious about the scar but until recently, massage therapy training did not include specific knowledge or clinical considerations about scar tissue. *Traumatic Scar Tissue Management: Massage Therapy Principles, Practice and Protocols* addresses this problem by synthesizing evidence into a comprehensive discussion on massage therapy principles for scar conditions.

The authors include pathological and clinical considerations to help readers absorb and apply new-found knowledge. They describe outcomes from a biopsychosocial perspective rather than adhering to a biomedical model, reflecting the truth about scars: once they become chronic, clients are the experts in how the scars feel, move and contribute to or impair function. The authors wisely emphasize the far-reaching consequences and life-altering effects of traumatic scarring that may result in clients feeling betrayed by their bodies. And they stress the importance of professionalism, boundaries and good communication skills when addressing clients with scars. Clients often share information about their scars that they may have not told anyone else. Indeed, many clients are grateful for the opportunity to discuss scar conditions because they might not have felt free enough to discuss them with any other person.

In addition, *Traumatic Scar Tissue Management: Massage Therapy Principles, Practice and Protocols* recognizes the need for client respect and choice. Since clients are often protective or concerned about their scars, therapists must educate the client about the possibilities for treatment and establish a clear informed consent before proceeding. The authors demonstrate the need for a transparent therapeutic process and discuss the complexities of the client–therapist partnership at length.

The authors draw upon decades of clinical experience and perspective. I have had the privilege of knowing Cathy Ryan for several years as both colleague and friend. I have read her cogent and thoughtful articles in both *Massage Therapy Canada* and *Touch U* with great interest. Our professional roles have intersected for many years and when discussions arise regarding how to move forward on a problem, Cathy's quiet and articulate presence helps to find practical and evidence-informed solutions. This book draws upon Cathy's passion for writing as well as her considerable knowledge about how fascia works and how it might impact the development and treatment of scarring.

I first had the pleasure to meet Nancy Keeney Smith after she presented her research at the 2013 Massage Therapy Foundation Research Conference in Boston. Nancy shared case reports based on over 10 years' work at Children's Burns Camp of North Florida. She told passionate, compelling and remarkable stories about how basic massage therapy skills were able to help camp survivors with a variety of scars and burns. I was fortunate to continue our conversations when we met again at another seminar in New Brunswick. Nancy understands the challenges of burn and scar survivors completely. Her finely tuned clinical and interpersonal skills reflect decades of hands-on care of this mostly hidden population.

This remarkable resource breaks new ground. It describes the wound healing process and considers how therapists' hands can reduce anxiety, pain, inflammation, and tissue tension. It stitches together the importance of manual therapies with collaborative therapeutic partnerships and therapist selfcare. It positions the profession's capacities to help clients with scars within an outcomes-based framework that may be employed by educators, massage therapists and researchers. To my knowledge, no other reference comprehensively combines the etiology, and factors associated with scars with massage therapy treatment guidelines and principles.

I hope that *Traumatic Scar Tissue Management: Massage Therapy Principles, Practice and Protocols* inspires massage therapists to look between its covers for answers to their questions and to seek evidence-informed treatment solutions for client scars.

Pamela Fitch, BA, RMT
Author, *Talking Body Listening Hands*
Faculty, Algonquin College
June 2015

FOREWORD

I am fond of saying that it takes a bushel basket full of knowledge and skill to intelligently apply a teaspoon of treatment. The more complex a client situation and story, the more you have to know to gently apply massage. This textbook, *Traumatic Scar Tissue Management: Massage Therapy Principles Practice and Protocols*, created by authors Nancy Keeney-Smith and Cathy Ryan, reflects these sayings in a logical, intentional and intuitive way. The text diligently but concisely presents the information and research necessary to intelligently and intuitively support successful scar tissue formation or to improve scar tissue function. A scar is a solution to the problem related to injury. Because the healing process involves scar formation, we need to respect how the body knits together and reforms the integrity of the body after tissue damage.

The use of massage and other forms of manual therapy introduces mechanical force by pushing and pulling on the tissue. Regardless of the style of massage this is what is done. Skilful pushing and pulling during massage loads soft tissue to produce a variety of strain patterns in the tissue to challenging the tissue to respond. Clear intent during the massage sends clear message to the tissues so the response is therapeutic. Therapeutic loading technique is the overarching term used by the authors. Readers should be pleased with the clear descriptions of methods in the assessment and treatment section of the text.

When working with soft tissue scars, we need to consider many factors and this book provides the necessary information to make informed decisions to best interact with the each individual who seeks our help. The authors skilfully weave together the various approaches used by massage and other manual therapists without promoting one particular style. Scar tissue management is an outcome and a process. Scar tissue management is not a method or a technique or even a modality.

A scar is part of the person and cannot be separated from the experiences related to the events that resulted in the scar. I have scars as many, if not all people do. Some scars involve soft tissue. Some scars function well. Some scars are complex. Some scars bind down and create limits. I had open heart surgery in 2006. I have a scar on my chest that I massaged using methods described in this text. It is a visible reminder that I am alive. Those that have scars have stories. With massage methods we can support and sustain a mobile and functioning scar. We can respectfully and compassionately listen to the story. The authors have wisely included content in the book to help us be therapeutic listeners. We need to understand and acknowledge the solution the scar provided and we can help the scar evolve as the tissue function changes and we heal.

If you are drawn to work with individuals and their scars, this book provides the information needed. You however will need to allow each story the scar tells teach you how to listen.

Sandy Fritz BS MS BCTMB
Lapeer, Michigan, USA
August 2015

PREFACE

More people are surviving traumatic events than ever before and sometimes survival can come with a *price*, in the form of detrimental scars.

Scars are not obligated to be problematic. In fact our bodies have an amazing, innate capacity to heal wounds. However, the process does not always unfold seamlessly and the end product is not always ideal. And sometimes scars can be disingenuous, on the surface all may look good however, below the surface the person's reality can be a whole other story.

We wrote this book to help the myriad of patients whose journey of healing and recovery doesn't stop when their wounds are stitched and *healed-over*.

Facilitating the healing of wounds and minimizing the aesthetic, emotional and functional impact of pathophysiological scars on the patient constitutes a central focus of the authors' clinical practice.

We have woven client stories, clinical anecdotes and relevant research into each chapter in an effort to give full credence to the scientific, technical and empathetic elements of the work.

In this book you will also find a robust chapter on communication and the therapeutic relationship, because we recognize that as a healing tool, establishing respectful connection, cultivating our patients' sense of trust, and our words can be every bit as therapeutic as our hands.

Whether you have a private practice, practice in a multi-modal clinical setting, are an urban or rural therapist and no matter where you are on this planet, the material covered in this book is relevant to your practice, because wounds and scars are universal. And scar tissue that interferes with structure and function and adversely impacts quality of life can be safely addressed by a professional, properly trained massage therapist.

Our aim is to provide other therapists with an evidence-informed guide that will assist with the development of their clinical expertise, enabling them to work safely and confidently with patients recovering from trauma of any kind whether accidental or surgical.

We hope you put this book to good use.

Nancy Keeney Smith LMT, MLD
Gainsville, Florida, USA
and
Catherine Ryan RMT
Telkwa, British Columbia, Canada
July 2015

ACKNOWLEDGEMENTS

A thank you to the extraordinary family I have – my husband, Forrest, daughter Daren and son Michael. Thank you for the eye rolling, the encouraging words and allowing me the space to always try something new.

To Cathy Ryan – thanks, chica, for not letting on that I am a clinician and not a writer. You, my friend, are exceptional at both.

Pam Fitch – see above.

To Diana Thompson for suggesting a presentation in Boston; to the wonderful and dedicated North Florida Children's Burn Camp volunteers at Camp Amigo for giving a massage therapist a chance to prove massage therapy does make a difference; to Rose Dean for her pursuit of making sure everyone she came in contact with knew that massage therapy changed her scars and quality of life; to Diane Garrison, Dana Ruben, Dr Annie Morien and Raquel Torres – many great memories from Camp in holding my hand through research; heartfelt thanks to Julie Speigel for her encouragement and compassion; hugs and much appreciation to Paul Davenport, Director and mentor from the best darn school in the world, The Florida School of Massage.

Much admiration to the entire staff at Handspring Publishing for the handholding, encouragement and guidance.

Thanks so much to all my wonderful clients that allowed me to 'explore' their treatment protocols and to the case managers and physicians that recognized massage therapy can be cost effective and beneficial to those with traumatic scarring.

We've only just begun …

NKS

My amazing partner and family, thank you for your love, support and encouragement and all of the ways you enrich my life and nourish my soul. Aleila, thank you for being the consummate role model of integrity, graciousness and working for the greater good – you inspire me daily.

Nancy Keeney Smith, thank you for boldly stepping into the world of massage therapy (MT) research and for having the courage to challenge the status quo. I am humbled by your knowledge, passion, compassion and dedication and all you do for those who grace your treatment table. You rock sister-friend.

Thank you to the lovely Mary Law who, serendipitously, brought Nancy and I together to collaborate on this book. And thank you to all the fine people at Handspring for their interest in and devotion to publishing bodywork, movement and manual therapy materials for the professional. Lynn Watt (our editor) – you are the bomb!

Over a lengthy career I have had the great privilege of being in the company of, and to learn from, outstanding educators, colleagues and students. A few that I acknowledge here have not only impacted me in significant ways but have also contributed, immeasurably, to progressing the profession: Andrew Lewarne, Annette Ruiten-beek, Donelda Gowan-Moody, Pamela Fitch and Rick Overeem – thank you all. Doug Alexander, thank you for your mentoring and for providing me with a garden to cultivate my writing. Susan Brimner, thank you for being the best MT teacher a fledgling could have ever hoped for and for introducing me to the world of scar tissue massage.

Thank you to all who support, promote and engage in MT research. I, like many, continually evolve and elevate my quality of care because of your efforts. RMTBC, I so appreciate your research efforts and research library.

Thank you to the Canadian Massage Therapy regulatory colleges for all you do to establish and ensure high professional standards and registrant delivery of safe, effective and ethical care.

To all who have graced my treatment table: it has been a privilege to facilitate care on your behalf. You have taught me and touched me in deeply meaningful ways.

Lastly, thank you, the reader; the true value of this book will be revealed through your hands ... off the page and on to the table.

CR

GLOSSARY AND KEY CONCEPTS

All the words defined in this Glossary are highlighted in color the first time they appear in the text

Active listening (aka paraphrasing)
The therapist's ability to recount the client's expressed thoughts and feelings in order to clarify the client-identified treatment goals and therapeutic needs.

Acute pain
Pain provoked by noxious stimuli in conjunction with injury and/or disease.

Acute stress disorder (ASD)
Characterized by the development of severe anxiety, dissociative, and other symptoms that occur within 1 month after exposure to an extreme traumatic stressor such as an injury, unplanned or planned (surgery).

Adhesions
Scar-like tissue that forms between articulating surfaces (e.g. muscle and adjacent muscle, epimysium and deep fascia of the limbs, viscera and adjacent structures).

Adipocytes (fat cells)
Play a role in heat preservation, storage, and provide fascia with protection from physical trauma. Abundant in superficial fascia, adipocytes also serve as a spacer. In some regions a layer of fascia is often separated from adjacent ones by a thin layer of adipocytes.

Allodynia
Pain due to a stimulus that does not normally provoke pain – a consequence of hyperexcitation.

Alphabet techniques
Cs, Js, and Ss – combinations of bending and torsion/rotation loading used to address superficial and deeper layers of tissue.

Alpha-smooth muscle actin
Contractile protein present in myofibroblasts (MFBs).

Altered body image
Changes in the way a person perceives his/her body, as is seen with disfiguring scars.

Alternating pump and stationary circles technique
A lymphatic technique commonly applied to the side of the thorax and extremites to facilitate lymph flow.

Angiogenesis
Growth of new blood vessels, including capillary beds – as seen during wound healing.

Anxiety
A state of unease, apprehension or dread.

Aponeuroses
Dense, sheet-like fascial expansions often serving as a means for muscle attachments, connecting/linking fascia; stabilizing/supporting, force transference and energy facilitation role.

Apoptosis
Cell death.

Autonomic balance
Homeostatic and complementary functioning of the sympathetic and parasympathetic nervous systems.

Autonomic discharge
Term used to describe sympathetic nervous system-mediated autonomic phenomena, such as fasciculation, tremor, shaking, tears, eye fluttering, skin colour changes, sweating, clamminess, and emotional responses such as: laughing, crying, expression of anger, irritation or aggression that can be triggered during panic and anxiety attacks, when under stress and sometimes during massage therapy treatments especially when a somatic memory occurs. Autonomic discharge can occur as a local or multisystem event.

Autonomic nervous system (ANS)
Mediates involuntary function of viscera, glands, smooth muscle, cardiac muscle and other structures. The ANS is subdivided into the parasympathetic (PSNS) and sympathetic nervous (SNS) systems.

Axillary web syndrome (AWS)
Also known as cording, is characterized by painful cording or strings of hardened lymph tissue in the axilla and can extend down the arm or into the chest wall. AWS is thought to be fibrosis of the fascial sheath surrounding lymph vessels and is likely triggered by axillary node dissection and subsequent disruption of lymphatic flow or physical insult of the tissue during the surgical procedure.

Barrier
Is defined as the point where the therapist perceives the first slight resistance to their manually applied tissue challenge. Engaging barrier is commonly used as both an assessment/evaluation and treatment method and barrier can be classified as either normal or pathological.

Bending technique
A therapeutic loading technique involving combined compression and tension loading. One side of the tissue is compressed as the other side is elongated, often performed cross fiber – intended to influence tissue length, tissue glide and fluid movement and mechanical cleavage/disengagement of undue cross-links.

Best research evidence
The best available clinical, client-centered research pertaining to accuracy, safety and efficiency of diagnostic/assessment procedures, prognostic markers and therapeutic interventions.

Bind
When assessing barrier, once barrier is reached or surpassed, tissues shift from a state of relative ease when challenged by therapist-applied motion/glide to a state of bind – essentially a stop-point or end-range of tissue mobility. Skin and fascia display increased bulk, firmness and tension when bind is reached.

Biotensegrity/tensegrity
Terms used to describe a bioarchitecture where structural integrity is maintained by continuous balance of tension and compression resistant forces. Biotensegrity supports the concept of anatomical and perceptive continuity vs segregated and functionally-isolated parts.

Body Awareness
Conscious, attentional focus on internal sensations, including consideration of the physical, physiological, psychological and existential aspects of self. Such perceptions are subjective and phenomenological aspects of proprio- and interoception and are considered modifiable by mental processes including attention, interpretation, appraisal, beliefs, memories, conditioning, attitudes and affect. Enhancing body awareness is considered a key mechanism of action in various therapeutic approaches such as yoga, body-oriented psychotherapy, various movement modalities and MT. Increased body awareness can assist with management of certain physiological and psychological symptoms (e.g. anxiety, tension and habitual stress-response patterns) associated with chronic pain, stress disorders and trauma.

Body Literacy
The ability to identify and articulate sensory experiences.

Bradykinin
Inflammatory mediator – a potent vasodilator, increases vascular permeability, stimulates pain receptors and causes contraction of extravascular smooth muscles (e.g. myofibroblasts).

Breast-conserving therapy (BCT)
Surgical removal of the least possible amount of breast tissue when removing a malignant tumor, and usually includes additional therapy after surgery (e.g. radiation).

Burnout
The physical and emotional exhaustion that an individual can experience when they have low job satisfaction or feel overwhelmed by their work or workload.

Calcitonin gene-related peptide (CGRP)
Neuropeptide, widely distributed throughout the central and peripheral nervous systems. CGRP, a potent vasodilator and sensitizing agent, plays a significant role in wound healing processes (e.g. angiogenesis and wound closure) and is implicated in chronic pain and migraine headaches.

Capsular contracture
Envelopment of an implanted device (e.g. silicone or saline breast implants, artificial joint, pacemaker) in a fibrous collagen capsule. The fibrous capsule can incapacitate the device by compressing/squeezing, distorting or causing the device to migrate or capsular contracture (fibrosis) can result in functional impairments and pain.

Central nervous system (CNS)
Comprises the brain, spinal cord, meninges (connective tissue membranes), cerebral spinal fluid (CSF) and cells, which collectively monitor and regulate biological activity.

Central sensitization
Increased responsiveness of nociceptive neurons in the CNS, typified by allodynia and hyperalgesia. Another hypothesis suggests heightened sensation may be due to neuroplastic changes resulting in the facilitated processing of pain messaging.

Chemokines
Small molecules released by cells at the site of injury or infection which bind to receptors on the surface of target cells, giving rise to intracellular signals that stimulate chemotaxis.

Chemotaxis
Migration of inflammatory and reparative cells to the wound site.

Chronic/persistent pain
Pain that persists for more than 6 months, often years, and may or may not be linked to a previous injury or body damage. Chronic pain is associated with significant functional, structural and chemical changes in the brain – termed sensitization, super or hypersensitization.

Chronic (pathophysiological) stress response
Occurs when stress stimulus exceeds our natural regulatory capacity and ability to return to homeostasis, characterized by the prolonged and/or elevated presence of stress hormones. The physical and psychological ramifications of chronic stress presents a host of clinical problems and the chronic propagation of stress response mechanisms have deleterious long-range effects.

Cicatrix
Another term for scar – the fibrous *replacement* tissue that is laid down following injury or disease.

Client-centered care
Therapeutic interaction that extends beyond the delivery of services to include client advocacy, empowerment and involvement in decision-making. Client-centered care is respectful of and responsive to individual patient preferences, needs, and values, and ensures that patient values guide all clinical decisions.

Clinical decision-making
Therapist ability to synthesize and analyze information in order to formulate and progress therapeutic interventions.

Collagen
Fibrous protein found in connective tissue, dermis, and fascia which provides tensile strength, guards against over extension and can store and release energy. Collagen's elastic-stiffening potential (viscoelastic property) is considered to be one of its defining features. Type I collagen is the fiber type typically *laid down* during tissue remodeling. Under normal, healthy circumstances collagen turnover (reconstruction phase of healing) lasts from 300 to 500 days, meaning it takes that length of time for collagen to fully mature – an important consideration in post-trauma recovery and rehabilitation.

Collagen crimp
The wavy formation seen in healthy/youthful collagen – this feature supports collagen's force transmission and energy facilitation roles. Aging, immobilization, lack of movement and injury can have a negative impact on collagen crimp.

Collagen cross-link
A chemical bond between adjacent collagen fibers. Physiological linkage augments mechanical stability. Excessive collagen cross-links can interfere with slide potential and contribute to mobility restrictions. Conversely, insufficient or unstable bonds can diminish tissue integrity and stability.

Collagenase
Enzymes that break down collagen peptide bonds (degrade/digest).

Compassion fatigue
The profound emotional and physical exhaustion that helping professionals and caregivers can develop over the course of their career.

Compensatory changes
Alterations in biomechanics associated with pain (antalgic shifts) or as a result of scar tissue.

Compression technique
A therapeutic loading technique involving downward-perpendicular pressure and approximation of two structures in the form of squeezing, grasping to increase pressure – intended outcomes include influencing fluid movement and endorphin release and mechanical cleavage/disengagement of undue cross-links.

Compression fascia
Forms a pressurized compartment to augment vascular function and enhances proprioception, muscular efficiency and coordination.

Connective tissue (CT)
The bodywide system that plays a well-identified role in integrating the functions of diverse cell types within each tissue in which it invests. CT presentation is variable, ranging from firm and dense to delicate and loose.

Consolidated edema
Chronic stage edema, where inflammatory exudate has transitioned to dense fibrous CT.

Contracture
Fibrosis of tissue resulting in unrelenting or permanent shortening of fascia, muscle, joint related tissues and skin.

Cortisol
Hormone released in response to stress and low blood sugar. Prolonged elevated levels of cortisol have been linked to blood sugar alterations, immune suppression, gastrointestinal issues, cardiovascular disease, insomnia, fatigue, depression and thyroid disorders.

Countertransference
The inability of the professional to separate the therapeutic relationship from personal feelings and expectations for the client, resulting in the professional's personalization of the therapeutic relationship.

Creep
A time-dependent response of viscoelastic tissues such as CT and fascia. Not an immediate or instant reaction to strain or force but a slow reaction that may result in the tissue not returning to its original state (length). For example, postural distortions and prolonged edema can keep tissues in a state of 'over-stretch' ultimately resulting in creep and diminished tissue integrity – also see hysteresis.

Cytokines
Cell-secreted proteins, peptides or glycoproteins that affect cell behavior, for example during wound healing, fibroblast proliferation, the expression of growth factors by macrophages and the migration of neutrophils to the wound site. Cytokines (e.g. tumor necrosis factor alpha (TNF-α) and interleukin-1 (IL-1) are released, mainly by polymorphonuclear leukocytes and macrophages, during episodes of inflammation and are crucial to the normal healing process.

Debridement
Removal of foreign material and dead or damaged tissue, especially in a wound.

Deep fascia (DF; aka fascia profunda)
Generally speaking, throughout the body DF presents as a multilayer organization – typically 2–3 dense collagen bundle layers interspersed with loose CT layers. The dense layers serve to augment force transmission and the loose layers augment slide/glide.

Deformation
Change in tissue shape in response to pressure or mechanical strain.

Degloving injury
A form of avulsion injury in which an extensive portion of skin and subcutaneous tissue detaches from the underlying fascia, and muscles or deeper tissues are avulsed from underlying bone or other structures. Injury classification ranges from limited avulsion with minimal tissue loss to circumferential multi-plane involvement of muscle groups and periosteum.

Densification
Term used in fascial manipulation (the Stecco method), used to describe the increased viscosity of ground substance in the loose connective tissue (CT) layers (*sliding layers*) due to aggregation of fragmented and entangled hyaluronic acid chains. Stecco suggests that such densification at specific points impacts CT and fascia's hydrodynamic and normal viscoelastic properties and subsequent increased viscosity negatively impacts sliding between adjacent tissues/structures, resulting in myofascial pain and altered proprioception.

Dermatome
Areas of skin supplied by a single nerve root.

Dermis
The CT layer of skin just beneath the epidermis which houses lymph and blood vessels, nerve endings, sweat glands, sebaceous glands and hair follicles.

Direct release technique
Commonly used in reference to myofascial techniques, where mechanical force is applied into the restriction barrier.

Dissociation
An abnormal sense of psychological, emotional, or physical detachment, experienced as a sense of unusual separation from the body (depersonalization) and/or unusual separation from the surrounding physical environment (derealization) – generally considered a psychological defense mechanism used as a means to cope with overwhelming traumatic events.

Double-crush injury
Term used to denote when an axon, compressed in one region, becomes susceptible to injury at another site (e.g. development of a cervical radiculopathy in conjunction with carpal tunnel syndrome. Mechanisms similar to those associated with sensitization are implicated.

Dry needling
A procedure involving insertion of an acupuncture needle into a myofascial trigger point. Although an acupuncture needle is used, this is not the same as acupuncture treatment of points along an identified meridian.

Edema (aka swelling)
Accumulation of fluid in cells, tissues or cavities as a result of vessel permeability and pressure changes and lymphatic flow obstruction. Physiological edema is considered part of the natural response of the body to injury or insult.

Elastin
Protein fiber that when underhydrated is susceptible to fraying or breaking, but when appropriately hydrated is highly flexible and extensible. Elastin fibers can be stretched up to 150% their resting length without causing any injury – 20 to 30 times more than collagen can withstand.

Empathy strain
A healthcare provider's overextension of psychological resources, contributing to burnout and, for some, even causing emotional pain.

Endomysium
Fascia surrounding and investing individual muscle fibers – the most delicate or thin layer of the myofascial coverings.

Endoneurium
Fascia surrounding individual nerve fibers.

Endotenon
Fascia surrounding and investing individual tendon collagen fibrils/fibers and primary, secondary and tertiary bundles.

Endothelial cells
Simple squamous cells that line the interior surface of blood and lymphatic vessels.

Endothelium
Interior lining of blood and lymphatic vessels.

Endoscope
An instrument that is used to look inside the body (images can be viewed in real-time or taped for repeat viewing).

Entrainment
Alteration of a biological rhythm in response to external stimuli; for example, the client's breath rhythm slowing to match the speed or rhythm of the therapists applied technique strokes. In MT, entrainment is a commonly employed and useful relaxation method.

Epidermis
The tough, outermost layer of the skin.

Epimysium
Outermost covering of fascia surrounding and investing an entire muscle – typically the densest and strongest of the myofascial coverings.

Epineurium
Outermost covering of fascia surrounding an entire peripheral nerve (including its blood and lymph vessels) – innervated by the nervi nervorum. Injury, compression and inflammation of the epineurium may be a source of neuropathic pain.

Epitenon
Outermost covering of fascia surrounding an entire tendon.

Epithelial cells
Cells that line the outer layer of the skin (epidermis), the surface of most body cavities, and the lumen of fluid-filled organs.

Epithelium
The outer layer of skin and outer lining of most body cavities, and lumen of fluid-filled organs, such as the stomach and intestines.

Evidence-based practice
Integrating best research with clinical expertise and client values to inform and guide treatment protocol and delivery of care.

Extracellular matrix (ECM)
The sum total of extracellular substance, mainly ground substance and protein fibers (goo and struts), within the extracellular space. Its form and composition help determine tissue characteristics.

Fascia
Fibrocollagenous CT, its morphology shaped by tensional loading. Fascia surrounds and interpenetrates all other soft-tissues, bones, nerves, circulatory vessels and organs. In its various forms, fascia serves to connect, separate and store/provide propulsion energy. Fascia is highly innervated and therefore is considered to play a significant role in proprioception and interoception and can be a potential pain generating tissue. By shifting its fluid dynamics (e.g. changes in ground substance viscosity), fascia can alter its viscoelastic properties, rendering fascia capable of instantly changing its properties in response to demand (e.g. mechanical strain). This feature of fascia is theorized to be the mechanism by which some of the tissue changes felt during and after manual therapy occurs (e.g. softening, improved pliability and mobility).

Fascicular fascia
Augments continuity and force transmission, provides proprioceptive feedback and protection of nerve, blood vascular and lymph vessels.

Fibrin
Fibrous protein involved blood clotting. Polymerized fibrin together with platelets forms a hemostatic plug or clot at wound sites.

Fibrinolysis
The break-down or dissolving of a hemostatic plug or clot. During wound healing and repair, fibrin deposition and lysis must be balanced to maintain temporarily and subsequently remove the hemostatic seal.

Fibroblasts
Synthesize the components of the ECM, secrete the precursors of the fibrous proteins and play a significant role in soft-tissue remodeling. These highly adaptable cells are noted for their ability to change shape and function (e.g. differentiate into MFBs) in response to a variety of signals including mechanical strain. This feature of fibroblasts provides a plausible explanation for the mechanism by which myofascial/fascial techniques produce therapeutic results.

Fibronectin
Glycoprotein found in plasma and tissue. Multifunctional fibronectins interact with many extracellular substances, including collagen, and with integrin receptors on cell surfaces, enabling fibronectin to play an important role in the transmission of communication signals between cells and components of the ECM.

Fibrosis
A process culminating in the replacement of the normal structural elements of tissue with excessive, distorted and non-functional collagen (e.g. aberrant fiber/bundle arrangement, density and reduced elastic-malleability). Fibrosis is commonly seen with unchecked/chronic inflammation as a result of cumulative trauma, soft-tissue over-use or repetitive strain/motion type impairments. Fibrotic tissue within an injured area can hinder muscle regeneration and lead to incomplete functional recovery (e.g. diminished contractile capabilities, and reduced elasticity), increasing the risk of re-injury.

Fluid dynamics
Neural-mediated mechanisms or neurobiological functions that impact the volume and constituent ratio of fluid in the ECM. These mechanisms have been identified as potential catalysts for tissue changes that occur as a result of manual manipulation (e.g. fascia's ability to change its fluid ratio and subsequently its stiffness/softness).

Fluid techniques
Techniques employed to facilitate the flow of lymph and venous blood.

Force transmission
The transference of muscular force across an array of tissue. Collectively, muscle fibers/bundles and the collagen-rich intramuscular CT (i.e. myofascial coverings) are now appearing (as a unit) to be functionally significant with regard to force transmission. A significant proportion of muscular force is simultaneously transmitted multi-directionally (e.g. obliquely, laterally, linearly) – on to adjacent fascia, synergists and antagonists.

Full-thickness skin grafts (FTSG)
Removal and transplantation of the entire thickness of the dermis.

Gentle circles technique
Circular motion loading technique used to target superficial tissues. This technique is also commonly used as a form of client self-massage for scar tissue.

Glycosaminoglycan (GAGs)
Are involved in a variety of biological processes. For example, during wound healing and childhood growth phases, hyaluronic acid is known to stimulate cytokine production by macrophages thereby promoting angiogenesis. Hydrophilic GAGs found in collagen and elastin play a role in tissue hydration, shock absorption and the reduction of friction during movement. The hydrophilic nature of GAGs causes a swelling pressure, or turgor, which enables the ECM to withstand compression forces. When healthy, the meniscus of the knee joint can support profound amounts of pressure due to its high GAG content.

Golgi receptors (GRs) and Golgi tendon organs (GTOs)
A type of mechanoreceptor found in dense fascia, joint related tissues and near myotendinous junctions – responsive to contractile tension and active–moderate, sustained stretch.

Granulation tissue
Soft pink fleshy projections that form during the wound healing process, consisting of many capillaries (hypervascularity) surrounded by fibrous collagen.

Ground substance (GS)
Amorphous gel-like medium of the ECM. GS is an important metabolic interface that fills the space between fibers and cells. The hydrophilic nature of GS constituents factors significantly into tissue viscoelasticity and slide potential.

Gross stretch technique
Combination of tension and compression loading utilized to engage broader areas of tissue. Gross stretch can be used when more intense, isolating or deeper techniques are uncomfortable for the client to receive. Gross stretch can also be used to pre-warm and soften tissue prior to applying more intense type of techniques. This technique can be used to address either superficial or deeper tissue layers.

Growth factors (GFs)
Diffusible signaling proteins that stimulate cell growth, differentiation, survival, inflammation, and tissue repair. Examples include epidermal growth factor (EGF), platelet derived growth factor (PDGF) and vascular endothelial cell growth factor (VEGF).

Half-moon or circle technique
Lymphatic technique involving the circular stretching the skin and SF to facilitate lymph flow.

Health psychology
The role of psychological factors in the development, prevention, and treatment of illness and includes such areas as stress and coping, the relationship between psychological factors and physical health, and ways of promoting health-enhancing behaviors.

Homeostasis
State of physiological equilibrium.

Hyaluronic acid (HA; aka hyaluronan)
Extremely hydrophilic, highly viscous lubricant (reduces friction/drag), found throughout skin, fascia, and neural tissue – a vital component of the sliding mechanism. It is suggested that alterations in HA amount and organization may play a role in tissue changes (e.g. tissue softening and improved slide/glide) following manual manipulation.

Hydrophilic
Water-loving, the ability of a compound to attract/bind water molecules.

Hyperalgesia
Heightened pain sensation from a stimulus that normally provokes pain, a consequence of hyperexcitation involving peripheral or central sensitization or both.

Hyperarousal
Term generally used to describe when the ANS is in a state of hypervigilance or hyperactivation.

Hyperexcitation

Neurons firing too easily or too often, which in turn can make something perceived as painful feel even worse (hyperalgesia), or it can make things hurt that should not (allodynia). Injury-induced hyperexcitability is not limited to nociceptors. Hyperexcitability can also develop in myelinated afferents that normally convey innocuous information (e.g. normal movement and touch) and under neuropathic conditions, mechanical allodynia can occur.

Hyperinnervation

Exaggerated, new, nerve growth seen in early wound healing. With normal wound healing, nerve density will normalize with scar maturation. Although densities may return to normal, normal responsiveness is not always re-established, as nerve end organs cannot regenerate and therefore sensory deficit or aberrancies may occur.

Hypertrophic scar

A thickened, red and raised scar that remains within the boundaries of the original incision or wound.

Hypervascularization

Exaggerated, new, capillary growth seen in early wound healing.

Hypothalamic–pituitary–adrenal (HPA) axis

A primary component in the stress response system, consisting of the hypothalamus, anterior pituitary, cortex, and the cortex of the suprarenal gland. The HPA axis regulates stress-related processes, including secretion of stress hormones (e.g. cortisol) and under normal circumstances orchestrates the eventual return to homeostasis.

Hysteresis

A property of systems (tissues) that do not immediately respond/react to forces applied to them, but react slowly or do not return to their original state – also see creep.

Impairment

Abnormality of body structures or loss of function that occur as a result of a medical condition or trauma, such as adherences, contractures, fibrosis, postural and movement adaptations, edema, pain, anxiety, SNS-hyperarousal, disturbed sleep and altered or impaired body awareness.

Indirect release technique

Mechanical force is applied away from the restriction barrier or client is moved away from the restriction barrier (e.g. positional release or counterstrain).

Indirect trauma

The cumulative response of exposure to other people's trauma. The indicators for indirect trauma resemble those of direct trauma (e.g. intrusive imagery, SNS stimulation, anxiety and over-whelm) and can impact the therapist's personal and professional relationships.

Informed consent

Process involving the therapist's explicit explanation of all relevant information about the proposed therapeutic interventions so that the client is able to fully understand and is able to provide or decline consent to proceed with a proposed treatment plan.

Integrins

Specialized cell membrane receptors that mediate cell-to-cell and cell-to-ECM communication. Via integrins, mechanical stimulus (e.g. loading in the form of tension and compression) can evoke biochemical responses which in turn can trigger a variety of cellular responses and activities.

Intense versus invasive

An important concept for the work provided in this book. It is the nature of this work to occur as intense at times but never invasive. **Intense**: precise, focused work that may elicit a tolerable level of discomfort which does not adversely affect the client's sense of comfort, feeling of safety or relaxed breathing. **Invasive**: that which occurs to the client as unproductive or overwhelming pain, feeling like the tissues are being forced or over-powered. Anything that is perceived by the client as invasive can trigger the SNS driven guarding/protection mechanism – which can negatively impact treatment effectiveness.

Interleukins

A group of cytokines with complex immunomodulatory functions, including cell proliferation, maturation, migration and adhesion. Interleukins also play an important role in immune cell differentiation and activation.

Interoception
Includes a wide range of physiological sensations including muscular effort, tickling, pain, hunger, thirst, warmth, cold, organ-distention, sensual and pleasant touch. Interoceptive activity is mediated by interstitial receptors that are known to influence the ANS. Interoception plays a fundamental role in the relationship between one's subjective state of well-being and physiological health.

Interstitial receptors (IRs)
Type of mechanoreceptor found in various presentations of fascia, including periosteum – are multi-modal in their function. In their role as mechanoreceptors they are responsive to tension, pressure, tissue stretch and ultra-light touch.

Keloid
Exuberant scar that forms at the site of an injury or an incision and spreads beyond the borders of the original lesion. The scar is made up of a swirling mass of collagen fibers and fibroblasts.

Keratin
A structural protein that protects epithelial cells from mechanical and non-mechanical stresses that cause cell rupture and death or rendering the skin more fragile and susceptible to injury and infection.

Keratinocytes
Predominant cell type of the epidermis – produces keratin.

Kinins
Peptides (e.g. bradykinin) produced and acting at the site of tissue injury or inflammation, stimulating a variety of effects including vasodilation, smooth muscle contraction, and influencing capillary permeability.

Lifting techniques
Are aimed at lifting and separating one component away from another, for example; muscle away from underlying bone or skin away from underlying SF. Lifting techniques can be combined with tension, bending, shear and torsion and can be utilized to address both superficial and deeper tissues/layers. Vertical lifts, a form of tension loading, can be used to treat scars/tissue that can be gripped between the thumb and fingers.

Linking fascia
Plays a role in augmenting bodywide functional and perceptive continuity.

Locomotor system
Comprises the bones, joints, capsules, ligaments, fasciae, aponeuroses and all the tissues surrounding and investing skeletal muscles and their tendinous expansions.

Lymph (aka lymphatic fluid)
When the interstitial fluid enters the lymphatic system, it is termed lymph. Lymph is generally clear and transparent, or milky in appearance when emulsified fats are present.

Lymph nodes
Filter and clean the lymph before it is returned to the circulatory system. Lymph nodes contain macrophages and lymphocytes that destroy bacteria, viruses and other substances. When inflammation is part of the protective process this sometimes results in the swelling commonly identified as *swollen glands*.

Lymphadenitis
An infection and inflammation of one or more lymph nodes.

Lymphangiogenesis
Formation of new lymph vessels either by outgrowth from pre-existing lymph vessels or via progenitor cells.

Lymphangitis
A bacterial infection in the lymphatic vessels.

Lymphatic drainage
The movement of fluid and molecules from the interstitium into the lymphatic capillaries.

Lymphatic load
Refers to total sum of substances (proteins, colloids, minerals, water, cells and fat) in the interstitium that cannot be absorbed by the hematic system.

Lymphatic return
Volume of lymph returned to the blood vascular system.

Lymphatic system
A low pressure, pump-less, one-way system directed toward the heart, that transports lymph and plays a significant role in homeostasis, immunity, and wound healing.

Lymphatic transport
The movement of lymph along a succession of vessels with eventual return to the blood vascular system.

Lymphatic transport capacity
The maximum amount of lymph the system can transport in a given time frame. A healthy lymphatic system is capable of transporting 10 times the volume of normal lymphatic loads, leaving ample room for accommodating fluctuations in lymphatic load volumes.

Lymphatic vessels
Tri-laminar vessels that transport lymph from the periphery, with eventual return of usable fluid to the blood vascular system. Lymphatic vessels contain more valves and more frequent anastomoses than blood vessels – thereby reducing back flow and creating an extensive, connected network of tubes.

Lymphedema
Abnormal accumulation of protein-rich lymph due to obstruction, destruction or hypoplasia of lymph vessels.

Lymphocyte
The main cell type found in lymph – constitute the three types of white blood cells: NK (natural killer), T and B cells.

Lymphoid organs
Include the spleen, tonsils, thymus glands and Peyer's patches of the intestine. The lymphoid organs contain phagocytes and lymphocytes, which support the immune system's ability to work in full vigor.

Macrophage
A type of phagocytic white blood cell active during the early stages of wound healing. Macrophages also secrete a variety of chemotactic and GFs.

Mast cell
A granulocyte found in CT that releases substances such as heparin and histamine in response to injury or inflammation of bodily tissues.

Mastectomy
Surgical removal of all breast tissue – may be performed as prevention/prophylactic or as treatment and is sometimes combined with chemo-, radio-, hormone and other targeted therapies.

Mechanoreceptor
Sensory receptors that respond to a variety of stimuli including touch, sound, pressure, tissue deformation and movement.

Mechanotransduction
The mechanism by which a mechanical stimulus is converted into a biochemical response.

Merkel cells
Type of mechanoreceptor found in superficial skin – responsive to localized pressure, sustained loading and tissue displacement.

Mixed/associated nerve fibers
Contain both sensory and motor nerve fibers.

Motor/efferent nerve fibers
Conduct motor impulses from the CNS to peripheral tissues/organs.

Mucosa-associated lymphatic tissue (MALT)
MALT works as sentinel, protecting the digestive tract and upper respiratory system from the constant barrage of foreign matter that enter these cavities. Peyer's patches and the tonsils are part of the MALT network.

Mucopolysaccharides
See GAGs.

Myofascial pain syndrome (MPS)
Chronic pain disorder associated with local or referred pain, limited ROM or pain/discomfort with movement, autonomic phenomena, local twitch response and muscle weakness without atrophy.

Myofascial trigger point (MTrP)
Hyperirritable, palpable localized hardening in the myofascia.

Myofibroblasts (MFBs)
Exhibit both fibroblast and smooth muscle characteristics, including the ability to contract in a smooth muscle-like manner. MFBs are seen in higher concentrations in fascia subjected to higher tensional demands (e.g. plantar fascia), perimysium and in injured fascia. MFB contraction plays a major role in wound healing/remodeling, contractures and fibrosis. Biomechanically, interactions between MFBs and the ECM contribute to whole body mobility and biotensegrity.

Myokinetic/myofascial chains or meridians
A grouping or sequence of muscles/motor units – fascially and neurologically linked together to support functional (movement) and perceptive continuity.

Myotome
Groups of muscles supplied by a single nerve root.

Nerve growth factor (NGF)
Neuropeptide released during wound healing – a potent neurotrophic agent and neuronal sensitizing agent that when uncontrolled, can lead to debilitating chronic pain syndromes and an excess of NGF during wound healing is implicated in pathophysiological scar formation.

Nerve receptors
Nerve terminations that provide a means by which our CNS can keep informed as to what is happening in our external and internal environment.

Nervi nervorum
The intrinsic innervation of nerve sheaths, are nociceptive and nocifensive, meaning that they are responsive to damaging stimuli by contributing to local inflammation, thus helping to defend and maintain the nerve's local environment.
Besides signaling pain from direct stimulation, nervi nervorum may play a role in initiating events leading to neuropathic and chronic pain. Stimulation of nervi nervorum may also play a role in maintaining CNS changes associated with chronic pain states.

Neurofascia
Tri-laminar, continuous fascial covering that surrounds and invests individual nerve fibers, bundles of fibers (fascicles) and the entire nerve.

Neuropathy
A disturbance of function or pathological change in a nerve.

Neuropathic pain
Pain due to damage to or pathological changes in the CNS or peripheral nervous system (PNS) (e.g. neuritis, Bell's palsy, hypersensitization). Paresthesia and heavy pain are often associated with neuropathic pain as are abnormal interactions between the somatic and SNS.

Neuroplasticity
An adaptation trait of the nervous system (NS) that enables modification of function and structure in response to demands via the strengthening, weakening, pruning, or adding of synaptic connections and by promoting neurogenesis. A key principle of neuroplasticity is that brain activity (increased or decreased) promotes brain adaptation and reorganization.

Neuropeptides
Signaling molecules that influence neuronal and brain activity. Neuropeptides released during wound healing modulate a number of important aspects of the process such as cell proliferation, cytokine and growth factor production, antigen presentation, mast cell degradation, increased vascular permeability and neovascularization.

Neutrophil
A type of phagocytic white blood cell active during the early stages of wound healing.

Nociception
Threatening stimuli activated by varying thresholds not activated during normal movement. In addition to sensitivity to tissue deformation, nociceptors are sensitive to endogenous chemicals (e.g. inflammatory and pain mediators) released as a result of disrupted tissue or by inflammatory cells. These nociceptive stimulants can have long-lasting effects and often potentiate one another.

Nociceptor
Threat detector responsive to various noxious stimuli that objectively can damage tissue (e.g. extreme hot, cold, swelling, tissue damage or prior tissue damage) and stimuli can subjectively be perceived as painful. Although there is a common tendency to identify nociceptors as pain receptors, not all nociceptive signals are interpreted as pain and not every pain sensation originates from a nociceptor.

Nociceptive pain
Pain that arises from actual or threatened damage to non-neural tissue – peripherally driven by chemical, thermal or mechanical insults to tissues housing nociceptors.

Non-collagenous cross-link proteins
Structural protein struts (fibrillin, fibronectin and laminin) providing flexible-stability and a pathway for transfer of mechanical strain/tensional loading information from cell to cell.

Oscillation technique
A form of shaking, movement back and forth and rocking of the tissue – effective in mobilizing tissue layers/disengaging stuck tissue and increasing the lubrication potential of HA in the sliding layers. Oscillations are commonly applied in combination with compression or lifting. Oscillations can be used to address superficial and deeper layers of tissue.

Oxytocin
Hormone that plays role in regulation of circadian homeostasis and is involved in social recognition, bonding and trust formation.

Pacini and paciniform corpuscles (PCs)
Type of mechanoreceptor found in deeper skin and deeper, dense fascia – responsive to vibration, mechanical pressure changes in tissue and light, brief tangential loading.

Pain
A complex and multi-etiological experience described as an 'unpleasant sensory and emotional experience associated with actual or potential tissue damage, or described in terms of such damage'.

Paresthesia
Altered sensations; e.g. burning, numbness, tingling.

Parasympathetic nervous system (PSNS)
In the absence of stress or under normal circumstances, the PSNS governs self-preservative functions, such as homeostasis and wound healing.

Pathological cross-link
Fibrotic collagen adherences that result dysfunction. Such links are noted as pathological indicating that the adherences are fibrotic vs chemical.

Pathophysiological scar
The result of prolonged, aberrant wound healing involving excessive fibroblast activity and collagen deposition. Regardless of etiology and size, pathophysiological scars display characteristics that differ from normal skin, viscera and fascia (e.g. thickened, dense, rough, lumpy, compromised elasticity and mobility, altered or abnormal neuro-functioning and discoloration).

Peripheral sensitization
Increased responsiveness of nociceptive neurons in the periphery.

Perimysium
Fascia surrounding and investing fascicles (i.e. bundles) of muscle fibers.

Perineurium
Fascia surrounding/investing bundles of nerve fibers.

Peyer's patches
Part of MALT, these tonsil-like looking patches embedded in the wall of the small intestine, place macrophages in the perfect position to capture and destroy bacteria in the intestine.

Phagocyte
Cells (e.g. macrophage and neutrophil) that are able to surround, engulf, and digest microorganisms and cellular debris.

Pitting edema
An edematous region where, upon compression or pressure, a dent or pit in the tissue persists – can be graded on a scale of 1–4 depending upon the depth and duration of the pit/dent.

Post-traumatic stress disorder (PTSD)
Pronounced psychological distress experienced following significant trauma exposure, such as threat of death or serious injury of self or another that persists for more than 1 month post-trauma exposure. PTSD is characterized by three predominant categories of symptoms: re-experiencing of symptoms, avoidance of triggering symptoms and hyperarousal. PTSD is associated with a wide range of psychiatric comorbidity, poor quality of life, and social dysfunction.

Primary lymphedema
A rare, hereditary condition resulting from a deficiency in the development, structure or the function of the lymphatic system (e.g. Milroy's, Meige's disease).

Proprioceptive disinformation
Receptors entrapped in dense, fibrosed tissue can under or overestimate mechanical stimuli, thereby dis-informing local, regional, or central nerve centers. Dis-informed centers may propagate altered proprioceptive signals out to the periphery which can result in abnormal biomechanics, aberrant movement patterns, muscle compensation, joint distress and subsequently increase the risk of injury (acute or over-use) and pain.

Proprioceptors
Mechanoreceptors involved in perception of movement and body position, location/orientation in space and coordination of movement along a kinetic chain or myofascial meridian.

Proteoglycan (PG)
Glycoproteins found primarily in CT and formed of subunits of glycosaminoglycans linked to a protein core. PGs retain water and form a gel-like substance (e.g. the viscous fluid of mucous and GS) through which ions, hormones and nutrients can move freely. Proteoglycans play an important role in the viscoelastic property of tissue/structures and also appear to play an important role in cell signaling and the binding of GFs and chemokines.

Provisional matrix
During the early stage of wound healing, a makeshift ECM that provides a structural framework for cellular attachment and subsequent cellular proliferation.

Pruritus
Itching sensation associated with a drug reaction, food allergy, kidney or liver disease, cancers, parasites, aging , dry skin, contact skin reaction, such as poison ivy, and pathophysiological scars.

Pumping technique
A lymphatic technique involving the use of the circle-shaped stretching and compressions of the skin to facilitate lymph flow.

Quality of Well-being Scale (QWS)
A general quality of life questionnaire which measures overall status and well-being over the previous 3 days in four areas: physical activities, social activities, mobility, and symptom/problem complexes.

Radiculopathy
Nerve or nerve root pathology that may result in pain or paresthesia felt in a corresponding dermatome, myotome or sclerotome.

Referred pain
Pain perceived at a location other than the site of the painful stimulus/ origin: a common occurrence in problems associated with the musculoskeletal system (e.g. MTrPs).

Remodeling (aka maturation stage of wound healing)
The final stage of wound healing during which stronger collagen fibers replace provisional ones and realign along tension lines. And cells that are no longer needed are removed by apoptosis.

Research literacy
The ability to find, understand, and critically evaluate research for the purpose of application into one's professional practice.

Retinaculae
Dense fascial bands that play an important proprioceptive and force transmission role.

Rotary technique
A lymphatic technique commonly applied to the thorax to facilitate lymph flow.

Ruffini organs (ROs)
A type of mechanoreceptor found in high concentrations in many forms of fascia and joint related tissues – responsive to slowly-applied and sustained, deeper pressure, slow/deep strokes and lateral/tangential mechanical stretch.

Scar
Mark left in various tissues or an internal organ following the healing of a wound, sore or injury. The bulk of the scar (replacement) tissue is made up of fibrous CT.

Scooping technique
Lymphatic technique used only on the extremities, involving half circle movements to facilitate lymph flow.

Secondary lymphedema
Occurs as a result of damage to the lymphatic system (e.g. infection, surgical removal of lymph nodes, postsurgical scarring or the use of radiation during cancer treatment).

Sedation techniques
Techniques that have a calming or tempering effect on the nervous system.

Self care
Those practices and activities we engage in: when healthy to prevent illness; during acute illness or injury to speed healing and decrease the incidence of complications or recurrence; and during chronic illness/injury to help manage and minimize the impact and support good quality of life.

Selfcare maintenance
Behaviors practiced by clients with chronic presentations to maintain physical and emotional stability.

Selfcare management
Response to sensations and/or changes when they occur. An important component of self-management, facilitated by somatic awareness, is the client's ability to reliably determine how his/her sensations change in response to MT treatment and/or selfcare practices and activities.

Selfcare monitoring
Comprises routine, vigilant body monitoring, surveillance, or *body listening* – the goal of self-monitoring is the ability to recognize that a change has occurred.

Sensitization
Changes in the PNS or CNS (adaptive or pathologic) that lead to heightened nociceptive responses and/or lower thresholds; i.e. a lower intensity stimuli results in increased responsiveness. Clinically, sensitization may only be inferred indirectly from presenting phenomena such as hyperalgesia or allodynia, and may include dysfunction of endogenous pain control systems. The process of sensitization involves noxious stimuli that results in prolonged pain or misinterpretation of non-noxious stimuli and explains how pain can exist in the absence of acute trauma or observable irritation of neuronal structures as is seen with some presentations of chronic pain.

Sensory/afferent nerve fibers
Conduct sensory information impulses from the periphery to the CNS.

Separating fascia
Limits the spread of infection, provides structural support, helps absorb shock, and augments sliding between articulating structures/surfaces.

Serotonin
Neurotransmitter involved in regulating mood, appetite, intestinal motility and sleep cycles.

Sclerotome
Area of bone or fascia supplied by a single nerve root.

Shear technique
A therapeutic loading technique involving oblique or laterally applied sliding type movement, of one tissue or layer in reference to another. Intended outcome is to influence fluid dynamics (e.g. GS and HA changes: shift GS viscosity and increase the lubrication potential of HA in the sliding layers), generate heat and mechanical cleavage/disengagement of undue cross-links.

Skin
The protective outer layer of covering of the body that creates a barrier to the outside world and plays an important role in homeostasis.

Skin graft
Medical procedure where a patch of skin is removed by surgery from one area of the body and is transplanted to another area – performed as a means of barrier and aesthetic restoration.

Skin rolling technique
A combination of lifting, tension and shearing loading, commonly used in the treatment of postsurgical scarring and scars associated with burns. Skin rolling has been shown to shift fluid dynamics, modify collagen density, improve tissue pliability and sedate SNS hyperactivity and therefore can be useful for ANS rebalancing. Skin rolling can be used to address various layers of tissue.

Sliding layers/mechanism
A delicate CT network, rich in HA, that allows for change and movement. The sliding layers/mechanism is found bodywide on both a macro and micro level.

Somatic/tissue memory
Memory stored in tissue and expressed as changes in the biological stress response. Pert asserts that cells

and neuropeptides hold and transport memories throughout the entire body. Such stored information may get triggered, resulting in reactions such as fear, panic, syncope (partial or complete loss of consciousness), and somatization.

Somatization
A tendency to experience and communicate psychological distress in the form of physical symptoms.

Somatoemotional response
In MT – used to describe an emotional response or release triggered by touch or movement of the client's body.

Split-thickness skin graft (STSG)
Removal and transplantation of the epidermis and only a portion of the dermis.

State anxiety
The experience of unpleasant feelings when confronted with specific situations, demands or a particular object or event. State anxiety is considered a temporary condition manifesting as an interruption of an individual's normal emotional state or change in equilibrium in response to a perceived threat such as following trauma or during a stressful event. The person's anxiety resolves when the stimulus/trigger perceived as threatening discontinues or goes away.

Stress
Any physical, physiological or psychological stimulus that disrupts homeostasis. Stress is further defined as the relationship between the person and the environment that is appraised by the person as taxing or exceeding his/her resources and endangering his/her well-being. Appraisal and coping are key to this definition and lead to the subjective experience of stress. Also, generally speaking, the degree of perceived threat (appraisal) influences the magnitude of the stress response.

Stress response adaptation
Any of the vast array of potential stress responses, such as fight, flight, freeze and tend/befriend.

Stress disorder
Severe or pathological stress reactions, wherein the various stress response mechanisms are sustained and remain active long after imminent danger is no longer present (e.g. PTSD, ASD and dissociation).

Stress response
Any cognitive, physiological, affective or behavioral response activated by real or perceived danger, injury or trauma. Stress response is innately intended to enhance coping, adaptation and chances of survival and normally terminates as soon as the danger has passed (i.e. return to homeostasis).

Structural proteins
Structural struts that while variably flexible, provide strength and stability (e.g. collagen and elastin).

Substance P
A neuropeptide acting as a neurotransmitter and as a neuromodulator, it is normally present in minute quantities in the NS and intestines and is found in higher concentrations in inflamed tissue. Substance P is a potent vasodilator and stimulator of smooth muscle contraction and plays a significant role in pain sensation and the transmission of pain impulses from peripheral receptors to the CNS. Substance P is also indicated in the regulation of depression and anxiety.

Superficial fascia (SF) (aka panniculus fascia)
Continuous with the dermis, the SF lies directly beneath the skin, supporting the skin's structural integrity. Essentially, the SF surrounds the entire torso and the extremities, surrounding organs, glands and (most but not all) neurovascular tissues – many of the larger circulatory, lymphatic and neural structures track through the SF.

Sympathetic nervous system (SNS)
Mediates activity associated with emergency or stress response. When activated, the SNS facilitates: acceleration of heart rate; elevation of blood pressure; constriction of peripheral blood vessels; and redirection of blood from the skin and intestines to the brain, heart and skeletal muscles.

Tension technique
A therapeutic loading technique involving tensile opposition of structures in the form traction, drag, glide, stretch, extension and elongation – intended outcome is lengthening tissue and mechanical cleavage/disengagement of undue cross-links.

Transforming growth factor beta-1 (TGF-β1)
Part of the superfamily of cytokines known to play a significant role in the remodeling stage of wound healing – stimulating collagen proliferation.

Therapeutic environment
Encompasses both the physical clinical space and MT demeanour.

Therapeutic loading techniques
A series of techniques that are intended to engage CT and fascia (SF and DF). Loading techniques (tension, compression, bending, shear and torsion/rotation) involve the application of mechanical strain and therefore have the potential to influence neurophysiological and integrin mediated responses. Manually applied strain is also thought to mechanically disengage fine pathological cross-links and cleave excessive/undue collagen cross-links.

Therapeutic relationship
Encompasses the professional and ethical working alliance and relationship that is established between client and therapist.

Thixotrophy
The process by which thermal or mechanical energy causes GS colloids to shift from a gel-like/gluey consistency to a more watery, liquid (sol) consistency. When energy (movement, mechanical strain of tissue) is present or initiated the colloids are more sol; when this energy is removed or is undisturbed the colloids are more gel.

Torsion/rotation
A therapeutic loading technique involving twisting-type loading; essentially a combination of compression and tension where there is simultaneous compression of some fibers with elongation of others. Outcomes are the same as those associated with compression and tension techniques.

Trait anxiety
A more intense degree anxiety toward a broader range of situations or objects – considered a perceptive personality characteristic rather than a temporary feeling.

Transdermal/transepidermal water loss (TWL or TEWL)
A measure of skin barrier function associated with dermatology and connected sciences, it is the measurement of the quantity of water that passes from inside a body through the epidermal layer to the surrounding atmosphere via diffusion and evaporation processes.

Transference
The personalization of the professional/therapeutic relationship by the client.

Trauma
Insult or injury to the physical body or psychological state.

Traumatic event
That which is outside the range of usual human experience that would markedly distress almost anyone. Such experiences can occur as actual or perceived and as a result of direct exposure to a traumatic event or indirectly in the form of learning about a traumatic event experienced by another.

Traumatic scar
Pathophysiological scar further compounded by traumatic emotional sequelae and other comorbidities.

Ultrasound elastography
A non-invasive imaging technology used to measure stiffness/strain of soft-tissue or provide images of tissue morphology and other biomechanical information.

Viscoelasticity
The ability of a medium (e.g. fascia) to be both mobile (elastic) and supportive (firm/viscous) when undergoing deformation.

Introduction

We are not just treating scars; we are treating people with scars

Pamela Fitch BA, RMT

In the developed world alone, a total of 100 million people develop scars each year as a result of 55 million elective operations and 25 million operations after trauma (Sund 2000). Current statistics estimate that over 50% of post-surgical patients will experience scar-related complications (Diamond 2012).

Millions of people worldwide are afflicted with non-fatal burn injuries. Although mortality and morbidity from burns have diminished significantly over the past several decades, these statistics do not reflect the overall impact on the burn survivor and how well they carry on with their life and manage post-burn deformities, contractures and other disabilities that collectively present with aesthetic and functional considerations (Goel & Shrivastava 2010).

The prevalence of occurrence, complications and sequelae associated with problematic scars, of varying etiology, present important clinical, economic and social considerations.

The occurrence of excessive scarring has been documented for centuries, dating back to the Smith papyrus around 1700 BC (Berman & Bicley 1995). The documented use of manual techniques in the treatment of wounds can be traced back to the 1550s; Paré, a French surgeon, administered massage to relieve joint stiffness and improve wound healing following surgery. It has also been documented that during the World Wars, military nurses and, sometimes, doctors provided massage as a component of scar treatment as a result of unplanned events and planned trauma (surgery).

Nowadays it is common to see *massage* noted in medical literature, as part of the recommended postsurgical care for scars, as a means to improve wound healing outcomes (e.g. better scar aesthetics and more pliant, less restrictive scars). However, ironically in the present day, specific protocols for the management of scars typically do not include massage therapy (MT) and specific referrals and patient accessibility to MT lag, presenting a paradoxical conundrum for the profession and those who could benefit from the treatment.

In part this *lag* falls to the responsibility of the MT profession itself. According to Cho and colleagues (2014):

> *Evidence to support the use of scar massage is inconclusive. There is much variability and inconsistency with regard to when treatment should be initiated, the appropriate treatment protocol and duration, and evaluation and measurement of outcomes.*

In order to improve the position of MT as a viable treatment consideration within the spectrum of mainstream medical care, the profession needs educational materials that guide the clinician's delivery of safe and effective care in order to achieve measureable, predictive and consistent clinical outcomes. This book is intended to support this initiative and be a go-to resource for manual scar tissue management, shaped to teach massage therapists how to work safely and confidently with *people with scars*.

Evolution is Fundamental

Health care is an ever-evolving environment. As healthcare providers within the field of manual therapy, we are continually learning new discoveries about the body's response to trauma, injury, healing and touch.

Newer technologies that aid imaging (e.g. high definition real-time ultrasound and endoscopy) and advances in research have been instrumental in expanding our understanding of important clinical considerations and in supporting the development of evidence-based practice guidelines. Additionally, the higher levels of educational preparation currently available to MT practitioners aid in the ability to find, critically evaluate and utilize best available evidence.

Evidence-based practice (EBP) emerges from evidence-based medicine (EBM), which Sackett et al. (1996) define as integrating client values with clinical expertise and the best available research evidence. Best research evidence encompasses best available clinical, client-centered research that examines the accuracy, safety, efficacy and cost effectiveness of diagnostic and assessment procedures, prognostic markers and therapeutic interventions. Clinical expertise encompasses the therapist's ability to use clinical skills and past experience to both identify each client's unique health status and the potential risks and benefits of the proposed interventions. Client values speak to the individual's unique preferences, goals and expectations within the therapeutic relationship (Andrade 2013). Evidence for massage is information on massage practice that researchers and therapists collect in a systematic manner (Sackett et al. 2000). In practice it is desirable to be as evidence-based as possible, and be evidence informed when definitive evidence does not exist (Fritz 2013).

Haraldsson (2006) states:

> *Patient Oriented Evidence (POE) asks the important question; 'Does this new evidence impact the patient by changing the prognosis of the illness/impairment or increase the quality of life?' As a profession, we need to come together and create evidence-based practice guidelines to improve our practices and keep up with the changing health care environment.*

A Reasonable Nexus

Precise etiologic factors driving excessive/abnormal scar formation remain somewhat elusive, with the exception of tissue trauma, further complicated by factors such as excessive or prolonged inflammation and excessive wound tension mediated by fibroblasts/myofibroblasts.

By better understanding the wound healing process (physiological and pathophysiological), what our hands can effect (e.g. anxiety, pain, inflammation and tissue tension) and how our hands can induce desired outcomes (mechanisms of action), we can better devise strategies for improved delivery of care and achieve improved and more reliable clinical outcomes.

Although it is widely accepted within health care that massaging a scar improves outcomes, there is a paucity of well-designed clinical trials to establish a solid evidence base for achieving productive results. And so, this book is written with the objective of establishing a reasonable nexus between available sound-science and achieving consistent clinical outcomes. In such this nexus, coupled with the authors' extensive clinical experience, will help shape guidelines for working with scar tissue and *people with scars*.

When properly developed, communicated and implemented, guidelines improve the quality of care that is provided and patient outcomes. Guidelines are intended to support the healthcare professional's critical thinking skills and judgment in each case.

In addition to guiding safer, more effective and consistent outcomes, the authors can only dare to dream that these guidelines will also support better constructed MT research methodology and designs, ultimately leading to the inclusion of MT professionals in mainstream interprofessional healthcare.

What Defines Traumatic Scarring?

The American Psychological Association defines trauma as an emotional response to a terrible event like an accident, sexual assault or natural disaster (APA 2015).

Scar or cicatrix, derived from the Greek *eschara* – meaning scab – is the fibrous *replacement* tissue that is laid down following injury or disease (Farlex 2012).

Scars are not obligated to be problematic – where would we be without our body's natural ability to heal itself following a wound? However, normal physiological processes can be altered in a variety of ways and, when altered, this constitutes what is termed pathophysiology.

Abnormal or pathophysiological scars can impact function within and beyond their physical borders and present considerations outside of the physical/physiological aspect of the scar tissue (Lewit & Olsanska 2004, Bouffard et al. 2008, Valouchová & Lewit 2012, Bordoni & Zanier 2014).

Problematic scarring following planned and unplanned trauma can be accompanied by serious physiological and psychological considerations and, as such, this brings us to traumatic scars as defined by the authors:

pathophysiological scars further compounded by traumatic emotional sequelae and other comorbidities.

Traumatic scars can occur as a result of accidents, acts of violence and other catastrophic events (e.g. disease, burn accident and surgery).

Over the last several decades, advancements in medical technology have led to improved surgical techniques and emergency care (Blakeney & Creson 2002). Simply put, more people are surviving injuries that would have been fatal 20 or 30 years ago, and an increase in survival rate means an increased need for professionals skilled in treating *people with scars*. Working successfully with traumatic scars requires expert navigation, not only of the physicality of the scar material but also inclusive of the whole clinical presentation. This book will provide the information needed to help guide the development of that expertise.

Given the complexity of traumatic scars, where such presentations and/or appropriate treatment fall outside of the MT profession's scope of practice, suggestions will be provided for appropriate referral resources to support the patient's best possible biopsychosocial outcomes.

It is the authors' intention that the end product will comprehensively cover both the physiological/physical and empathetic elements of MT and in doing so honour both the art and science of the work. Like interprofessional collaboration, integration of art and science are essential for excellence in contemporary healthcare and achieving the best possible patient-focused outcomes for *people with scars*.

Overview of Chapters

Individual chapters will cover normal/abnormal scar formation; the role of various systems in wound healing; the impact of pathophysiological scars and associated sequelae; the biochemical and emotional impact of trauma; communication skills (including interprofessional communication); assessment and treatment protocols; client/therapist self care and shared experiences from therapists and *people with scars*.

In order to assist with research translation, throughout this book pathophysiological and clinical considerations will be interspersed as Boxes where it makes sense to do so.

The views expressed in these pages are founded on the result of several years of close observation, study, and experiment. It is possible some of my deductions are erroneous, but at least they are capable of being argued and are not merely arbitrary.

J.B. Mennell (1920)

References

Andrade CK (2013) *Outcome-based massage: putting evidence into practice.* 3rd edn Baltimore Md: Lippincott Williams & Wilkins.

APA (2015) American Psychological Society. Available at: https://apa.org/topics/trauma/index.aspx [Accessed 16 February 2015].

Berman B, Bieley HC (1995) Keloids. Journal of American Academy of Dermatology 33: 117–23.

Blakeney P, Creson D (2002) Psychological and physical trauma: treating the whole person. Available at: http://www.jmu.edu/cisr/journal/6.3/focus/blakeneyCreson/blakeneyCreson.htm [Accessed 10 December 2014].

Bordoni B, Zanier E (2014) Skin, fascias, and scars: symptoms and systemic connections. Journal of Multidisciplinary Healthcare 7: 11–24.

Bouffard NA, Cutroneo KR, Badger GJ et al (2008) Tissue stretch decreases soluble TGF-β and type I procollagen in mouse subcutaneous connective tissue: evidence from ex vivo and in vivo models. Journal of Cellular Physiology 214: 389–395.

Cho YS, Jeon JH, Hong A et al (2014) The effect of burn rehabilitation massage therapy on hypertrophic scar after burn: a randomized controlled trial. Burns 40(8): 1513–20.

Diamond M (2012) Scars and adhesions panel. Third International Fascia Research Congress, Vancouver.

Farlex (2012) Medical Dictionary for the Health Professions and Nursing. © Farlex 2012.

Fritz S (2013) Mosby's Fundamentals of therapeutic massage, 5th edn. St Louis, Elsevier, p 45.

Goel A, Shrivastava P (2010) Post-burn scars and scar contractures. Indian Journal of Plastic Surgery: official publication of the Association of Plastic Surgeons of India 43(Suppl): S63.

Haraldsson BG (2006) The ABCs of EBPs. How to have an evidence-based practice. Massage Therapy Canada. Available at: http://www.massagetherapycanada.com/content/view/1402/[Accessed 7 December 2014].

Lewit K, Olsanska S (2004) Clinical importance of active scars: abnormal scars as a cause of myofascial pain. Journal of Manipulative and Physiological Therapeutics 27(6): 399–402.

Mennell JB (1920) Physical treatment by movement, manipulation and massage, 2nd edn. Philadelphia: Blakiston.

Sackett DL, Rosenberg W, Gray JA et al (1996) Evidence based medicine: what it is and what it isn't. BMJ 312(7023): 71–72.

Sackett DL, Strauss SE, Scott Richardson W et al (2000) Evidence-based medicine: how to practice and teach EBM, 2nd edn. New York, Churchill Livingstone.

Sund B (2000) New developments in wound care. London, PJB Publications.

Valouchová P, Lewit K (2012) In: Schleip R, Findley T, Chaitow L, Huijing P (eds) Fascia the tensional network of the human body. Edinburgh: Churchill Livingstone Elsevier, p 343.

Skin and fascia

Nothing in life is to be feared, it is only to be understood. Now is the time to understand more, so that we may fear less

Marie Curie

The delivery of safe and effective scar tissue management requires an understanding of the structure and function of the organs and systems we are working with and of the wound-healing process.

The aim of this chapter is to provide a solid base for understanding skin and fascia sciences (structure and function). The role of skin and fascia in wound healing and the impact of abnormal wound healing on them will be covered in greater detail in Chapters 5 and 6.

Skin and Fascia: Overview

Skin and fascia are highly complex and diverse systems. This book provides an overview of each, favoring relevance to massage therapy (MT) and is comprehensive enough to guide treatment protocol and clinical best practice.

Although we will explore these systems individually, the various layers of the skin and underlying fascia are connected, support each other structurally and functionally, and continuously engage in the exchange of information. We begin with an overview of the extracellular matrix (ECM) as it constitutes the sum total of extracellular substance within skin and fascia.

General Histology

Extracellular Matrix Structure and Function

The extracellular matrix structure (ECM) is a complex blend of structural and functional macromolecules (see Table 2.1).

The ECM comprises (*covered in more detail):

- *Structural proteins, e.g. collagen and elastin (covered in greater detail on pp. 15–16)

- *Non-collagenous/cross-link proteins, e.g. fibrillin, fibronectin and laminin

ECM constituents	Examples and function
Structural proteins	Collagen and elastin: structural struts that while flexible, provide strength and stability
Non-collagenous cross-link proteins	Fibrillin, fibronectin and laminin: structural struts providing flexible-stability and a pathway for transfer of mechanical strain/tensional loading information from cell to cell
GS	Amorphous, hydrophilic gel, comprised of PGs and GAGs: an important metabolic interface that fills the space between cells and fibers
GAGs and PGs	Glucosamine, chondroitin, HA: highly negatively charged macromolecules that attract water and perform a variety of physiological and mechanical functions, such as lubrication to improve slide/glide between various structural proteins
Polysaccharides	Starch, glycogen, cellulous: an important class of biological polymers that provide primarily a storage or structure related function

Table 2.1

The extracellular matrix (ECM)

- *Ground substance (GS)

- *Ionized water

- Glycosaminoglycans (GAGs, e.g. chondroitin, *hyaluronan) and proteoglycans (PGs)

- Polysaccharides play a role in energy, storage and ECM structure.

Non-collagenous/cross-link proteins

Non-collagenous/cross-link proteins, where normal, healthy cross-link proteins bind collagen fibers to the cell membrane, creating the pathway for mechanical strain/tensional loading information to transfer from the tissues to the cell. Additionally, normal cross-link proteins augment collagen fiber stability.

Clinical Consideration

Vitamin C has been identified as an important component in the formation of healthy cross-links. Here we can see the importance of adequate intake during tissue remodeling following exercise and trauma (Boyera et al. 1998).

Pathophysiological Consideration

Abnormal or pathological cross-links, instigated by various pathophysiological circumstance (e.g. diminished GS), can adversely impact tissue mobility and lead to tissue contracture and shortening (Van den Berg 2010, 2012). Changes to the ECM (adhesions between microfilaments, i.e. pathological cross-links) are seen in scarred fascia (Kozma et al. 2005, Chirasatitsin & Engler 2010).

Ground substance

Ground substance (GS), the amorphous gel-like component of the ECM, is an important metabolic interface that fills the space between cells and fibers. GS influences tissue development and cellular migration, proliferation, shape and metabolic functions.

Constituents within the GS (e.g. GAGs and PGs) perform a variety of functions that can influence tissue development and cellular migration, proliferation, shape and metabolic functions (Van den Berg 2012). One important feature of these constituents is their ability to attract and bind water, which factors significantly into fascia's viscoelastic properties and in lubrication, thereby reducing friction between moving or sliding fibers, tissues and layers.

Water

Water plays an important role in viscoelasticity and lubrication. Water also serves as a transport system and solvent. Up to 80% of the human body is water (in bound and unbound states).

Pathophysiological Consideration

In addition to tissue dehydration seen with trauma, our water volume tends to diminish as we age. Under-hydration may play a role in age-related collagen changes and the pain and dysfunction that accompanies such changes (Purslow & Delage 2012). The clinical significance of the impact of tissue dehydration is discussed further throughout this chapter.

Pathophysiological Consideration

Age-related changes seen in fascia show some similar characteristics to those seen in injured fascia such as tangled pathological cross-links, less coherent collagen fiber arrangement, under-hydrated and less wavy or crimped collagen ('collagen crimp'). Such changes can impact tissue slide and glide,

Hyaluronan

This hydrophilic, viscous lubricant is found throughout fascia, skin and neural tissue. Hyaluronan (HA) is involved in a variety of physiological and mechanical functions such as wound healing, lubrication, cellular signaling, maintaining osmotic balance and tissue hydration (Liao et al. 2005, Matteini et al. 2009).

HA helps reduce the impact of compressive forces in synovial-joint related tissues and improves slide/glide between various structural proteins and layers of adjacent tissue (e.g. between various layers of fascia and between muscle fibers) (McCombe et al. 2001, Stecco et al. 2011). HA and the sliding mechanism will be covered in greater detail later in this chapter.

Collectively the ECM defines the shape and form of our cells. It provides a framework to which the cells can adhere, move about in and communicate through. The ECM creates a medium by which appropriate balance can be maintained between porosity, hydration and ionic environment, thus allowing nutrients and metabolites to diffuse freely into and out of our cells. The ECM acts as an immune barrier. It is also a repository for metabolites and toxins, and for storing fat.

The ECM plays an important role in wound healing and repair. It serves as a repository for signaling molecules and mediates signals from other cells to promote cell proliferation and differentiation.

The ECM is responsive to mechanical strain and tensional loading (tissue deformation). Mechanical forces exert influence on the tissue structural elements (microfilaments) and the molecular composition of the ECM (Benjamin & Ralphs 1998, Milz et al. 2005). Strain type, degree, direction and duration can influence ECM composition and impact fibroblast functions that guide healing and adaptation responses (Purslow 2002, Ingber 2003, Standley & Meltzer 2008, Stecco et al. 2009, Blechschmidt & Gasser 2012). The clinical relevance of this feature of the ECM will be noted throughout this book.

One of the mechanisms by which cells sense changes in mechanical strain/tensional load is via specialized (matrix adhered) transmembrane receptors (integrins). Integrins play a role in defining cellular shape, mobility, regulating the cell cycle and mediating cell-to-cell and cell-to-ECM signals. Via integrins, mechanical stimulus can evoke a biochemical response, which, in turn, can trigger a variety of cellular responses and activities. Conversion of mechanical stimulus into biochemical response is called mechanotransduction. The integrin–mechanotransduction communication system works much faster than neurally transmitted signals, allowing cells to make rapid and flexible responses. In addition to evoking biochemical responses, the internal to external and cell-to-cell linkage mechanism provides the means by which the organism can sense and respond to mechanical demand or forces placed upon it – monitoring and regulating 'enough tension' to ensure the shape and integrity of any given cell and the entire musculoskeletal/myofascial system.

Skin Structure and Function

In order to better understand the formation of scar tissue, we need to look at the marvelous organ that is our skin.

Along with the glands, hair and nails, skin makes up the integumentary system. On average, skin

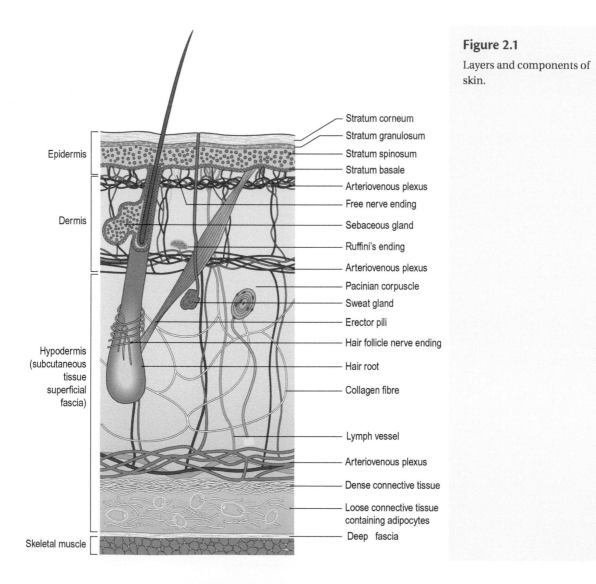

Figure 2.1

Layers and components of skin.

Epidermis

Dermis

Hypodermis (subcutaneous tissue superficial fascia)

Skeletal muscle

Stratum corneum
Stratum granulosum
Stratum spinosum
Stratum basale
Arteriovenous plexus
Free nerve ending
Sebaceous gland
Ruffini's ending
Arteriovenous plexus
Pacinian corpuscle
Sweat gland
Erector pili
Hair follicle nerve ending
Hair root
Collagen fibre

Lymph vessel
Arteriovenous plexus
Dense connective tissue
Loose connective tissue containing adipocytes
Deep fascia

constitutes 10% of human body mass. Skin acts as a barrier to the outside world and plays an important role in homeostasis. The skin, our outer layer of protection, is susceptible to infections, injuries, growths, rashes, cysts, boils, discoloration, burns, adhesions and *scars*.

Skin Histology

The skin comprises:

- Epithelium
- Connective tissue (CT).

Epithelium

There are three basic types of epithelial tissue: squamous, cuboidal and columnar – arranged in either a one-layer (simple) or multilayer (stratified) configuration. Epithelium forms many glands and lines the cavities and surfaces of structures throughout the body (e.g. the epidermis consists of stratified squamous keratinizing epithelium) (Marieb et al. 2012).

CT

Considered a system, CT consists of several different types of cells (e.g. fibroblasts and adipocytes), protein fibers (elastin and collagen) surrounded by the gelatinous ECM (Schleip et al. 2012a, Andrade 2013).

CT is a continuous bodywide system that plays a well-identified role in integrating the functions of diverse cell types within each tissue it invests (c.g. skeletal muscle, tendon, bone, viscera (Langevin 2006)). CT is highly variable in its presentation. Various terms are used to describe CT typology, for example:

- Dense and loose are used to describe how dense, tightly or spread out the fibers are packaged within an array of tissue
- Regular, irregular, unidirectional, multidirectional, parallel ordered and woven are used to

describe fiber orientation and configuration within a particular sheet, layer or area of tissue (Terminologia Histologica 2008).

Clinical Consideration

As CT is intimately associated with other tissues and organs it may influence the normal or pathological processes in a wide variety of organ systems (Findley et al. 2012).

CT, fascia and the sliding mechanism

One of the more recent discoveries in the world of fascia research is the sliding/gliding that occurs throughout the CT and fascial systems, which facilitates unimpeded, frictionless movement (McCombe et al. 2001, Guimberteau & Bakhach 2006, Stecco et al. 2008, Wang et al. 2009). Some suggest that sliding layers are interspersed between CT and fascial layers; however, Guimberteau suggests that rather than separated or superimposed layers there exists a singular, highly hydrated, tissular architecture which can maintain the necessary space between structures to facilitate optimal sliding and tissue excursion (Guimberteau & Bakhach 2006, Guimberteau 2012) – see Figure 2.2.

Whether the presentation is layers between layers or a singular architecture, the sliding mechanism comprises loose CT – consisting of predominantly fine collagen strands, adipocytes and an abundance of HA.

The sliding mechanism occurs bodywide on both a macro and micro level; between interfascial planes, endofascial fibers, endomuscular fibers and intracellular fibers (Guimberteau et al. 2005, Ingber 2008, Stecco et al. 2008, Wang et al. 2009, Langevin 2010). The impact of traumatic scarring on the sliding mechanism and clinical considerations will be noted throughout this book.

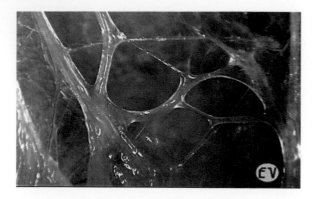

Figure 2.2

The delicate, well-hydrated, loose network of connective tissue that augments tissue excursion and movement. The sliding mechanism/system comprises a continuous structure composed of billions of microvacuolar components (polyhedron 'bubbles') that allow for structures to move freely without anything else moving around them. Collagen and elastin fibrils form the framework of the microvacuolar bubbles. (Reproduced from Guimberteau and Armstrong: *Architecture of Human Living Fascia*, 2015, published by Handspring Publishing with kind permission from Dr J-C Guimberteau & Endovivo Productions.)

Skin layers and Functions (Marieb et al. 2012)

The skin comprises two primary layers:

- Epidermis
- Dermis.

Epidermis

As thin as a sheet of paper, the epidermis is the tough, outermost layer of the skin. Most of the cells in the epidermis are keratinocytes, which constitute the first immune barrier, acting essentially as sentinels. Keratinocytes produce the structural protein keratin, which supports the skin's ability

to protect the rest of the body. Other cells include melanocytes and immune cells (e.g. Langerhans and T-lymphocytes) (Adameyko et al. 2009, Sidgwick & Bayat 2012, Bordoni & Zanier 2014).

The outermost portion of the epidermis is pretty much waterproof and helps to keep most bacteria, viruses and other foreign substances from entering the body. The epidermis, working in concert with the other skin layers, also protects our internal organs, muscles, nerves, and blood vessels against trauma.

Dermis

The dermis is made up of layers of fibrous and elastic fibers (collagen and elastin). Collagen supports and stabilizes while elastin allows for stretch and absorbs tensile forces – collagen and elastin will be covered in greater detail further on in this chapter.

The dermis is often described as the workhorse of the skin because it contains lymph vessels, nerve endings, sweat glands, sebaceous glands, hair follicles, and blood vessels.

Nerve endings in skin sense pain, touch, pressure and temperature and relay information to the brain (Kiernan & Rajakumar 2013, Bordoni & Zanier 2014). Mechanoreceptors in skin provide information on posture, positioning and movement (Macefield 2005, Bordoni & Zanier 2014, Mouchnino & Blouin 2013). As with all systems of the body, nerve receptors in skin and fascia can evoke sympathetic nervous system (SNS) responses that can impact each other and all the other systems.

The sweat glands produce sweat in response to heat and stress. Sweat is composed mainly of water and salt. When sweat evaporates, it helps to cool the body. There are specialized sweat glands in the armpits and the genital region that secrete a thick, oily sweat that produces body odor when the sweat is digested by the skin bacteria.

The sebaceous glands secrete oil called sebum into hair follicles. Sebum keeps the skin moist and pliable and helps create a barrier against foreign substances.

The hair follicles produce various types of hair found throughout the body. Hair contributes to a person's appearance, helps regulate body temperature, provides protection from injury and enhances sensation. At the base of each hair follicle are sensory nerve fibers that wrap around the hair bulb. Moving or bending the hair stimulates the nerve endings, which allow a person to feel their hair has been moved. A portion of the follicle also contains stem cells capable of regenerating a damaged epidermis.

Functions of the skin: Summary

Collectively, the layers of the skin perform a variety of functions (Marieb 2003):

- The skin provides a protective barrier against microorganisms, pathogens, most bacteria and viruses and protection from the elements (e.g. rain, cold, heat)

- Thermoregulation is carried out through sweating and regulation of blood flow

- The skin prevents fluid loss, distributes essential nutrients to the body and provides a medium for absorption (e.g. the outermost layer of skin cells are almost exclusively supplied by external oxygen, and various medications or agents can be administered topically)

- Salts and small amounts of wastes can be excreted through the skin (e.g. ammonia and urea)

- The skin provides a storage reservoir for lipids and water and synthesizes vitamin D

- The skin houses sensory receptors that provide information to the brain pertaining to pain and movement perception, non-verbal communication and convey indicators of state of well-being and health (e.g. mood, emotions and pigmentation changes – as is seen with jaundice).

The number of sweat glands, nerve endings, sebaceous glands, hair follicles and blood vessels vary throughout the body. These variations serve a functional role; for example, the palms of our hands have less hair than the top of our head. As the head is generally more exposed, hair can provide warmth and UV protection. Another example would be the concentration of sensory nerve endings – a high concentration is found on the fingertips to assist with dexterity (Marieb 2003).

Fascia Structure and Functions

In the field of MT, the terms fascia and myofascia are commonly used to describe the various tissues that play a significant role in locomotion (Chaitow 1980, Schleip et al. 2012a).

In human biological sciences the skin and CT proper have been studied in great detail; however, fascia has been largely unconsidered. Historically, fascia has been viewed as an inert shaping and binding tissue. More recent research has shown that fascia plays a significant role in human locomotion and may be a source of soft-tissue pain and dysfunction.

Clinical Consideration

The fascial system is now recognized as a pain-generating tissue and significant proprioceptive organ (Mitchell & Schmidt 1977, Yahia et al. 1992, Schleip 2003, Stecco et al. 2008, Benjamin 2009, Taguchi et al. 2009, van der Wal 2009, Findley et al. 2012)

Current (mainstream) protocols for assessment, treatment and recovery time for 'musculoskeletal' issues (including scarring) do not take the fascia into consideration. This oversight will be addressed throughout this book.

The International Fascia Research Congress (FRC) has been instrumental in shedding light on this long overlooked tissue. The research presented at and generated by this initiative provides the world of MT with some foundational knowledge needed to work safely and effectively with the impact of scars and burns on this tissue.

In order to better facilitate understanding of this section, the following key terms/concepts are briefly described:

- What is fascia? Definitions vary; this book offers an amalgam of the most current. Fascia is described as all fibrocollagenous CT whose morphology is influenced by mechanical strain/tensional loading (Schleip et al. 2012a). The term 'fascia' is inclusive of various presentations (e.g. dense and loose) that are innervated, vascularized and continuous (fascia envelops and invests all other soft tissues, bones, nerves, circulatory vessels and organs), functioning as an organ of stability and locomotion (Findley & Schleip 2007, Schleip et al. 2012a, Kumka & Bonar 2012). Fascia can present in many forms depending upon its location, density, fiber orientation or configuration, required role and relationship with other structures or tissues (Terminologia Histologica 2008). Different terms are used to describe more accurately fascia's various histological, mechanical, topographical and functional properties (e.g. epimysium, perineurium, periosteum, aponeuroses, retinaculae, viscera membranes) (Langevin & Huijing 2009, Schleip et al. 2012a). Although in the world of fascia there is much debate, it is universally agreed upon that fascia's fundamental characteristic is its continuity – an uninterrupted, viscoelastic network that three-dimensionally envelops and invests all structures of the body from head to toe (Chaudhry et al. 2008, Grinnell 2008, Benjamin 2009, Stecco & Stecco 2009, van der Wal 2009, Schleip et al. 2012a). Fascia is a highly innervated tissue and is considered to be the most extensive mechanosensitive organ in the human body (Benjamin 2009, Hoheisel et al. 2011, Schleip et al. 2012a).

- Viscoelasticity: a viscoelastic material (e.g. collagen) can both resist strain or deformation and return to its original state following deformation. The viscoelastic nature of fascial collagen provides a means by which this tissue can be both mobile (elastic) and supportive (firm/more viscous) at the same time. Fascia is the only tissue that can instantly change its property in response to demand (e.g. mechanical strain). Fascia's viscoelastic properties can be rapidly modified by shifting its fluid dynamics; this is mediated by the nervous and vascular systems and specialized cells within fascia (e.g. fibroblasts and MFBs) (Klingler et al. 2004, Barnes 1997, Pischinger 1991, Reed et al. 2010).

Pathophysiological Consideration

The viscoelastic nature of fascia can only be observed in hydrated tissue, which underscores the importance of adequate hydration and the potential pathophysiological consequences of dehydration.

- Locomotor system (Chaitow 1980): constitutes the bones, joints, capsules, ligaments, fasciae, aponeuroses and all the tissues surrounding and investing skeletal muscles and their tendinous expansions. So as to aid functional understanding, Myers (2014) subdivides the tissues of the locomotor system into outer and inner layers. The outer constitutes the myofascial layer that surrounds and invests the 600 or so muscles in the human body. The inner layer consists of joint capsules, ligaments and periostea. The outer and inner layers are not segregated but are a continuous, organized network that serves to augment force transmission and regulate movement.

- Force transmission: collectively, muscle fibers/bundles and the collagen-rich intramuscular CT (myofascial envelopes) are now appearing (as a unit) to be functionally significant with regard to force transmission. A significant proportion of muscular force is simultaneously transmitted multidirectionally (e.g. obliquely, laterally, linearly) in a shearing fashion onto adjacent fascia and associated muscular synergists and antagonists (Huijing 2007, 2009, Maas & Huijing 2009, van der Wal 2009, Maas & Sandercock 2010).

- Biotensegrity or tensegrity (Myers 2014, Chaitow 2011, Levin & Martin 2012): fascia, considered a biotensegrity system, displays a particular bioarchitecture composed of two primary elements – compressional and tensional.

  - *Compressional*: described as struts, non-continuous structures that exhibit the fundamental behavior of resisting compression (bones).

  - *Tensional*: described as bands or sheets, continuous tissues capable of transferring forces across the vast network of all other bands/sheets (fascia) (Fuller 1961, Kumka & Bonar 2012).

  Although each element exhibits a fundamental behavior, compression and tensional properties co-exist in bones and fascia such that structural integrity is maintained by continuous balance of tension and compression forces. The ability to support (resist compression) and share the load (distribute/transfer forces) is seen on a macro (bodywide) and micro (ECM and cellular) level (Ingber 2008, Levin & Martin 2012). In a biotensegrity system, loading of one segment of the structure effects *the whole*. It is with this concept in mind that bodywork and movement modalities are considered most effective when considered and applied globally in addition to locally. Biotensegrity properties and functional capabilities differ in healthy verses unhealthy tissues (Levin & Martin 2012).

- Myokinetic/myofascial chains or meridians: terms used to describe a grouping or sequence of tissues/structures – structurally and neurologically linked together to support functional and perceptive continuity. According to Richter (2012), '*the locomotor system is to be considered one continuous unit that functions as a whole*'. The linkage of various tissues and structures is supported by the work and/or research of many (for example Benjamin, Busquet, Cantu, Huijing, Ingber, Kabat, Mass and Sundercock, Mazieres, Myers, Pilat, Rolf, Stecco and van der Wal) and is well illustrated in Myers' *Anatomy Trains* (2014) and in Stecco's *Fascial Manipulation for Musculoskeletal Pain* (Stecco 2004) and *Fascial Manipulation - the Practical Part* (Stecco & Stecco 2009).

Clinical Consideration

Pain referral patterns associated with myofascial trigger points will sometimes distribute along the myokinetic or myofascial chain associated with the involved muscle.

Histology

Fascia comprises:

- ECM (covered previously)
- Cells
- Fibrous proteins.

Cells

The most prominent cellular components of fascia include:

- Mast cells and macrophages
- Adipocytes
- Fibroblasts.

Mast cells and macrophages play a role in wound repair and immune response.

Adipocytes play a role in heat preservation, storage, protection from physical trauma and also serve as a 'spacer' separating adjacent layers of fascia (Stecco et al. 2008).

Fibroblasts, the predominant cell type, are highly adaptable and noted for their ability to:

– remodel in response to mechanical strain

– produce biochemical responses, and

– differentiate into various cell types (e.g. myofibroblasts) (Eagen et al. 2007, Mammoto & Ingber 2009, Stecco et al. 2009, Meltzer et al. 2009).

Fibroblasts synthesize the components of the ECM and play a significant role in soft-tissue remodeling.

Clinical Consideration

Changes in fibroblast shape and subsequently function occurs in response to a variety of signals, including mechanically applied tension or strain (Eagen et al. 2007, Mammoto & Ingber 2009, Stecco et al. 2009, Meltzer et al. 2009). This feature of fibroblasts enables fascia to alter its fiber configuration in response to mechanical demands or stress placed upon it (e.g. movement, exercise, posture, work-related activities). Additionally, this provides a plausible explanation for the mechanism by which fascial specific therapies (e.g. structural integration/Rolfing, myofascial massage and acupuncture) produce therapeutic results (Langevin et al. 2004).

Clinical Consideration

Manual therapy techniques treat the fascial layers by altering density, tonus, viscosity and the arrangement of fascia (Findley et al. 2012).

Myofibroblasts (MFBs): differentiation of fibroblasts into MFBs is triggered in response to mechanical strain/tensional loading and certain cytokines (e.g. transforming growth factor beta-1; TGF-β1). MFBs play an important role in inflammation, remodeling and fibrosis (Cathie 1974, Powell et al. 1999, Tomasek et al. 2002, Hinz & Gabbiani 2003, Schleip et al. 2007, Nekouzadeh et al. 2008, Hinz 2013).

Clinical Consideration

Fascia plays a significant role in conveying mechanical tension, in order to control an inflammatory environment (Bordoni & Zanier 2014).

Clinical Consideration

Transforming growth factor beta-1 (TGF-β1) is known to stimulate collagen synthesis and proliferation. Collagen is the predominant fiber found in fascia and the predominant type of fiber laid-down during soft-tissue repair/remodeling – more on this in Chapter 5.

MFBs can contract in a smooth muscle-like manner providing fascia with contractile capabilities independent of muscle contraction (Spector 2002, Schleip et al. 2005, Schleip et al. 2006).

MFB contraction plays a major role in wound healing/remodeling, pathological fascial contractures and fibrosis (e.g. Dupuytren disease, plantar fibromatosis, frozen shoulder, ChLBP and abnormal scar formation) (Gabbiani 2003, Langevin et al. 2009). Therefore higher than normal concentrations of MFBs are typically present in injured or traumatized fascia.

Clinical Consideration

The presence of *higher than normal* concentration of MFBs in injured and scarred fascia further

It is suggested that MFBs also play a role in issues associated with decreased myofascial tension or hypermobility (e.g. peri-partum pelvic pain due to pelvic instability, sacroiliac joint force closure dysfunction or back pain due to spinal segmental instability) (Schleip et al. 2012).

MFBs are also present in normal healthy fascia implying a valid – homeostatic –functional purpose (Wilson & Dahners 1988, Murray & Spector 1999, Ralphs et al. 2002). For example, MFBs provide fascia with the ability to remodel itself in response to normal daily movement and activity demands (adaptation). Recall from page 12: fibrocollagenous tissue morphology is shaped by tensional loading. Demand (mechanical/tensile forces) invokes MFB proliferation and therefore (normally) higher concentrations of MFBs are typically present in dense presentations of fascia commonly subjected to higher tensional demands (e.g. those that play a significant role in stability and support, fascia lata, plantar, crural and thoroacolumbar fascia, perimysium).

Biomechanically, interactions between MFBs and the ECM contribute to whole body mobility and tensional integrity or biotensegrity (Schleip et al. 2005, Guimberteau 2007, Ingber 2008, Levin & Martin 2012).

Fibrous Proteins

Fascia is constructed from two predominant fiber types:

- Collagen
- Elastin.

Collagen

Collagen is the most abundant fiber type found throughout fascia. Various types of collagen occur in the human body (Type I is the most predominant) (Gelse et al. 2003, Gartner & Hiatt 2007, Gordon & Hahn 2010, Ross & Pawlina 2011, Kumka & Bonar 2012).

Collagen cross-linking, a chemical bond between adjacent collagen fibers, plays a significant role in tissue integrity. Physiological linkage augments mechanical stability, however excessive (pathological) cross-links can interfere with slide potential and contribute to mobility restrictions. Conversely, insufficient or unstable bonds can result in diminished tissue integrity.

Collagen provides tensile strength, guards against over extension and can 'store and release' energy (can store and release an equal amount of energy while stretching only 100th the amount of elastin) (Zorn 2011). This is often referred to as catapult or rebound effect. Collagen fibers are somewhat firm yet pliant and able to yield to force (e.g. they can bend, twist and lengthen). Collagen's elastic-stiffening potential (viscoelastic property) is considered to be one of its defining features (Zorn & Hodeck 2011). Normal healthy collagen fibers display a distinctive 'wavy/crimped' formation which factors into normal healthy functioning (e.g. force transmission and energy facilitation).

Adequate hydration is vital to collagen health and functioning. Dehydration has been identified as an initiator of inflammatory response in collagen and once present, inflammatory mediators can contribute to tension held in collagenous tissues (e.g. skin and fascia). As previously noted, dehydration also decreases the fluid-bulk of GS which can result in pathological collagen cross linking, diminished lubrication and reduced tensile strength.

Type I collagen is the fiber type typically *laid-down* during tissue remodeling. Under healthy normal circumstances, collagen turnover (reconstruction phase of healing) lasts from 300 to 500 days, meaning it takes that length of time for collagen to fully mature – an important consideration in post-trauma recovery and rehabilitation (van den Berg 2010).

Kumka and Bonar (2012) note that if function changes (e.g. increased mechanical strain, insufficient mechanical strain or prolonged immobilization), pro-collagen in the fibroblasts will change types (e.g., collagen type I into collagen type III), or undifferentiated cell types may adapt towards a more *functionally* appropriate lineage (e.g. chondrocyte) (Benjamin & Ralphs, 1998, Bank et al. 1999, Jarvinen et al. 2002, Milz et al. 2005, Mammoto & Ingber 2009). Therefore, a tissue that is exposed to unusual demand may remodel into a form or presentation that is atypical to its fundamental nature.

Clinical Consideration

Significant compression can ultimately culminate in tissues changing their morphology (e.g. tissue that was once populated with fibroblasts, becomes invested predominately with chondrocytes – forming cartilage, along with its mineral deposition (Benjamin & Ralphs 1998, Bank et al. 1999). These adaptations have been demonstrated in the supraspinatus tendon (aka calcific tendonitis), transverse acetabular ligament, transverse ligament of atlas, as well as various other ligaments and tendons throughout the body (Bank et al. 1999, Milz et al. 2005). What once was pliant mobile tissue exhibits entirely different functional capabilities and palpable feel (Kumka & Bonar 2012). Here we can envision the potential for unfavourable outcomes as a result of improperly stimulated tissue during the repair/remodeling stage of healing.

Timing is everything – more on this in Chapter 05.

Elastin

Elastin, which are stretchy, rubber-like fibers, vary in prevalence and amount throughout skin and fascia depending upon functional demand.

Elastin fibers tend to branch, creating a net-like architecture (Van den Berg 2012). When placed under tensional force, these fibers lengthen and when the force is removed they enable tissue to return to its normal, resting length. When dehydrated, elastin becomes brittle but when well hydrated it is elastic and flexible. Elastin fibers can be stretched up to 150% their resting length without causing any injury (20 to 30 times more than collagen can withstand) and like collagen can store or release energy. When placed under sustained stretch-demand, elastin has been shown to lose some of its recoil potential.

Within the tissues of the locomotor system, collagen and elastin are often intertwined.

Fascia Layers and Functions

Fascia taxonomy varies almost as widely as fascia itself. Which is likely why (at least in part) at the FRC 3 in 2012, Dr Paul Standley proclaimed, *'We need a Rosetta Stone of manual therapy.'*

In an attempt to simplify functional understanding and create a conceptual visual, favoring relevance to MT, this book will briefly cover two of the most current classification systems: Willard's (2012a, 2012b) layer/structural classification system and Kumka and Bonar's (2012) functional classification system.

Layer Classification

Willard (2012a) suggests four primary categories: superficial/panniculus (loose), deep/axial (investing), meningeal and visceral (Swanson 2013). Only the superficial and axial layers will be covered in more detail – as the techniques covered in subsequent chapter predominantly target the superficial and deep fascial layers. The meningeal layer will be covered (in some detail) in Chapter 4, the visceral layer will not be covered in much detail in this book. For more information on visceral work please see the recommended references and reading suggestions provided at the end of the chapter.

Superficial/panniculus fascia (SF)

Although not a universally accepted term, in many textbooks superficial fascia is used to describe the subcutaneous loose CT layer (Platzer 2008, Standring 2008, Netter 2011, Tank 2012).

Continuous with the dermis, the SF lies directly beneath the skin, supporting the skin's structural integrity. Essentially, the SF surrounds the entire torso and the extremities and mostly comprises loose CT and adipocytes.

According to Langevin and colleagues (Langevin et al. 2009), there are two typical presentations of SF:

- Loose/areolar CT often embedded with adipocytes

- A fine mesh of dense irregular CT with areolar CT and adipocytes within the mesh.

There is often an abundance of elastin fibers in SF which augments its recoil capabilities (i.e. its ability to expand and return to its previous state). The SF is the intermediary between the skin and the deep fascia – interspersed sliding layers allow for independent motion of the various layers (e.g. skin, superficial and deep fascia).

The SF serves as an insulator, a reservoir for fat storage, and provides a passageway for larger nerves, blood and lymphatic vessels. The SF supports the patency (openness) of these passageways (i.e. neurovascular tracts) and the neurovascular structures within (Stecco et al. 2009). Many nerves track through the SF and Pacinian corpuscles (i.e. deep pressure receptors) and nociceptors are found within it.

Clinical Consideration

Superficial and deep layers of the thoracolumbar fascia may be a source of nociceptive input in low back pain (Yahia et al. 1992, Bednar et al. 1995, Taguchi et al. 2009, Tesarz et al. 2011).

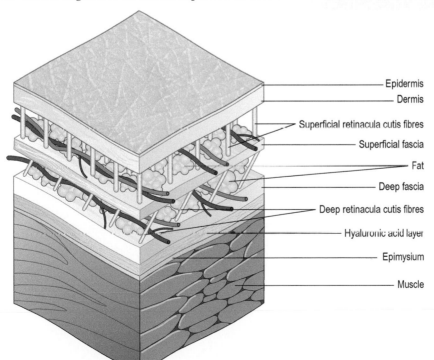

Epidermis
Dermis
Superficial retinacula cutis fibres
Superficial fascia
Fat
Deep fascia
Deep retinacula cutis fibres
Hyaluronic acid layer
Epimysium
Muscle

Figure 2.3

Fascial membranes and rentinacula cutis fibers. Cross-section from the skin to musculature, showing fascial membranes and retinacula cutis fibers (RCF). (Adapted from Stecco et al. 2013.)

Retinacula cutis fibers (RCF)

Fibrous strands that invest and are continuous throughout the skin, superficial and deep fasciae layers. RCF play a role in tissue connectivity and mobility.

Clinical Consideration

When thickened, as a result of injury or trauma, these vertical septa can restrict and impact function. Any undue 'tugging' of bound tissue (e.g. during 'normal' movement) can lead to hypersensitization and consequent pain (Stecco 2004, 2009, Muscolino 2012).

Deep/axial fascia (DF)

Deeper scars (e.g. following surgery or due to penetrating puncture wounds) will impact the deep fascia layer and, potentially, the underlying muscular fascia (epi, peri and endomysium).

Generally speaking, DF presents throughout the body as a multilayer organization, typically 2–3 dense collagen bundle layers interspersed with loose CT layers that contain collagen, adipocytes and are rich in HA. The dense layers serve to augment force transmission and the loose layers augment slide/glide.

In each dense layer the collagen bundles are arranged in parallel with adjacent (above or below) layers arranged at a 78° angle to one another. This configuration (interspersed with sliding layers) allows for multidirectional movement and the ability of fascia to counter/resist tension multidirectionally (see Fig. 2.4).

DF displays some distinct regional differences:

- Trunk/torso: the superficial layer of the DF is thinner than that found in the limbs (except for the thoracolumbar fascia – TLF). In some

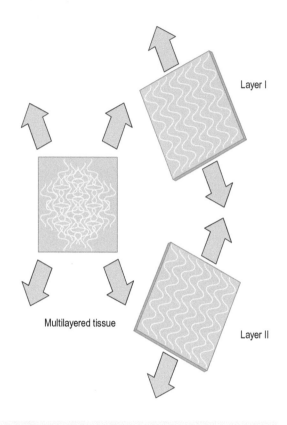

Layer I

Multilayered tissue

Layer II

Figure 2.4

The multilayer organization of deep axial fascia (DF). (Adapted from Stecco C et al. 2009.)

areas this thin layer envelops the underlying muscles (meaning there is no distinct epimysium). This presentation is seen in conjunction with the pectoralis major, latissimus dorsi, trapezius, deltoid and gluteus maximus and functionally serves as a means to connect the limbs to the trunk/torso. In this presentation the fascia and muscles move (or not) together (hence the greater potential for undifferentiated movement patterns in the trunk/torso).

- Limbs: in general the DF of the limbs is not very elastic, although the upper limb contains more elastin than the lower (providing greater tissue compliance or a wider range of movement). In the limbs there is a sliding layer between the DF and underlying epimysium. The DF and underlying muscles can therefore move independently of one another and when they do not – pain/dysfunction often ensue. This particular presentation supports force transmission and perhaps the greater variety of movement potential seen in the limbs (in comparison to the trunk/torso) (Stecco et al. 2008, Stecco et al. 2011).

Functional Classification

According to Kumka and Bonar (2012), the functional properties of fascia are reliant on the composition of the ECM, specific cells and filaments, including but not limited to the ratio of collagen types.

Kumka and Bonar (2012) suggest four primary functional categories: linking; fascicular; compression; and separating (see Table 2.2).

Linking

Linking fascia is sub-divided into dynamic and passive components:

- Dynamic fascia can contract autonomously (embedded with MFBs) and plays a role in locomotion, force transmission and biotensegrity.

- Passive fascia displays noci and proprioceptive capabilities and can only transmit forces when it is stretched/loaded.

- Linking fascias play a primary role in augmenting bodywide functional and perceptive continuity.

Classification	Functional role and examples
Linking	Connects various tissues/structure for the purpose of augmenting bodywide functional and perceptive continuity. Dynamic presentation can contract autonomously and plays a role in locomotion, force transmission and biotensegrity. Passive presentation displays noci and proprioceptive capabilities and can only transmit forces when it is stretched or loaded. Examples include tendon, ligament, retinaculae and aponeuroses. Note: some forms of linking fascia facilitate energy generation and/or storage
Fascicular	Augments continuity and force transmission, provides proprioceptive feedback and protection of nerve, blood vascular and lymph vessels. Examples include vascular tunics, neurofascia and myofascia
Compression	Forms a pressurized compartment to augment vascular function and enhances proprioception, muscular efficiency and coordination. Examples include compartments such as in the lower leg
Separating	Provides structural support, helps absorb shock, limits the spread of infection and creates space which reduces friction and augments slide/glide between articulating structures/surfaces. Examples include the loose/well-hydrated sliding layers

Table 2.2

Summary of fascia's functional classifications and roles

Fascicular

Fascicular fascia augments continuity and force transmission, provides proprioceptive feedback and protection of nerve, blood vascular and lymph vessels.

Clinical Consideration

Perimysium plays a significant role in force transmission. Perimysium is commonly thicker in postural muscles, tends to display a higher concentration of MFBs and can adapt more readily to changes in mechanical tension. The driving force behind long-term, sustained contracture and pronounced muscular 'stiffness' could be explained in part by the presence of MFBs in fascia – in particular in the perimysium. Surgical reconstruction processes (e.g. distraction osteogenesis, psoas lengthening) are frequently accompanied by increased muscle stiffness, shown to correlate with a significant increase in perimysial thickness – a response to the (sudden) increased tissue stretch (Schleip et al. 2005, Huijing 2007).

Clinical Consideration

Muscle spindles are embedded in the endomysium. If the enveloping fascia is too rigid (e.g. fibrosis, contracture), this may alter the stretch of the muscle spindle and adversely affect its normal firing (Stecco 2004).

Compression

Compression fascia forms a pressurized compartment to augment vascular function (e.g. venous return) and enhances proprioception, muscular efficiency and coordination.

Separating

Separating fascia provides structural support, helps absorb shock, limits the spread of infection and reduces friction and augments movement between articulating structures and surfaces. The loose well-hydrated sliding layers also fall into this category.

Functions of Fascia: Summary

Fascia physiology in brief: as a component of the locomotor system, fascia performs essentially three mechanical functional roles: separation, connection and energy facilitation.

Fascia as a tissue of separation: creates space which serves as an interface for ease of sliding and gliding of structures and tissues in relation to one another. Spatial separation supports unimpeded motion and motion ensures the healthy functioning of tissues and structures and the sliding–gliding interface.

Fascia as a tissue of connection: links together various anatomical components (bones, joints, muscles etc.) thereby creating an architecture that augments the transfer of forces across a broader array of tissues/structures. Connection enhances strength, stability and efficient coordinated movement. Bodywide perceptive and functional continuity affords linked tissues the ability to function and, potentially, dysfunction together.

Fascia as an energy facilitator: healthy, springy or crimped collagen is a potential energy generator or storehouse rather than an energy consumer, such as muscle. When stretched, collagen will rebound, augmenting propulsion (especially flatter, sheet-like fascia and tendons, e.g. Achilles tendon and Achilles aponeurosis) (Schleip & Müller 2013). Ultrasound-based measurements indicate that fascial tissues are commonly used for a dynamic energy storage (catapult action) during oscillatory movements, such as walking, hopping or running, and during such movements the supporting skeletal muscles contract more isometrically while the loaded fascial elements lengthen and shorten like elastic springs (Fukunaga et al. 2002). The rebound/catapult potential of fascia decreases the need for muscular energy – resulting in greater efficiency and endurance.

Myokinetic/Myofascial Chains and Meridians

The continuity seen throughout the fascial system is a key functional characteristic. It is agreed upon by many that dysfunction (scarring, densification, fibrosis) anywhere along the chain or meridian can impact function in other regions.

When challenged by stretch or movement dense and/or restricted fascia may alter proprioceptive afferent signals that lead to eventual abnormal biomechanics, aberrant movement patterns, muscle compensation, joint distress and pain (Bouffard et al. 2008).

In the absence of normal physiological elasticity, receptors embedded within the fascia may also be in an active state even at rest. Any further stretching, even that produced by normal muscular contraction, could cause excessive stimulation with consequent propagation of nociceptive afferents. Furthermore, over a certain threshold (i.e. consistent stimulus over time), all receptors can potentially become algoceptors (pain receptors) in response to consequent propagation of nociceptive signals (Ryan 2011).

Chain/meridian clinical considerations will be covered in greater detail in Chapter 9.

Clinical Consideration

Fascia supports and functions in tandem with our skin and all of our soft and hard tissues. Therefore it is reasonable to suppose that some degree of fascial involvement may be seen in conjunction with any functional loss and pain associated with scarring – as well as the milieu of compensatory *musculoskeletal* disorders that often accompany burns and problematic scars (e.g. cumulative trauma/overuse syndromes, chronic low back pain (ChLBP) and/or dysfunction and compression syndromes).

Clinical Consideration (Cont.)

In the field of MT we commonly encounter fascial changes associated with acute injury and trauma, chronic strain (physical or emotional), immobilization and the spectrum of subsequent sequelae (e.g. adhesions, fibrosis, myofascial trigger points, diminished gliding within the sliding layers, neural and circulatory consequences).

Clinical Consideration

According to Lewit and Olsanska (2004), scars may contribute to the formation of myofascial trigger points in adjacent tissues along with the potential for pain in other regions (e.g. low back pain associated with appendectomy).

As the impact of a scar can reach far beyond its physical borders, in addition to the degree or depth of the scar – from a MT perspective – it is also important to consider how a scar in one region of the body can impact functioning in distant (seemingly unrelated) tissues or areas.

According to Bordoni and Zanier (2014):

Every element or cell in the human body produces substances that communicate and respond in an autocrine or paracrine mode, consequently affecting organs and structures that are seemingly far from each other. This applies to the skin and subcutaneous fasciae. When the integrity of the skin has been altered, or when its healing process is disturbed, it becomes a source of symptoms that are not merely cutaneous. Additionally, the subcutaneous fasciae is altered when there is a discontinuous cutaneous surface. The consequence is an ample symptomatology, which is not limited to the body area where the scar is located.

In this light it is also prudent to consider the impact of scarring on the circulatory, lymphatic and neural structures servicing and travelling throughout the skin and fascia.

References

Adameyko I, Lallemend F, Aquino JB et al (2009) Schwann cell precursors from nerve innervation are a cellular origin of melanocytes in skin. Cell 139(2): 366–379.

Andrade C-K (2013) Outcome-based massage: putting evidence into practice, 3rd edn. Baltimore: Lippincott Williams and Wilkins.

Bank R, TeKoppele J, Oostingh G, Hazleman B, Riley G (1999) Lysylhydroxylation and non-reducible crosslinking of human supraspinatus tendon collagen: changes with age and in chronic rotator cuff tendinitis. Annals of the Rheumatic Disease 58: 35–41.

Barnes MF (1997) The basic science of myofascial release: morphologic change in connective tissue. Journal of Bodywork and Movement Therapies 1: 231–238.

Bednar DA, Orr FW, Simon GT (1995) Observations on the pathomorphology of the thoracolumbar fascia in chronic mechanical back pain: A microscopic study. Spine 20(10): 1161–1164.

Benjamin M (2009) The fascia of the limbs and back – a review. Journal of Anatomy 214: 1–18 doi: 10.1111/j.1469-7580.2008.01011.x.

Benjamin M, Ralphs JR (1998) Fibrocartilage in tendons and ligaments – an adaptation to compressive load. Journal of Anatomy 193: 481–494.

Blechschmidt E, Gasser RF (2012) Biokinetics and biodynamics of human differentiation: principles and applications. Berkeley: North Atlantic Books.

Bordoni B, Zanier E (2014) Skin, fascias, and scars: symptoms and systemic connections. Journal of Multidisciplinary Healthcare 7:11.

Bouffard NA, Cutroneo KR, Badger GJ et al (2008) Tissue stretch decreases soluble TGF-β and type I procollagen in mouse subcutaneous connective tissue: Evidence from ex vivo and in vivo models. Journal of Cellular Physiology 214: 389–395.

Boyera N, Galey I, Bernard B (1998) Effect of vitamin C and its derivatives on collagen synthesis and cross-linking by normal human fibroblasts. International Journal of Cosmetic Science 20(3): 151–158.

Cantu R, Grodin A (1992) Myofascial manipulation. Gaithersburg, MD, Aspen Publications.

Carano A, Siciliani G (1996) Effects of continuous and intermittent forces on human fibroblasts in vitro. European Journal of Orthodontics 18(1): 19–26.

Cathie A (1974) Selected writings - Academy of Applied Osteopathy Yearbook 1974. Colorado Springs: Academy of Applied Osteopathy.

Chaitow L (1980) Soft Tissue Manipulation. Wellingborough: Thorsons.

Chaitow L (2011) Learning about fascia. Journal of Bodywork and Movement Therapies 15(1): 1–2.

Chaudhry H, Schleip R, Ji Z et al (2008) Three-dimensional mathematical model for deformation of human fasciae in manual therapy. Journal of the American Osteopathy Association 108: 379–390.

Chirasatitsin S, Engler AJ (2010) Detecting cell-adhesive sites in extracellular matrix using force spectroscopy mapping. Journal of Physics: Condensed Matter 22(19). Doi:10.1088/0953–8984/22/19/194102.

David-Raoudi M, Tranchepain F, Deschrevel B et al (2008) Differential effects of hyaluronan and its fragments on fibroblasts: relation to wound healing. Wound Repair and Regeneration 16: 274–287.

Eagan TS, Meltzer KR, Standley PR (2007) Importance of strain direction in regulating human fibroblast proliferation and cytokine secretion: a useful in vitro model for soft tissue injury and manual medicine treatments. Journal of Manipulative and Physiological Therapeutics 30(8): 584–592.

Evanko SP, Wight TN (1999) Intracellular localization of hyaluronan in proliferating cells. Journal of Histochemistry and Cytochemistry 47: 1331–1342.

Findley TW, Schleip R (2007) Fascia research: basic science and implications for conventional and complementary health care. Munich: Elsevier Urban and Fischer.

Findley TW (2012) Fascia science and clinical applications: a clinician/researcher's perspectives. Journal of Bodywork and Movement Therapies 16(1): 64–66.

Findley T, Chaudhry H, Stecco A, Roman M (2012) Fascia research – A narrative review. Journal of Bodywork and Movement Therapies 16(1): 67–75.

FitzGerald MP et al (2009) Randomized Multicenter Feasibility Trial of Myofascial Physical Therapy for the Treatment of Urological Chronic Pelvic Pain Syndromes. Journal of Urology 182(2): 570–580.

Fukunaga T, Kawakami Y, Kubo K, Kanehisa H (2002) Muscle and tendon interaction during human movements. Exercise and Sport Sciences Reviews 30: 106–110.

Fuller B (1961) Tensegrity. Portfolio and Art News Annual 4: 112–127.

Gabbiani G (2003) The myofibroblast in wound healing and fibrocontractive diseases. Journal of Pathology 200: 500–3.

Gartner L, Hiatt J (2007) Color textbook of histology, 3rd edn. Edinburgh: Saunders Elsevier, pp 1–592.

Gelse K, Poschl E, Aigner T (2003) Collagens—structure, function, and biosynthesis. Advanced Drug Delivery Reviews :55: 1531–1546.

Gordon M, Hahn R (2010) Collagens. Cell Tissue Research 339(1): 247–257.

Grinnell F (2008) Fibroblast mechanics in three-dimensional collagen matrices. Journal of Bodywork and Movement Therapies 12(3): 191–193.

Guimberteau JC (2007) Human subcutaneous sliding system. The basic stone: the microvacuolar concept. Plea for a new perception of the human anatomy of the living matter architecture. In: Fascia Research. Basic Science and Implications for Conventional and Complementary Health Care (eds Findley TW, Schleip R). Munich: Urban and Fischer, pp 237–240.

Guimberteau (2012) Scars and Adhesion Panel. Lecture notes from The 3rd International Fascia Research Congress, Vancouver, March 28–30.

Guimberteau JC, Bakhach J (2006) Subcutaneous tissue function: the multimicrovacuolar absorbing sliding system in hand and plastic surgery. Tissue Surgery 1: 41–54.

Guimberteau JC, Sentucq-Rigall J, Panconi B et al (2005) Introduction to the knowledge of subcutaneous sliding system in human. In: Annales de Chirurgie Plastique et Esthetique 50(1): 19–34.

Hinz B (2013) It has to be the [alpha] v: myofibroblast integrins activate latent TGF-[beta] 1. Nature Medicine. 19(12): 1567–1568.

Hinz B, Gabbiani G (2003) Mechanisms of force generation and transmission by myofibroblasts. Current Opinion in Biotechnology 14: 538–546.

Huijing PA (2007) Epimuscular myofascial force transmission between antagonistic and synergistic muscles can explain movement limitation in spastic paresis. Journal of Electromyography and Kinesiology 17(6): 708–724.

Huijing PA (2009) Epimuscular myofascial force transmission: a historical review and implications for new research. International Society of Biomechanics Muybridge Award Lecture, Taipei, 2007. Journal of Biomechanics 42(1): 9–21.

Ingber DE (2003) Tensegrity I. Cell structure and hierarchical systems biology. Journal of Cell Science 116(Pt 7): 1157–1173.

Ingber D (2008) Tensegrity and mechanotransduction. Journal of Bodywork and Movement Therapies 12(3): 198–200.

Jarvinen TA, Jozsa L, Kannus P et al (2002) Organization and distribution of intramuscular connective tissue in normal and immobilized skeletal muscles. An immunohistochemical, polarization and scanning electron microscopic study. Journal of Muscle Research and Cell Motility 23(3): 245–254.

Kiernan J, and Rajakumar R (2013) Barr's the human nervous system: an anatomical viewpoint. Ch. 3, p.35. Baltimore: Lippincott Williams & Wilkins.

Klingler W, Schleip R, Zorn A (2004) European Fascia Research Project Report. 5th World Congress Low Back and Pelvic Pain, Melbourne.

Kozma EM, Olczyk K, Wisowski G et al (2005) Alterations in the extracellular matrix proteoglycan profile in Dupuytren's contracture affect the palmar fascia. Journal of Biochemistry 137: 463–476.

Kumka M, Bonar B (2012) Fascia: a morphological description and classification system based on a literature review. Journal of the Canadian Chiropractic Association 56(3): 179–191.

Langevin H (2010) Presentation: Ultrasound imaging of connective tissue pathology associated with chronic low back pain. 7th Interdisciplinary Congress on Low Back and Pelvic Pain, Los Angeles.

Langevin HM, Huijing PA (2009) Communicating about fascia: history, pitfalls, and recommendations. International Journal of Therapeutic Massage Bodywork 2: 3–8.

Langevin H, Sherman K (2006) Pathophysiological model for chronic low back pain integrating connective tissue and nervous system mechanisms. Medical Hypotheses 68(1): 74–80.

Langevin H, Cornbrooks C, Taatjes D (2004) Fibroblasts form a body-wide cellular network. Histochemistry and Cell Biology 122(1): 7–15.

Langevin HM, Stevens-Tuttle D, Fox JR et al (2009) Ultrasound evidence of altered lumbar connective tissue structure in human subjects with chronic low back pain. BMC Musculoskeletal Disorders 10: 151.

Levin S (2003) The tensegrity-truss as a model for spine mechanics. Journal of Mechanics in Medicine and Biology 2(3): 374–388.

Levin S, Martin D (2012) Biotensegrity The mechanics of fascia. In: Schleip R, Findley T, Chaitow L, Huijing P (eds) Fascia. The tensional network of the human body. Edinburgh, Elsevier, pp 137–142.

Lewit K, Olsanska S (2004) Clinical importance of active scars: abnormal scars as a cause of myofascial pain. Journal of Manipulative and Physiological Therapeutics 27(6): 399–402.

Liao YH, Jones SA, Forbes B, Martin GP, Brown MB (2005) Hyaluronan: pharmaceutical characterization and drug delivery. Drug delivery 12(6): 327–342.

Maas H, Huijing PA (2009) Synergistic and antagonistic interactions in the rat forelimb: acute effects of coactivation. Journal of Applied Physiology 107(5): 1453–1462.

Maas H, Sandercock TG (2010) Force transmission between synergistic skeletal muscles through connective tissue linkages. Journal of Biomedicine and Biotechnology 12: 575672.

Macefield VG (2005) Physiological characteristics of low threshold mechanoreceptors in joints, muscle and skin in human subjects. Clinical and Experimental Pharmacology and Physiology 32(1-2): 135–144.

Mammoto A, Ingber D (2009) Cytoskeletal control of growth and cell fate switching. Current Opinion in Cell Biology 21(6): 864–870.

Marieb EN (2003) Human anatomy and physiology, 5th edn. Redwood City, CA, Benjamin/Cummings Publishing, p 5.

Marieb EN, Reece JB, Urry LA et al (2012) Essentials of Human Anatomy and Physiology with Essentials of Interactive Physiology CD-ROM, 10/E.

McCombe D, Brown T, Slavin J, Morrison WA (2001) The histochemical structure of the deep fascia and its structural response to surgery. Journal of Hand Surgery (British) 26: 89–97 doi:10.1054/ jhsb.2000.0546.

Matteini P et al (2009) Structural behavior of highly concentrated hyaluronan. Biomacromolecules 10(6): 1516–22.

Meltzer K et al (2009) In vitro modelling of repetitive motion injury and myofascial release. Journal of Bodywork and Movement Therapies 14: 162–171.

Milz S, Benjamin M, Putz R (2005) Molecular parameters indicating adaptation to mechanical stress in fibrous connective tissue. Advances in Anatomy Embryology and Cell Biology (Vol. 178). Berlin, Springer-Verlag.

Mitchell JH, Schmidt RF (1977) Cardiovascular reflex control by afferent fibers from skeletal muscle receptors. In: Shepherd JT et al. (eds) Handbook of Physiology, Sect 2, Vol III, Part 2. Bethesda, MA: American Physiological Society, pp 623–658.

Mouchnino L, Blouin J (2013) When standing on a moving support, cutaneous inputs provide sufficient information to plan the anticipatory postural adjustments for gait initiation. PLOS One. DOI: 10.1371/journal.pone.0055081.

Muscolino J (2012) Body mechanics – fascial structure. Available at: http://www.learnmuscles.com/MTJ_SP12_BodyMechanics%20copy.pdf [Accessed 14 June 2015].

Murray MM, Spector M (1999) Fibroblasts distribution in the anteromedial bundle of the human anterior cruciate ligament: the presence of a-smooth actin-positive cells. Journal of Orthopaedic Research 17(1): 18–27.

Myers T (2014) Anatomy trains: myofascial meridians for manual and movement therapists, 3rd edn. Edinburgh: Elsevier.

Nekouzadeh A, Pryse KM, Elson EL, Genin GM (2008) Stretch activated force shedding, force recovery, and cytoskeletal remodeling in contractile fibroblasts. Journal of Biomechanics 41(14): 2964–2971. doi:10.1016/ j.jbiomech.

Netter FH (2011) Atlas of human anatomy, professional edn (5th edn). Philadelphia: Saunders Elsevier.

Pilat A (2009) Myofascial induction approaches for headache. In: Fernández-de-las- Peñas C, Arendt-Nielsen L, Gerwin RD (eds). Tension type and cervicogenic headache: pathophysiology, diagnosis and treatment. Boston: Jones and Bartlett Publishers.

Pischinger A (1991) Matrix and matrix regulation: basis for a holistic theory in medicine. Brussels: Haug International.

Platzer W (2008) Color atlas of human anatomy, 6th edn, vol. 1. New York: Thieme.

Powell D, Mifflin R, Valentich J et al (1999) Myofibroblasts. I. Paracrine cells important in health and disease. American Journal of Physiology-Cell Physiology 277(1): C1-19, July.

Purslow PP (2002) The structure and functional significance of variations in the connective tissue within muscle. Comparative Biochemistry and Physiology, Part A, 133: 947–966.

Purslow P, Delage J-P (2012) General anatomy of the muscle fasciae. In: Schleip R, Findley T, Chaitow L, Huijing P (eds). Fascia: the tensional network of the human body. Edinburgh: Churchill Livingstone, Elsevier.

Ralphs JR, Waggett AD, Benjamin M (2002) Actin stress fibres and cell–cell adhesion molecules in tendons: organisation in vivo and response to mechanical loading of tendon cells in vitro. Matrix Biology 21(1): 67–74.

Reed RK, Liden A, Rubin K (2010) Edema and fluid dynamics in connective tissue remodelling. Journal of Molecular and Cell Cardiology 48(3): 518–523. doi: 10.1016/j.yjmcc.2009.06.023.

Richter P (2012) Myofascial chains. In: Schleip R, Findley T, Chaitow L, Huijing P (eds) Fascia. The tensional network of the human body. Edinburgh, Churchill Livingstone Elsevier, pp 123–130.

Rolf I (1962) Structural dynamics. British Academy of Applied Osteopathy Yearbook 1962. London: BAAO.

Ross M, Pawlina W (2011) Histology: a text and atlas, 6th edn. Philadelphia: Lippincott Williams and Wilkins, p 218.

Ryan C (2011) The story of fascia – Interview with Julie Day. In: Ryan C. Massage Matters Canada Magazine, Summer issue.

Schleip R (2003) Fascial plasticity: a new neurobiological explanation, Parts 1 and 2. Journal of Bodywork and Movement Therapies 7(1): 11–19.

Schleip R, Müller DG (2013) Training principles for fascial connective tissues: Scientific foundation and suggested practical applications. Journal of Bodywork and Movement Therapies 17(1): 103–115.

Schleip R, Naylor IL, Ursu D et al (2006) Passive muscle stiffness may be influenced by active contractility of intramuscular connective tissue. Medical Hypotheses 66(1): 66–71.

Schleip R, Vleeming A, Lehmann-Horn F et al (2007) Letter to the Editor concerning 'A hypothesis of chronic back pain: ligament sub-failure injuries lead to muscle control dysfunction' (M. Panjabi). European Spine Journal 16: 1733–35.

Schleip R, Jäger H, Klingler W (2012a) What is 'fascia'? A review of different nomenclatures. Journal of Bodywork and Movement Therapies 16(4): 496–502.

Schleip R, Findley T, Chaitow L, Huijing P (2012b) Fascia: the tensional network of the human body. Edinburgh: Churchill Livingstone Elsevier.

Schleip R, Klingler W, Lehmann-Horn F (2005) Active fascial contractility: fascia may be able to contract in a smooth muscle-like manner and thereby influence musculoskeletal dynamics. Medical Hypotheses 65(2): 273–277.

Sidgwick GP, Bayat A (2012) Extracellular matrix molecules implicated in hypertrophic and keloid scarring. Journal of the European Academy of Dermatology and Venereology 26(2): 141–152.

Spector M (2002) Novel cell-scaffold interactions encountered in tissue engineering: contractile behavior of musculoskeletal connective tissue cells. Tissue Engineering 8(3): 351–357.

Standley PR, Meltzer KR (2008) In vitro modeling of repetitive motion strain and manual medicine treatments: potential roles for pro- and anti-inflammatory cytokines.

Journal of Bodywork and Movement Therapies 12: 201–203.

Standley PR (2012) Fluid dynamics - Clinical Implications Panel. Lecture notes from The 3rd International Fascia Research Congress, Vancouver, March 28–30.

Standring S (2008) Gray's Anatomy, 40th edn. The anatomical basis of clinical practice. Edinburgh: Elsevier.

Stecco A, Macchi V, Stecco C et al (2009) Anatomical study of myofascial continuity, anterior upper limb. Journal of Bodywork and Movement Therapies 13: 53–62.

Stecco C, Pavan PG, Porzionato A, et al (2009) Mechanics of crural fascia: from anatomy to constitutive modelling. Surgical and Radiologic Anatomy 31(7): 523–529.

Stecco C, Porzionato A, Lancerotto L et al (2008) Histological study of the deep fasciae of the limbs. Journal of Bodywork and Movement Therapies 12(3): 225–230.

Stecco C, Stern R, Porzionato A et al (2011) Hyaluronan within fascia in the etiology of myofascial pain. Surgical and Radiologic Anatomy 33(10): 891–6.

Stecco C, Tiengo C, Stecco A, et al (2013) Fascia redefined: anatomical features and technical relevance in fascial flap surgery. Surgical and Radiologic Anatomy 35(5): 369-376.

Stecco L (2004) Fascial manipulation for musculoskeletal pain. Padova, Piccin.

Stecco L, Stecco C (2009) Fascial manipulation: practical part. Padova: Piccin.

Swanson RL (2013) Biotensegrity: a unifying theory of biological architecture. Journal of the American Osteopathic Association 113(1): 34–52.

Taguchi T, Tesarz J, Mense S (2009) The thoracolumbar fascia as a source of low back pain. In: Huijing PA, Hollander P, Findley TW, Schleip R (eds) Fascia research II – basic science and implications for conventional and complementary health care. Munich: Elsevier GmbH.

Tank PW (2012) Grant's dissector, 15th edn. Philadelphia: Lippincott Williams and Wilkins.

Terminologia Histologica (2008) International terms for human cytology and histology/ Federative International Committee on Anatomical Terminology (FICAT). Baltimore: Wolters Kluwer/Lippincott Williams and Wilkins, pp 1–207.

Tesarz J, Hoheisel U, Wiedenhofer B and Mense S (2011) Sensory innervation of the thoracolumbar fascia in rats and humans, Neuroscience 194:3020308. doi: 10.1016/j.neuroscience.2011.07.066.

Tomasek JJ, Gabbiani G, Hinz B et al (2002) Myofibroblasts and mechano-regulation of connective tissue remodelling. Nature Reviews Molecular Cell Biology 3: 349–363.

Van den Berg F (2010) Angewandte physiologie – Band 1: Das bindegewebe des bewegunfsapparates;verstehen und beeinflussen [Applied physiology, vol. 1, The connective tissue of the locomotor apparatus; understanding and influencing]. Stuttgart, Thieme Verlag.

Van den Berg F (2012) The physiology of fascia: an introduction. In: Schleip R, Findley T, Chaitow L, Huijing P (eds) Fascia. The tensional network of the human body. Edinburgh: Churchill Livingstone Elsevier, pp 149–155.

Van der Wal J (2009) The architecture of the connective tissue in the musculoskeletal system – an often overlooked functional parameter as to proprioception in the locomotor apparatus. International Journal of Therapeutic Massage and Bodywork 2(4): 9–23.

Wang N, Tytell J, Ingber D (2009) Mechanotransduction at a distance: mechanically coupling the extra cellular matrix with the nucleus. Science 10: 75–81.

Willard F (2012a) Somatic fascia. In: Schleip R, Findley T, Chaitow L, Huijing P (eds) Fascia. The tensional network of the human body. Edinburgh: Churchill Livingstone Elsevier, pp 30–36.

Willard F (2012b) Visceral fascia. In: Schleip R, Findley T, Chaitow L, Huijing P (eds) Fascia. The tensional network of the human body. Edinburgh: Elsevier, pp 53–56.

Wilson CJ, Dahners LE (1988)) An examination of the mechanism of ligament contracture. Clinical Orthopaedics and Related Research (227): 286–291.

Yahia LH, Rhalmi S, Newman N, Isler M (1992) Sensory innervation of human thoracolumbar fascia: an immunohistochemical study. Acta Orthopaedica 63(2): 195–197.

Zorn A, Hodeck K (2011) Walk with elastic fascia. In: Dalton E (ed) Dynamic body. Oklahoma City, OK: Freedom From Pain Institute, pp 96–123.

Resources and Further Reading

Barral Institute: http://www.barralinstitute.com/

Charter Society of Physiotherapy: http://www.csp.org.uk/events/manual-therapy-abdominal-viscera

Upledger Institute: http://www.upledger.com/

The lymphatic system

'Milk me'

Client statement upon entering the clinic room ready for her second Manual Lymph Drainage session

The lymphatic system is a lesser known yet important system of the body that chugs along, quietly assisting the blood vascular and immune systems. In brief, it is a low pressure, pump-less system that transports lymphatic fluid (lymph).

Lymph is formed in the digestive system and is taken up by the specialized lymph vessels known as lacteals (Choi et al. 2012). When functioning normally, it is the squeeze–release action of the skeletal muscles and the changes in pressure during breathing that pushes or 'milks' the lymph toward its destination (Marieb 2003).

While the blood vascular system has been studied extensively, the lymphatic system has had little scientific and medical attention, likely due to its elusive morphology and mysterious pathophysiology. Over the past decade a number of new studies have begun to change the misconception that the lymphatic system is secondary to the more *essential* blood vascular system and, indeed, substantiate the view that the lymphatic system is an integral and equal partner in supporting homeostasis, immunity, and wound healing (Choi et al. 2012).

Utilizing the information that is currently available, the aim of this chapter is to provide a solid understanding of the lymphatic system. Particular relevance to this book is the lymphatic system's role in creating a favorable environment for wound healing and healthy scar formation and the consequences associated with impaired lymphatic function (Marieb 2003).

Discovery of the Lymphatic System

The lymphatic system has been documented since early recorded history:

- Hippocrates (460–377 BC) talked about vessels containing 'white blood'

- Aristotle (384–322 BC) described vessels containing a 'colorless fluid', or 'white blood'

- The French anatomist Marie Sappey (1810–1890) used subcutaneous mercury injections to graphically represent the anatomy of the lymphatic system.

Hippocrates spoke of white blood cells, introduced the term chyle and defined a lymphatic temperament (Chikly 2002). Chyle – a milky-colored fluid – consists of lymph, emulsified fats and free fatty acids.

In 1627 Gasparo Aselli discovered lymphatic vessels, calling them *lacteae venae*, or milky veins. In 1652 Thomas Bartholin, a Danish physician and anatomist, called the vessels *vasa lymphatica* and is credited with giving the lymphatic system its name.

Early comprehensive study of the intricate and complex lymphatic system began at the beginning of the twentieth century but slowed significantly because of the lack of specific lymphatic markers, and the histogenetic origin of lymphatic vessels remains a controversial issue (Oliver & Detmar 2002).

The most accepted understanding of the development of the lymphatic system was put forth by Dr Florence Sabin in the early twentieth century (Sabin 1902, Sabin 1904). Sabin injected ink into the lymphatic system of pig embryos and cataloged the results. Sabin concluded that isolated primitive lymph sacs originate from endothelial cells that bud from the veins during early development. It was proposed that the two jugular lymph sacs developed in the junction of the subclavian and anterior cardinal veins by endothelial budding from the anterior cardinal veins (Sabin 1902, Sabin 1904). According to Sabin, the remaining lymph sacs originate from the mesonephric vein and those in the dorsomedial edge of the Wolffian bodies in the junction of the subclavian and anterior cardinal veins. Sabin's early findings have been validated through more recent research (Wilting et al. 2003).

Lymphatic, Hematic and Immune Systems

The lymphatic, hematic (blood vascular) and immune systems play a shared role in supporting homeostasis, defending the body against disease and helping wound repair and healing.

Homeostasis is a continual balancing act of the body systems to provide a 'steady state' – an internal environment that is compatible with life. The two liquid tissues, blood and lymph, have separate but interrelated functions in maintaining this balance and function in tandem with the immune system to protect the body against pathogens that could threaten the organism's viability.

Only a brief overview of the hematic and immune systems will be provided in this book as these systems are extensively studied and ample resources are available.

Hematic System

The heart, blood vessels and blood constitute the main components of this closed-loop system with the heart as its central pump.

The part of the hematic system that delivers blood to and from the lungs is known as the pulmonary circulation, and the flow of blood throughout the rest of the body is administered by the systemic circulation. The hematic system plays an integral role in the removal of waste products associated with metabolism and the transportation of gases (oxygen and carbon dioxide), chemical substances (e.g. hormones, nutrients, salts), and cells that defend the body. Additionally, this system helps regulate the body's fluid and electrolyte balance, pH and body temperature, and helps protect the body from infection and loss of blood by the action of clotting.

As noted in Chapter 2, the hematic system plays an important role in wound repair and healing. In the early stages of wound healing angiogenesis, the formation of capillary-sized microvessels ensure the delivery of blood-borne cells, nutrients and oxygen to areas undergoing remodeling.

Immune System

The immune system is a collection of cells (e.g. mast cells, macrophages, neutrophils), tissues and organs (e.g. skin, bloodstream, lymph nodes, thymus, spleen, mucosal tissue) with the skin constituting the first 'line-of-defense'.

All immune cells originate from precursors in the bone marrow and develop through a series of changes that occur in various tissues and organs.

Immune response protects the body against pathogens that could threaten the organism's viability. As noted in Chapter 2, the immune system plays an important role in wound repair/healing.

Lymphatic System Structure and Function

The lymphatic system consists of fluid (lymph) and structural components (vessels, tissues, nodes, organs) (Marieb 2003).

Lymph

When the interstitial fluid enters the lymphatic system, it is termed lymph. Lymph is generally clear and transparent, or milky in appearance when emulsified fats are present (chyle) (Zuther 2011). Before returning to the blood vascular system, lymph travels through a successive number of lymph nodes, which filter out impurities.

Lymphatic Vessels (Chikly 2002, Zuther 2011)

The lymphatic system develops in parallel with the blood vascular system. Lymphatic vessels are typically not present in avascular structures such as epidermis, hair, nails, cartilage and cornea, nor in some vascularized organs such as brain and retina (Oliver & Detmar 2002).

The general structure of lymphatic vessels is similar to that of blood vascular vessels presenting in various sizes (lymph capillaries, lymphatic collectors). Additionally, larger lymphatic vessels are trilaminar:

- **Tunica intima**: the innermost layer consists of endothelial cells and is equipped with valves that direct the flow of lymph, preventing *back flow.*

- **Tunica media**: the intermediate layer consists of smooth muscle and elastin.

- **Tunica adventitia**: the outermost layer consists of collagen and elastin. Lying on the exterior surface of the adventitia are the vasa vasorum, a petite collection of arteries, veins, lymphatics and nerves that service the vessels themselves.

Clinical Consideration

Nerves, blood vascular and lymphatic vessels are wrapped in layers of connective tissue (CT) or fascia – considered to be a form of CT. Recent stud-

Clinical Consideration (Cont.)

ies indicate that CT can dynamically regulate its tension (Langevin et al. 2013) suggesting that changes in tissue tension could affect the functioning of the surrounding enveloped structures. Releasing undue tension may improve neural function and fluid flow.

Lymphatic vessels contain more valves and more frequent anastomoses than blood circulatory vessels, thereby reducing back flow and creating an extensive, connected network of tubes (Marieb 2003, Macdonald et al. 2008). The smaller, thin-walled lymph capillaries are slightly larger than those seen in the blood vascular system. Unlike the tightly joined endothelial cells lining blood vascular capillaries, lymph capillary endothelial cells loosely overlap, augmenting porosity thereby facilitating the collection of larger molecules.

Afferent lymphatic vessels: carry unfiltered lymph into the nodes, where waste products and some of the fluid is filtered out.

Efferent lymphatic vessels: carry the filtered lymph out of the node to continue its return to the circulatory system.

Lymph Nodes

The lymph node (see Fig. 3.2) is part of the many types of lymphoid organs in the body. There are between 600 and 700 lymph nodes present in the average human body. It is the role of these nodes to filter the lymph before it can be returned to the circulatory system. Although these nodes can increase or decrease in size throughout life, any nodes that have been damaged or destroyed do not regenerate.

Lymph nodes contain macrophages that destroy bacteria, viruses and other substances before the lymph is returned to the blood vascular system (Marieb 2003).

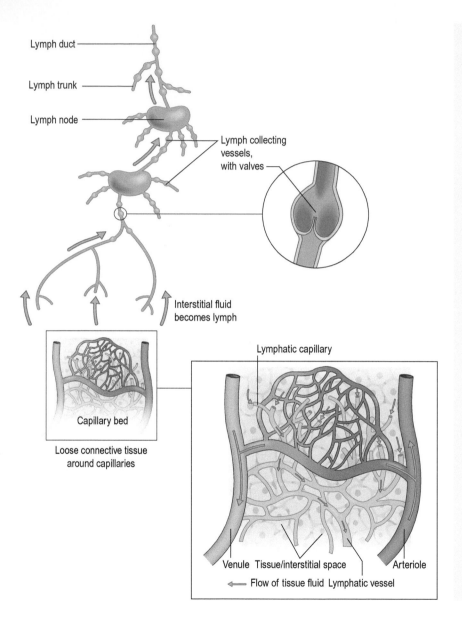

Figure 3.1
Lymph tissue structure.

In another section of the node, lymphocytes, specialized white blood cells (WBCs), kill pathogens that may be present. When inflammation is part of the protective process this sometimes results in the swelling commonly identified as *swollen glands*. Lymph nodes also trap cancer cells, with the ability to slow the spread of the cancer, until the system becomes overwhelmed.

Lymph nodes are typically kidney shaped and less than an inch (2.5 cm) in diameter but can

Figure 3.2
Lymph node structure.

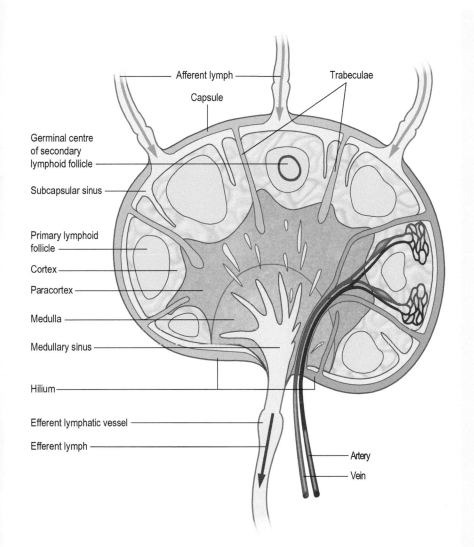

Afferent lymph

Trabeculae

Capsule

Germinal centre of secondary lymphoid follicle

Subcapsular sinus

Primary lymphoid follicle

Cortex

Paracortex

Medulla

Medullary sinus

Hilium

Efferent lymphatic vessel

Efferent lymph

Artery

Vein

fluctuate in both shape and size. Lymph nodes are embedded within the fascia and are surrounded by trabeculae – fibrous CT that divides the capsule into numerous compartments and provides structural support (Marieb 2003).

The lymph system is present throughout the body. Common areas where enlarged lymph nodes can be felt (palpable nodes) include: the popliteal, inguinal, axilla and neck regions; under the jaw and chin; behind the ears; and over the occiput. There are also non-palpable lymph nodes in the abdomen, pelvis and chest regions. Their function is the same regardless of their location.

The lymph passes through numerous lymph nodes where the cleaning and filtering process is carried out (Marieb 2003).

Lymphoid Organs

The lymphoid organs include the spleen, tonsils, thymus glands and Peyer's patches of the intestine. There is commonality between each of these organs: namely, a high proportion of reticular CT and lymphocytes. The lymphoid organs contain the phagocytes and lymphocytes, which are crucial for the immune system to work in full vigor (Marieb 2003).

Organ Types and Functions

Peyer's patches

Peyer's patches are a little like tonsils in appearance. They are embedded in the wall of the small intestine, placing associated macrophages in the perfect position to capture and destroy bacteria in the intestine.

Peyer's patches and the tonsils are just one part of the smaller lymph tissues known as mucosa-associated lymphatic tissue (MALT) (Marieb 2003). MALT works as a sentinel, protecting the digestive tract and the upper respiratory system from the constant barrage of foreign matter that enters these cavities.

Tonsils

The tonsils are made up of little collections of lymphatic tissue encased in mucosa that encircle the pharynx. The tonsils remove bacteria and foreign pathogens that enter through the throat. Tonsillitis results when the nodes become overwhelmed with bacteria and become red, edematous and sore.

Thymus

The thymus is a lymphoid gland comprised of two identically sized lobes, located behind the sternum and in front of the heart. The thymus functions mainly during our youth as it produces hormones and thymosin that assist certain lymphocytes in the programing of their immune defense roles in the body.

Spleen

The spleen is located on the left side of the abdominal cavity and spreads to the anterior aspect of the stomach. The spleen is a blood-rich organ that filters out bacteria, viruses and other cellular debris from the blood.

The spleen also destroys depleted red blood cells and returns waste products to the liver. The spleen also stores platelets and takes on the role of a blood reservoir (Marieb 2003).

Lymphatic Drainage and Transport

In order to better facilitate understanding of the next section, the following key terms, concepts and mechanisms are briefly described:

- Lymphatic drainage: the movement of fluid and molecules (e.g. proteins) from the interstitium into the lymphatic capillaries.

- Lymphatic transport: the movement of lymph along a succession of vessels with eventual return to the blood vascular system (lymphatic return).

- Lymphatic load: the term 'lymphatic load' was coined by renowned lymphologists, Drs Michael and Etelka Földi. Lymphatic load refers to total sum of substances (proteins, colloids, minerals, water, cells and fat) in the interstitium that cannot be absorbed by the hematic system (Földi et al. 1989).

- **Protein**: within a 24-hour period, at least half of the proteins in the blood will leave the capillaries and make a home in the interstitial spaces (Zuther 2011).These proteins provide cell nutrition, immune defense, transportation of hormones, fats, minerals and waste products, and coagulate the blood. Proteins are generally too large to reenter the bloodstream through the blood capillaries. Through intercellular openings in the capillaries of the lymph node, large protein molecules can be 'taken-up' or collected.

- **Fluid/water**: approximately 10–20% of the water that leaves the blood capillary system makes up the water in the lymphatic load. It is returned to the blood system through the thoracic duct, the right lymphatic duct and venous angles. It is estimated that 2–3 liters is recirculated per day (Zuther 2011). The blood capillaries in the node reabsorb most of the remaining fluid. This action reduces the lymphatic load returning through the thoracic duct and the right lymphatic duct into the venous system.

- **White and red blood cells (WBC, RBC)**: by continuously leaving the blood capillaries, WBCs and RBCs are absorbed by the lymphatic system. When the lymphocytes are circulated back into the bloodstream it results in an important immune response in the body. The lymphatic system also transports cell fractions (debris) that can be caused by trauma or tissue neoformation (regeneration). Bacteria and cancer cells are also carried through the lymphatic system. Additional particles that enter the body through digestion, inhalation (e.g. mold spores, dust, dirt) or injury are absorbed by the lymphatic vessels and delivered to the lymph nodes. Once inside the node, the immune response is activated (Zuther 2011).

- **Fat**: if fat is part of the lymph, the usually clear lymph takes on a cloudy, milky color. Fat compounds that cannot be absorbed into the small intestines are absorbed by the chylous vessels (lymph vessels of the small intestines). It is through the chylous vessels that fatty acids and other compounds reenter the bloodstream (Zuther 2011).

- Lymphatic transport capacity: is the maximum amount of lymph the system can transport in a given time frame (Földi et al. 1989). A healthy lymphatic system is capable of transporting 10 times the volume of normal lymphatic loads. This leaves ample room for accommodating fluctuations in lymphatic load volumes – when the system is healthy. With either primary or secondary lymphedema (described further on in this chapter), transport capacity cannot handle the lymphatic load; this constitutes mechanical insufficiency (Zuther 2002).

Transport and Drainage Structures

The drainage and transport of lymph involves the capillaries, nodes and vessels dispersed throughout the body. This collection of lymph structures are divided into two separate and distinct layers: superficial and deep (Zuther 2011).

Superficial

The superficial layer is responsible for the drainage of the epidermis, dermis and subcutaneous tissue. The superficial transport of lymph is a system that is embedded in the subcutaneous tissue or superficial fascia.

Deep

The deeper layer of the lymphatic system drains lymph from tendon sheaths, muscle tissue, nerves, the periosteum and most joint structures – with the exception of a few distal joints of the extremities that drain via the superficial nodes (Zuther 2011). The deeper lymphatic transport vessels are usually grouped together in the same fascial tunnel with blood vessels and nerves.

Perforating vessels connect the deep lymphatic system with the superficial lymphatic system (Zuther 2011). Internal organs, such as the spleen, are in a subcategory of the deep lymphatic system.

Primary upper lymphatic structures

The thoracic duct is the largest lymphatic structure in the body and constitutes the terminal end of the lymphatic transport system. The thoracic duct is positioned between the 11th thoracic and the 2nd lumbar vertebrae just anterior to the vertebral column. The thoracic duct is between 10 and 18 inches (25 and 45 cm) long and contains

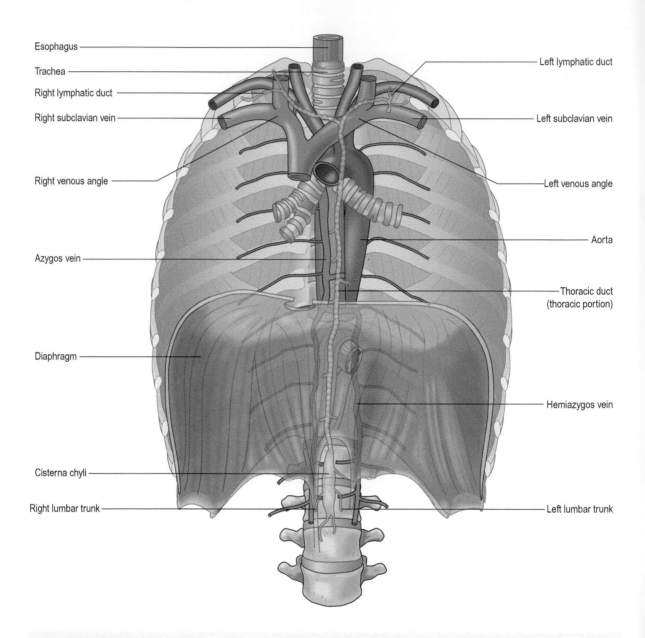

Esophagus

Trachea

Right lymphatic duct

Right subclavian vein

Right venous angle

Azygos vein

Diaphragm

Cisterna chyli

Right lumbar trunk

Left lymphatic duct

Left subclavian vein

Left venous angle

Aorta

Thoracic duct
(thoracic portion)

Hemiazygos vein

Left lumbar trunk

Figure 3.3
Torso and pelvic anatomy.

a large number of valves. It perforates the diaphragm and continues to run upward to connect with the left venous angle.

The left venous angle is an area located behind the left clavicle and is made up by the connection of the left subclavian and internal jugular veins (Fig. 3.3). Approximately 2–3 liters of lymph are returned to the venous blood via the thoracic duct within a time period of 24 hours.

Primary lower lymphatic structures

The lymph coming from the lower extremities drains into the inguinal lymph nodes. Inguinal lymph nodes are located in the medial femoral triangle, which is outlined by the inguinal ligament (proximal border), the sartorius muscle (lateral border) and the gracilis muscle (medial border). Dissection and/or radiation of these lymph nodes could result in secondary lymphedema. The more common reason for the onset of lymphedema in the lower extremity is congenital malformations of the lymphatic system, resulting in primary lymphedema (discussed in more detail later in this chapter).

Right side lymphatic drainage

The right side of the body has the smallest drain field. The right side drainage route transports lymph from the right side of the head and neck, the right arm and upper right quadrant of the body (see Fig. 3.4).

Lymph from this area flows into the right lymphatic duct (see Fig. 3.3). This duct empties the lymph into the right subclavian vein (see Fig. 3.3).

Left side lymphatic drainage

The left side drain field is extensive (see Fig. 3.4). The left side drainage route transports lymph from of the left side of the head and neck, the left arm and the left upper quadrant, the bilateral lower trunk and legs.

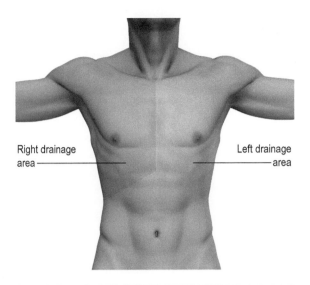

Right drainage area

Left drainage area

Figure 3.4

Lymphatic drainage areas.

The cisterna chyli (see Fig. 3.3) temporarily stores lymph as it moves upward from the lower areas of the body. The thoracic duct (see Fig. 3.3) transports lymph upward to the left lymphatic duct. The left lymphatic duct empties the lymph into the left subclavian vein.

Lymphatic System Functions

A brief overview and summary:

- Cleanses the cellular environment

- Collects proteins and tissue fluids, returning them to the blood circulation

- Provides a pathway for the absorption of fats and fat-soluble vitamins into the bloodstream

- Helps defend the body against disease and invaders.

The primary function of the lymphatic system is to collect and transport fluid, larger molecules and cellular waste and debris. Via the extensive

Clinical Consideration

Lymph is the new blood

Readily visible, blood and its associated vessels have been studied for centuries, garnering much attention including detailed, shiny color plates in health science textbooks. However, a recent stunning discovery challenges current textbooks, calling for more in-depth study and an extreme make-over for anatomy and physiology editions.

Generally presumed by manual lymph therapists but *unverified*, researchers have now discovered that the meningeal linings of brain have a lymphatic vessel network that connects to the systemic lymphatic system. Until now, lymphatic vessels in the central nervous system (CNS) have remained elusive (i.e. no shiny color plates), but the development of better imaging methods has changed all that (Aspelund et al. 2015, Louveau et al. 2015, University of Helsinki 2015, University of Virginia Health System 2015).

Vessels displaying all the molecular hallmarks of lymphatic vessels have been discovered and mapped, running parallel to the dural sinuses, arteries, veins and cranial nerves. It is suggested that they serve as a direct clearance route for the brain and cerebrospinal fluid macromolecules out of the skull and into the deep cervical lymph nodes (Aspelund et al. 2015, Louveau et al. 2015, University of Helsinki 2015, University of Virginia Health System 2015).

As is known, the lymph system clears fluids and macromolecules and plays an important role in immune function. Previously, the CNS has been considered devoid of lymphatic vasculature, leaving immunologists puzzled as to how lymphocytes access and exit the brain (Aspelund et al. 2015, Louveau et al. 2015, University of Helsinki 2015, University of Virginia Health System 2015).

The extensive lymph network found in the brain changes our understanding of how the brain is cleared of excess fluid and calls for the rethinking of brain disease etiology and treatment approaches. This discovery has also raised several new questions concerning some fundamental brain functions and changes how we look at the relationship between the CNS and immune system (Aspelund et al 2015, Louveau et al. 2015, University of Helsinki 2015,

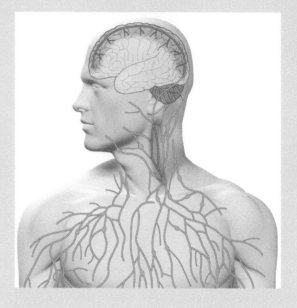

Fig 3.5
Brain lymphatic vessels.

University of Virginia Health System 2015).
Researchers find it highly possible that brain–lymph connection will prove important in neuro-immunological diseases as well as in diseases characterized by the pathological accumulation of misfolded proteins or fluid into the brain parenchyma (e.g. Alzheimer's disease, MS and autism). In Alzheimer's for example, there are accumulations of big protein chunks in the brain and it has been suggested that these chunks may be accumulating because they're not being efficiently removed by the CNS lymph system (Louveau et al. 2015).

Given the lymph and immune systems role in wound healing, one can surmise that future work in this area may reveal significant considerations for scar management.

collection of lymph capillaries, reusable products (e.g. fluid, larger proteins, viable blood and immune cells) can be collected and then recirculated back into the blood vascular system, whereas excess fluid, waste, debris, dead blood cells, pathogens, cancer cells and toxins can be removed – ridding the body of undesirables or potentially harmful agents. The lymphatic system also works with the circulatory system to deliver nutrients, oxygen and hormones from the blood to the cells that make up the tissues of the body. Additionally, the lymphatic system plays an important role in immunity, inflammation and wound healing.

Lymph flow is a one-way system directed toward the heart. The lymphatic system begins out in the tissues as small lymphatic vessels (lymph capillaries) and continues with successively larger lymphatic vessels (collectors and trunks), which ultimately connect to the venous part of the blood vascular system.

There is no central pump; lymph vessels produce their own propulsion system with a network of smooth musculature located in the walls of lymph collectors and trunks. In addition to phasic contraction of smooth muscle, lymph flow is also assisted by pressure gradients, skeletal muscle contraction, intestinal motility, respiration, extrinsic compression forces, movement (active and passive) and manual lymphatic techniques (Rockson 2001, Knott et al. 2005, Hodge et al. 2007 & 2010, Macdonald et al. 2008, Quick et al. 2008, Davis et al. 2009, Huff et al. 2010, Hodge & Downey 2011).

Clinical Consideration

Manual lymphatic techniques improve lymph flow, reduce edema and boost immunity (Knott et al. 2005, Hodge & Downey 2011).

Since the lymph vessels work according to the one-way principle and not as a closed circulatory system, it is more appropriate to speak of lymph transport rather than lymph circulation. While the flow of blood through the blood vessels is uninterrupted, the transport of lymph through the lymph vessel system is interrupted by lymph nodes, where the lymph is filtered, cleaned and concentrated (see Fig. 3.6).

Immunity

Lymph nodes play an important part in the body's defense against infection. Many immune reactions occur in the lymph nodes. Swelling might occur even if the infection is trivial or not apparent.

The lymphatic system aids the immune system in destroying pathogens and filtering waste so that the lymph can be safely returned to the circulatory system.

Lymphocytes – the main cell type found in lymph – constitute the three types of WBCs: NK (natural killer), T and B cells. Lymphocytes are a part of the immune system, directly attacking foreign bodies with T cells and macrophages and indirectly with B cell that produce antibodies (Zuther 2011). Antibodies produced in lymph nodes travel in the lymph to the bloodstream for distribution in the body. Lymphocytes in the nodes and the spleen attack foreign invaders in the system.

In tissues affected by lymphedema, the lymph is unable to drain properly. Instead, the protein-rich lymph becomes stagnant within these swollen tissues. When bacteria enter this fluid through a break in the skin, they thrive on this protein-rich fluid. This is why lymphedema-affected tissues are prone to infections.

Lymphadenitis is an infection and inflammation of one or more of the lymph nodes and usually results from an infection that begins near a lymph node. Often caused by *Staphylococcus aureus* bacteria, this condition affects the nodes in the neck, groin

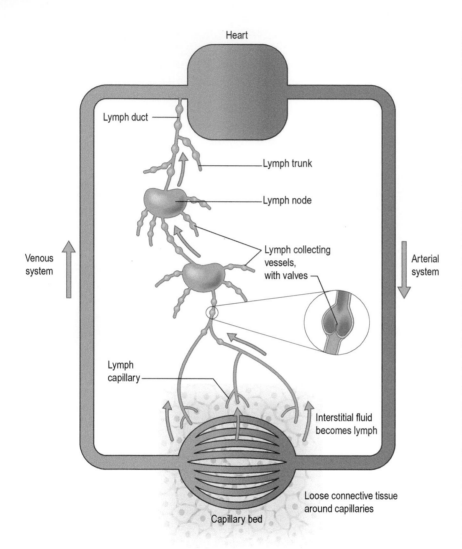

Heart

Lymph duct

Lymph trunk

Lymph node

Lymph collecting
vessels,
with valves

Venous
system

Arterial
system

Lymph
capillary

Interstitial fluid
becomes lymph

Loose connective tissue
around capillaries

Capillary bed

Figure 3.6

Blood vascular
circulation loop and
lymph transport flow.

and armpit. It sometimes strikes individuals who have had coronary artery bypasses using a saphenous vein from the leg: the removal of this vein is accompanied by removal of related structures of the lymphatic system, lowering immunity to infection.

Acute lymphangitis is a bacterial infection in the lymphatic vessels, which is characterized by painful, red streaks below the skin surface. This is a potentially serious infection that can rapidly spread to the bloodstream and be fatal.

Lymph nodes are filters that can catch malignant tumor cells or infectious organisms. When they do, lymph nodes increase in size and are easily felt.

While lymph nodes are the most common cause of a lump or a bump in the neck, there are other, much less common causes, e.g. cysts from abnormalities of fetal development or thyroid gland enlargement.

Wound Healing

As with the blood vascular system, successful tissue repair requires the regrowth and reconnection of lymphatic structures. In the early stages of wound healing, the formation of lymphatic vessels in circumferential wounds helps bridge the margins of a newly forming scar (Bellman & Oden 1958, Oliver & Detmar 2002).

In full-thickness skin wounds angiogenesis in newly formed granulation tissue largely dominates the delayed and comparatively less pronounced formation of new lymphatic vessels (lymphangiogenesis) (Paavonen et al. 2000, Oliver & Detmar 2002).

During tissue repair, lymphatic vessels reconnect with lymphatic vessels – not with blood vessels – and cultured lymphatic endothelial cells remain separate from blood vascular endothelial cells during tube formation in vitro (Kriehuber et al. 2001).

It is known that in adults lymphangiogenesis can occur by outgrowth from pre-existing lymph vessels (Clark & Clark 1932, Paavonen et al. 2000) but it is unclear if during tissue repair lymphangiogenesis involves progenitor cells, as in angiogenesis.

Impact of Trauma and Pathophysiological Scars on the Lymphatic System

Trauma and scars can disrupt the network of lymph capillaries, which can hinder fluid drainage and negatively affect the healing process.

The development of scar tissue that hinders the flow of lymph can have various causes:

- Surgical procedures that interrupt normal lymphatic function, such as surgery for cancer in the breast or groin areas, may prevent lymph flowing naturally through its system (Zuther 2011)

- Radiation therapy can damage an otherwise healthy lymphatic system by causing scar tissue to form, subsequently interrupting the normal flow of lymph (Zuther 2011)

- Traumatic scars may affect the lymphatic system, damaging the normal flow of lymph.

Clinical Consideration

Four continuous minutes of abdominal lymph pumping (1 pump/sec) has been shown to increase immune cell release from mesenteric lymph nodes. Specialized T cells primed in the gut are faster-acting/ superior-performing immune cells. Recent studies suggest that abdominal lymphatic pumping may inhibit solid tumor development and bacterial pneumonia (Hodge et al. 2010, 2013).

Pathophysiological Consideration

Abdominal scarring may interfere with the effectiveness of local lymph pump techniques (Hodge et al. 2010, 2013).

In addition, repeated episodes of infection can cause progressive closure of the lymphatic system, thus worsening the condition.

If the transport pathway becomes congested, blocked, damaged or severed, fluids can accumulate in the surrounding tissues leading to edema and fibrosis. Eventually cell pathology may occur. If the lymph system is incapacitated in any way (e.g. burns, ulceration, chronic inflammation, hematoma), wound healing processes can be impaired (e.g. transport of damaged cells and inflammatory byproducts away from the injury site). Healing and recovery can be assisted by supporting healthy lymphatic function.

Lymphatic Inadequacy

Inadequacy in the lymphatic system occurs if the lymphatic load is more than the transport capacity can handle. When lymphatic tissues or lymph nodes have been damaged, destroyed or removed, lymph cannot drain normally from the affected area. When this happens excess lymph accumulates and results in the swelling that is characteristic of edema and lymphedema (Zuther 2011).

Clinical Consideration

Compression bandages promote reduction in capillary hypertension and lymphatic load – creating a massaging effect to influence venous and lymphatic hemodynamics resulting in reduction of edema (Földi et al. 2005, Williams 2005).

There are three types of inadequacies which may result in lymphedema or edema: dynamic, mechanical and combined (Zuther 2011).

Dynamic

Dynamic inadequacy occurs when the active and passive edema protective measures are depleted and results in edema.

Mechanical

Mechanical inadequacy occurs when the transport capacity of the lymphatic load slows due to functional or organic causes, such as surgery, radiation, and trauma, or to a response from certain drugs or toxins. Due to the pressure exerted and leakage of proteins into the lymphatic wall structure, fibrosis may occur.

The stagnation of water, proteins, waste products and cell debris in the tissue can cause damage to the tissue. It also reduces the ability of the immune response due to the lack of circulation of the macrophages and lymphocytes. This can lead to a high incidence of infections such as cellulitis (Zuther 2011).

Combined

Combined inadequacy results from the lymphatic load being slowed due to the stagnation of the transport capacity. In other words, the system is very sluggish and not moving the fluid at a normal rate. When this occurs, the combination can lead to necrosis (severe tissue damage) and chronic inflammation (Zuther 2011).

Edema

Edema – the medical term for swelling – is considered to be a symptom. Edema can occur as a natural response of the body to injury or insult. Increased fluid in the affected area can be beneficial by assisting the delivery of immune cells to the area to fight an infection and assist with debris cleanup.

Edema can be isolated to a small area (localized) or can affect the entire body (generalized).

Pregnancy (preeclampsia or toxemia), tissue trauma, infections, medications and various conditions can result in edema; for example, venous insufficiency, obstruction of flow (e.g. thrombosis, tumor), low albumin, allergic reactions, congestive heart failure, liver and kidney disease, and critical illness (WebMD 2015).

Medications known to result in lower extremity edema include non-steroidal anti-inflammatory drugs (NSAIDs), corticosteroids and some medications used for hormone replacement, diabetes, depression and high blood pressure (WebMD 2015).

Discussion of the role of edema in critical illness, such as a burn or surgery, will be discussed in Chapter 5.

How the Body Responds to Edema

When there is an increase in the lymphatic load of water and proteins, the lymph system responds protectively with either active or passive edema.

Passive edema protection (Zuther 2011) is an increase in the volume of water leaving the blood capillaries. This is followed by an increase in the volume of fluid in the interstitial tissue, which creates pressure in the tissue. This pressure increases net reabsorption pressures, which assists edema protection.

In active edema protection (Zuther 2011), the lymphatic system responds to the increase in the lymphatic load of water and protein by elevating the contraction frequency in the lymph collectors and lymph trunks. The increase in fluid pressure stimulates the smooth muscle inside the wall of the node, which increases contraction frequency and volume in the node.

Lymphedema

Lymphedema is an abnormal accumulation of protein-rich lymph in the interstitial spaces (Zuther 2011). Lymphedema – considered to be a disease – can present as acute or chronic and if left untreated can evolve into a permanent, disfiguring condition. Most common areas for lymphedema are the extremities (arms and legs) but it may also develop in the breast, head, neck, trunk or genitals.

Causes of lymphedema include trauma in the form of infection, cancer, scar tissue from radiation therapy or surgical removal of lymph nodes and inherited conditions in which lymph nodes or vessels are absent or abnormal (Zuther 2011, National Lymphedema Network 2014).

Lymphedema is classified as primary and secondary:

- Primary lymphedema: a rare, hereditary condition results from a deficiency in the development, structure or the function of the lymphatic system (e.g. Milroy disease, Meige lymphedema) (Poage et al. 2008)

- Secondary lymphedema occurs as a result of damage to the lymphatic system (e.g. infection, surgical removal of lymph nodes or the use of radiation during cancer treatment).

Early indications of lymphedema include self-reported sensations of heaviness in the affected limb, edema, tingling, fatigue or aching. Lymphedema may initially be dismissed as edema, discomfort and inflammation after surgery. Axillary paresthesia and pain in the breast, chest and arm have been reported as symptoms of lymphedema. (Poage et al. 2008). Lymphedema associated with breast cancer treatment will be covered in greater detail in Chapter 6.

When the collection of protein-rich fluid remains in a specific area, it usually attracts more fluid and increases the inflammation response. This inflammatory reaction results in scar tissue called *fibrosis* in the affected area. The increase in viscous fluid (consolidated edema) and resulting fibrosis prevents oxygen and other essential nutrients reaching the area. This process slows down healing and creates an environment where bacteria can thrive and cause infections on or under the skin.

Lymphatic treatment protocols will be covered in detail in Chapter 9.

References

Aspelund A, Antila S, Proulx ST et al (2015) A dural lymphatic vascular system that drains brain interstitial fluid and macromolecules. The Journal of Experimental Medicine 212(7): 991–999.

Bellman S, Oden B (1958) Regeneration of surgically divided lymph vessels. An experimental study on the rabbit's ear. Acta Chirurgica Scandinavica 116: 99–117.

Chikly B (2002) Silent waves: theory and practice of lymph drainage therapy: with applications for lymphedema, chronic pain, and inflammation. Scottsdale, AZ: IHH Publishing.

Choi I, Lee S, Hong YK (2012) The new era of the lymphatic system: no longer secondary to the blood vascular system. Cold Spring Harbor Perspectives in Medicine 2(4): a006445.

Clark ER, Clark EL (1932) Observations on the new growth of lymphatic vessels as seen in transparent chambers introduced into the rabbit's ear. American Journal of Anatomy 51: 49–87.

Davis MJ, Davis AM, Lane MM et al (2009) Rate-sensitive contractile responses of lymphatic vessels to circumferential stretch. Journal of Physiology 587: 165–82.

Földi E, Földi M, Clodius L (1989) The lymphedema chaos. Annals of Plastic Surgery 22: 505–15.

Földi E, Jünger M, Partsch H (2005) The science of lymphoedema bandaging. EWMA Focus Document: Lymphoedema Bandaging in Practice.

Hodge LM, King HH, Williams AG, Jr et al (2007) Abdominal lymphatic pump treatment increases leukocyte count and flux in thoracic duct lymph. Lymphatic Research and Biology 5: 127–33.

Hodge LM, Bearden MK, Schander A et al (2010) Abdominal lymphatic pump treatment mobilizes leukocytes from the gastrointestinal associated lymphoid tissue into lymph. Lymphatic Research and Biology 8: 103–10.

Hodge LM, Downey HF (2011) Lymphatic pump treatment enhances the lymphatic and immune systems. Experimental Biology and Medicine (Maywood) 236(10): 1109–15.

Hodge LM, Bearden MK, Schander A et al (2013) Lymphatic pump treatment mobilizes leukocytes from the gut associated lymphoid tissue into lymph. Lymphatic Research and Biology 8(2): 103–110.

Huff JB, Schander A, Downey HF, Hodge LM (2010) Lymphatic pump treatment enhances the lymphatic release of lymphocytes. Lymphatic Research and Biology 8: 183–7.

Langevin HM, Nedergaard M, Howe AK (2013) Cellular control of connective tissue matrix tension. Journal of Cellular Biochemistry 114(8): 1714–9.

Louveau A, Smirnov I, Keyes TJ et al (2015) Structural and functional features of central nervous system lymphatic vessels. Nature; 1 June. Doi: 10.1038/nature14432.

Knott EM, Tune JD, Stoll ST, Downey HF (2005) Increased lymphatic flow in the thoracic duct during manipulative intervention. The Journal of the American Osteopathic Association 105: 447–56.

Kriehuber E, Breiteneder GS, Groeger M et al (2001) Isolation and characterization of dermal lymphatic and blood endothelial cells reveal stable and functionally specialized cell lineages. Journal of Experimental Medicine 194: 797–808.

Macdonald AJ, Arkill KP, Tabor GR et al (2008) Modeling flow in collecting lymphatic vessels: one-dimensional flow through a series of contractile elements. American Journal of Physiology – Heart and Circulatory Physiology 295: H305–13.

Marieb EN (2003) Human anatomy and physiology, 6/e. Upper Saddle River, NJ: Pearson Benjamin Cummings.

National Lymphedema Network (NLN) (2014). FAQ: What is lymphedema? Available at: http://www.lymphnet.org/le-faqs/what-is-lymphedema [Accessed 22 May 2014].

Oliver G, Detmar M (2002) The rediscovery of the lymphatic system: old and new insights into the development and biological function of the lymphatic vasculature. Genes and Development 16(7): 773–783.

Paavonen K, Puolakkainen P, Jussila L et al (2000) Vascular endothelial growth factor receptor-3 in lymphangiogenesis in wound healing. American Journal of Pathology 156: 1499–1504.

Poage E, Singer M, Armer J et al (2008) Demystifying lymphedema: development of the lymphedema putting evidence into practice card. Clinical Journal of Oncology Nursing 12(6): 951–964.

Quick CM, Venugopal AM, Dongaonkar RM et al (2008) First-order approximation for the pressure-flow relationship of spontaneously contracting lymphangions. American Journal of Physiology – Heart and Circulatory Physiology 294: H2144–9.

Rockson SD (2001) Lymphedema. American Journal of Medicine 110: 288–95.

Sabin FR (1902) On the origin of the lymphatic system from the veins and the development of the lymph hearts and thoracic duct in the pig. American Journal of Anatomy 1(3): 367–389.

Sabin FR (1904) On the development of the superficial lymphatics in the skin of the pig. American Journal of Anatomy 3(2): 183–195.

University of Helsinki (2015) Unraveling the link between brain, lymphatic system. ScienceDaily. Available at: www.sciencedaily.com/releases/2015/06/150615094258.htm [Accessed 9 July 2015].

University of Virginia Health System (2015) Missing link found between brain, immune system – with major disease implications. Public release: 1-Jun-2015. Available at: http://www.eurekalert.org/pub_releases/2015-06/uovh-mlf052915.php [Accessed 9 July 2015].

WebMD (2015) Edema overview. Available at: http://www.webmd.com/heart-disease/heart-failure/edema-overview [Accessed 19 March 2015].

Williams AF, Franks PJ, Moffatt CJ (2005) Lymphoedema: estimating the size of the problem. Palliative Medicine 19(4): 300–313.

Wilting J, Tomarev SI, Christ B, Schweigerer L (2003) Lymphangioblasts in embryonic lymphangiogenesis. Lymphatic Research and Biology 1(1): 33–40.

Zuther J (2002) Traditional massage therapy in the treatment and management of lymphedema. Massage Today June 2(6).

Zuther JE (2011) Lymphedema management: the comprehensive guide for practitioners, 2e. Stuttgart: Thieme.

Resources and Further Reading

Chikly Health Institute: http://www.chiklyinstitute.org/

Földi E, Földi M (2011). Manual lymph drainage (Földi method). In: Lymphedema. London: Springer, pp 237–243

Harris R (2015). Manual lymphatic drainage. Modalities for Massage and Bodywork, In: Stillerman, E. *Modalities for Massage and Bodywork.* 2nd edn, ch 7. Philadelphia: Mosby Elsevier.

The Vodder School: http://www.vodderschool.com/health-care-professional

Wittlinger H (2003) Textbook of Dr. Vodder's manual lymph drainage: basic course. Stuttgart: Thieme

Neurology

Each human nervous system is unprecedented. The work of each (expressed or hidden) is unpredictable, ever-different, surprising, startling, at times horrifying, but not infrequently magnificent

J.B. Angevine Jr (2002)

The nervous system (NS) comprises a collection of cells, tissues and organs that regulate the body's responses to internal and external stimuli. In addition to neurological biochemical and electrical activity, there is also the whole of the human being and each individual's life experiences to consider in contemplating the workings of this highly complex system.

Only a brief overview of the NS will be provided in this book as this system has been extensively studied and ample resources are available. Of particular relevance to this book is the role of the NS in wound healing, scar innervation and the impact of pathophysiological scars on the functioning of this system and consequent sequelae associated with neuropathy. Additionally, the integrin-mediated cell-signaling system will also be covered in brief detail as this system also plays a role in wound healing.

Although some of the techniques we use are intended to achieve physical tissue changes, such as disengagement of pathophysiological collagen cross-bindings, many of the outcomes we hope to achieve are mediated by the NS and the integrin-mediated system operating in the biotensegrity matrix. In essence the quality and clarity of the *conversation*, imparted through our hands to the receiver's neural receptors and integrins, can influence desirable clinical outcomes. To be effectively articulate in the *conversation*, one must be fluent in the language. And so the primary aims of this chapter are to lay a solid foundation for understanding the workings of the NS and how to safely and effectively influence our client's nervous and matrix systems. And this speaks to the very core of mastering the art and science of massage therapy (MT).

NS Structure

The human NS comprises the brain, spinal cord, nerves, ganglia and parts of the receptor and effector organs, and is organized into two main parts: the central nervous system (CNS) and the peripheral nervous system (PNS) (see Fig. 4.1).

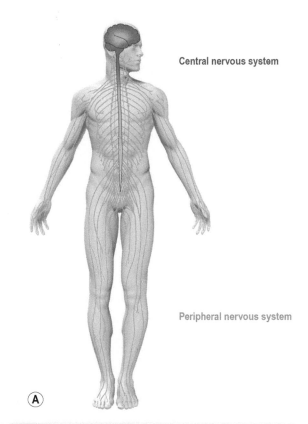

Central nervous system

Peripheral nervous system

Ⓐ

Figure 4.1

A Major anatomical components of the CNS and PNS.

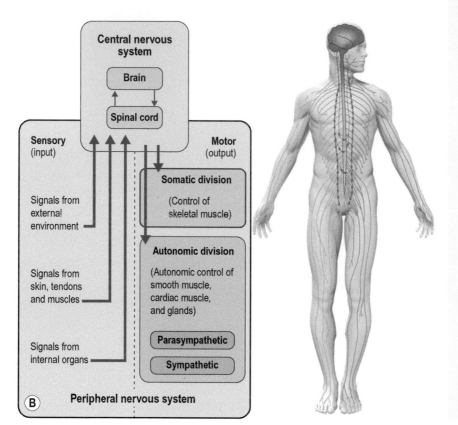

Figure 4.1

B Functional composition of the CNS and PNS.

CNS

The primary structures of the CNS include the brain, spinal cord, meninges (connective tissue (CT) membranes), cerebral spinal fluid (CSF) and cells.

Brain

Thousands of discernable brain areas can be identified based on fine distinctions of neural structure, chemistry and connectivity (Kandel et al. 2000). Each area serves as a dedicated processing, integrating and control center; however, as neuroplasticity research has shown, this marvelous organ can adapt and compensate in the most remarkably peculiar of ways, which is of significant consideration in terms of trauma and injury.

Pathophysiological Consideration

When one brain hemisphere has been damaged, the intact hemisphere may take over some of its functions. Compensation can also occur via reorganization and formation of new connections between intact neurons. The 'rewiring' of neuronal connection is stimulated by activity. For neurons to form beneficial connections, they must be correctly stimulated. Inappropriately stimulated, bored or unstimulated neurons will disengage or find something else to do. Neuroplasticity can also result in an impairment or harmful compensation; for example, some who are deaf may experience tinnitus, thought to be the result of the rewiring of brain

Spinal Cord

The spinal cord propagates nerve impulses between the spinal nerves and the brain, primarily functioning as a conduit for motor and sensory information, and as a center for coordinating certain reflexes, which it can independently control.

Each of the 31 segments of the spinal cord comprises one pair of dorsal and ventral horns:

- Ventral components: groups of efferent (out-going) motor neurons
- Dorsal components: groups of afferent (in-coming) sensory neurons (Zigmond et al. 1999) (Fig. 4.2).

The spinal cord also contains interneurons which modulate bidirectional information from the sensory and motor components.

Meninges and CSF

The meninges, a tri-laminar connective tissue membrane (dura, arachnoid and pia mater), surrounds and protect the brain and spinal cord. The choroid plexus, within the pia mater, produces CSF.

The CNS is nourished by blood which is filtered through the blood–brain barrier and by CSF. A clear liquid-filtrate of blood, CSF:

- Is produced in the ventricles of the brain
- Is found in the subarachnoid space and central canal of the spinal cord
- Provides mechanical and chemical protection and plays a role in homeostasis.

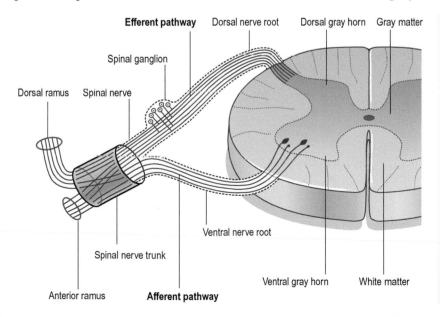

Figure 4.2

Dorsal and ventral components/afferent and efferent pathways.

Chapter 4

Cells

Neurons and neuroglia are the two main cell types found in the CNS.

Neurons

- Excitable nerve cells and their processes (dendrites and axons), which transmit information in the form of electrical signals to other neurons and other cells of the body (Fig. 4.3).

- Sensory neurons provide information about the body's internal and external environment.

- Motor neurons assist with reaction or response to the environment.

- Interneurons form connections between neurons and function as a relay station; for example, in the spinal cord a fast-track connection between a sensory and motor neuron creates a reflex arc which speeds reaction time as it cuts out the middle man … the brain.

Neuroglia (glia)

- Specialized connective tissue cells

- Ensure the health of neurons and support their function (e.g. create the blood–brain barrier, marshal immune responses, transport of nutrients, clean up debris, help secure neurons in place and produce myelin).

In addition to the two main cells, the CNS comprises extracellular matrix (ECM), gray and white matter. ECM within the CNS is histologically similar to the presentation outlined in Chapter 2.

CNS gray matter comprises the cell bodies, neuronal dendrites and axons and synapses between neurons. Synapses facilitate communication between neurons and other tissues. Neuronal dendrites are covered with synapse terminations that communicate with the terminations of adjacent axons. Each neuron can communicate with roughly 10 000 other neurons. Some axons can synapse directly onto:

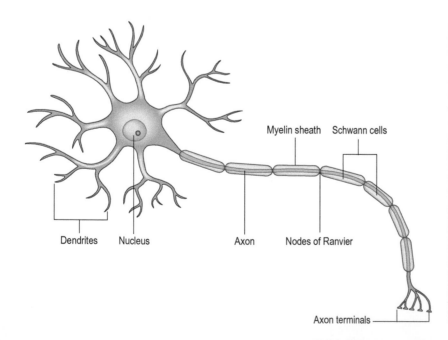

Dendrites Nucleus Axon Nodes of Ranvier Myelin sheath Schwann cells Axon terminals

Figure 4.3

Neuron anatomy: most neurons comprise a cell body, an axon and dendrites. The cell body contains the nucleus and cytoplasm. The axon extends from the cell body and often gives rise to many smaller branches before ending at nerve terminals. Dendrites extend from the neuron cell body and receive messages from other neurons.

- The cell bodies of other neurons

- Another axon or axon terminal

- Into the bloodstream

- Or diffusely into the adjacent nervous tissue (Fig. 4.4).

Synapses can relay information either electrically or chemically. In an electrical synapse, the presynaptic and postsynaptic cell membranes are connected by gap junctions which are capable of conducting an electric current across the synaptic cleft to the adjacent or postsynaptic cell. In chemical synapses, electrical activity on the presynaptic side triggers the release of neurotransmitters, endogenous chemicals housed in synaptic vesicles. Once released into the synaptic cleft, neurotransmitters diffuse across to the postsynaptic side where they bind to specific receptors initiating an electrical response or a secondary messenger pathway that may either excite or inhibit the postsynaptic neuron. Each synapse is managed by roughly 250 000 000 uniquely different proteins that turn over every couple of days (Schuman 2013).

CNS white matter contains axons and many axons are sheathed in myelin, which accelerates signal transmission. Fatty myelin is responsible for the light color of the 'white' matter (Goodman & Fuller 2012).

PNS

The primary structures of the PNS include Schwann cells, peripheral nerves and neural pathways (Fig. 4.5). Functionally, the PNS is divided into the somatic NS, which controls voluntary activity, and the autonomic NS, which controls involuntary activity – covered in greater detail later in this chapter.

Schwann Cells

Schwann cells, the principle glial cells of the PNS, produce myelin which surrounds axons and assists with conductivity.

Peripheral Nerves

Nerves are commonly classified into categories based on the presence or absence of myelin (e.g. myelinated and non-myelinated fibers), composition or function (sensory, motor and

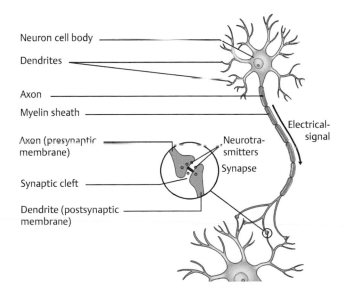

Neuron cell body

Dendrites

Axon

Myelin sheath

Axon (presynaptic membrane)

Synaptic cleft

Dendrite (postsynaptic membrane)

Neurotransmitters

Synapse

Electrical-signal

Figure 4.4

Classic axon to dendrite synapse and components of a synaptic cleft.

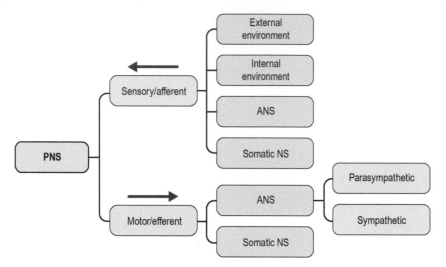

Figure 4.5

PNS: organization and functional divisions.

mixed/associated) and origin (cranial or spinal) (Fig. 4.6).

- Sensory/afferent nerve fibers conduct impulses from sense organs to the CNS

- Motor/efferent nerve fibers conduct nerve impulses from the CNS to peripheral tissues

- Mixed/associated nerve fibers, containing both sensory and motor nerve fibers, conduct sensory impulses from sense organs to the CNS and motor impulses from the CNS to effector organs.

The PNS comprises 12 pairs of cranial nerves, 31 pairs of spinal nerves and their associated ganglia.

At each intervertebral foramen, the anterior and posterior roots unite to form a spinal nerve, consisting of both motor and sensory fibers. As a spinal nerve exits the foramen it divides into a large anterior ramus and a smaller posterior ramus.

- Anterior ramus:

  - Supplies the muscles and skin over the anterolateral torso and all the muscles and skin of the extremities.

- Posterior ramus:

  - Supplies the muscles and skin of the posterior torso (Magee 2008).

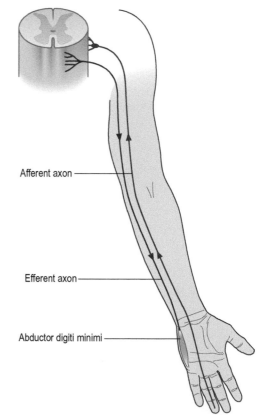

Figure 4.6

PNS efferent (motor) and afferent (sensory) pathways.

Autonomic Nervous System (ANS)

The ANS is connected to higher brain centers, including the medulla oblongata and hypothalamus, which integrates the activities of the autonomic and neuroendocrine systems.

The ANS mediates involuntary function of viscera, glands, smooth muscle, cardiac muscle and other structures. The ANS is subdivided into the parasympathetic nervous system (PSNS) and the sympathetic nervous system (SNS), both of which contain afferent and efferent nerve fibers (Fig. 4.7). The PSNS and SNS are considered to have a complementary rather than antagonistic relationship.

PSNS

The PSNS mediates homeostatic activities (conserving and restoring energy, control of normal heart, peristalsis, intestine and glandular activity, sphincter and lumen dilation and constriction). Commonly referred to as the 'rest

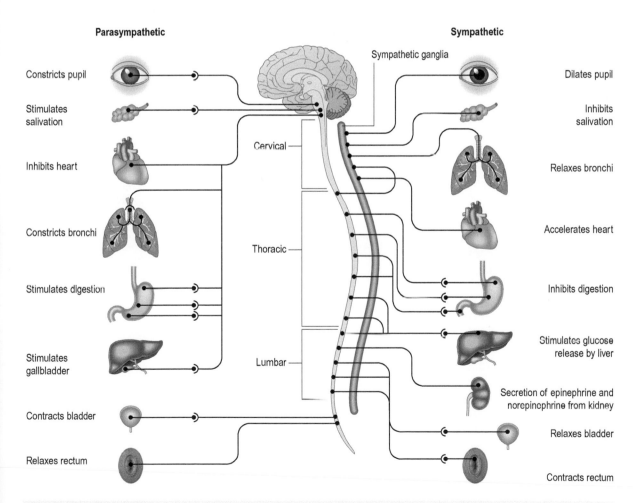

Figure 4.7

PSNS and SNS control.

and digest' or 'feed and breed' aspect of the nervous system as it controls sexual arousal, salivation, lacrimation, urination, digestion and defecation. The primary neurotransmitter associated with the PSNS is acetylcholine (ACH).

Clinical Consideration

PSNS afferent myelinated fibers travel from the viscera to their cell bodies located either in the sensory ganglia of the cranial nerves or in the posterior root ganglia of the sacrospinal nerves. The central axons then enter the CNS and take part in the formation of local reflex arcs or pass to higher centers of the ANS. The location of the sensory ganglia gives rise to the basic anatomical principle of craniosacral work – with intended outcomes mediated by the PSNS (Upledger 1987, Frymann 1988, Schleip 2003a, 2003b, Dorko 2003, Minasny 2009).]

SNS

The SNS mediates activity associated with emergency or stress response, commonly referred to as the fight, flight or freeze aspect of the nervous system. The SNS facilitates activity such as accelerated heart rate, elevated blood pressure and constriction of peripheral blood vessels when the need arises. Blood from the skin and intestines is redirected to the brain, heart and skeletal muscle to enhance chances of survival (e.g. fight or flight). The primary neurotransmitter associated with the SNS is norepinephrine. Norepinephrine can stimulate the adrenal medulla, triggering the release of noradrenalin and adrenalin, which are known to prolong the effects of sympathetic stimulation. The impact of prolonged sympathetic stimulation associated with trauma will be covered in greater detail in Chapter 7.

Clinical Consideration

Stress and the myofascial system – psychological distress or anxiety – has clearly been identified as a source of 'unnecessary' muscular tension: the confusing intermediate between a non-voluntary muscle contraction (spasm) and viscoelastic tension (a fascial property) showing no electromyography (EMG) activity (Simon & Mense 2007). According to Chaitow (2007):

the shortened fibers of the soft tissues may be the result of a combination of structural anomalies, trauma, and/or **physical or emotional stress**, and are always influenced by underlying nutritional and behavioral elements. Some of these shortened fibers and tender spots (i.e. trigger points) may be the source of reflex symptoms and pain. Such soft tissue dysfunctions respond to manual pressure in the form of modalities like MT.

Clinical Consideration

SNS activation may lead to increased fascial tonus, mediated by MFB contraction (Staubesand & Li 1996, Schleip et al. 2006, Bhowmick et al. 2009). Conversely, SNS sedation can lead to a decrease in fascial tone.

Neural Pathways

Collectively the neural pathways link the CNS to the various body parts (muscles, glands and sense organs). Each spinal nerve within the pathway is connected to the spinal cord via the anterior and posterior roots.

- Anterior root:
  - Consists of bundles of nerve fibers carrying nerve impulses away from the CNS – termed descending or efferent fibers.

Efferent, motor fibers, connected to skeletal muscle mediate contraction.

- Posterior root:
  - Consists of bundles of nerve fibers that carry impulses to the CNS – termed ascending or afferent fibers. Afferent, sensory fibers, convey information such as touch, pain, temperature, and vibration.

Each nerve root comprises a somatic component, which innervates the skeletal muscles and provides sensory input from the skin, fascia, muscles, and joints, and a visceral component, which is part of the ANS (Magee 2008).

Dermatomes, Myotomes and Sclerotomes

During embryonic development, mesodermal tissue that forms along the neural tube gives rise to the various hard and soft tissues of the body (e.g. bone, muscle, skin and CT). Nerves make early connections with the developing tissues establishing segmental innervation patterns or divisions. Segmental divisions include:

- **Dermatomes:**
  - Areas of skin supplied by a single nerve root. Regional representations of dermatome distribution vary from person to person and also exhibit a great deal of overlap (Lee et al. 2013).

- **Myotomes:**
  - Groups of muscles supplied by a single nerve root.

- **Sclerotomes:**
  - An area of bone or fascia supplied by a single nerve root. As with dermatomes, sclerotomes can show a great deal of variability among individuals (Magee 2008).

Dermatomes, myotomes and sclerotomes provide a means by which referred pain can be felt

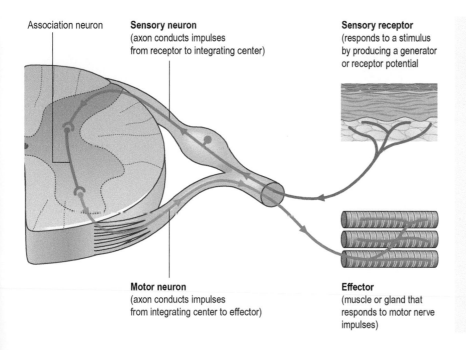

Association neuron

Sensory neuron
(axon conducts impulses from receptor to integrating center)

Sensory receptor
(responds to a stimulus by producing a generator or receptor potential)

Motor neuron
(axon conducts impulses from integrating center to effector)

Effector
(muscle or gland that responds to motor nerve impulses)

Figure 4.8

Anterior and posterior divisions of the spinal cord and afferent/sensory and efferent/motor neurons.

in areas of the body a distance from the trauma-tized or originating tissue. Referred pain will be discussed in more detail later in this chapter.

Neurofascia

Fascia forms a tri-laminar, continuous struc-ture that surrounds and invests individual nerve fibers, bundles of fibers (fascicles) and the entire nerve, thus constituting the three lev-els of organization (Fig. 4.9): 50% of peripheral nerves consist of CT (Sunderland & Bradley 1949, Coppieters & Nee 2012).

Epineurium

- The outermost layer that surrounds the entire nerve comprises mostly areolar tissue and houses the nerve's blood and lymphatic ves-sels, which have feeder vessels that branch off to supply all inner parts of the nerve.

- Epineural blood vessels are slightly coiled, rendering them adaptable of nerve mobil-ity within a 'normal' range. The loose areo-lar matrix allows for unimpeded nerve fiber growth changes (Bove 2008, Magee 2008).

Perineurium

The perineurium:

- Is the intermediate layer that surrounds bun-dles or fascicles of nerve fibers. Thin yet dense, it provides tensile strength and protects the nerve from over extension trauma.

- Maintains the blood–nerve barrier and if cut into, the axon may herniate due to traumatiz-ing pressure changes (Bove 2008).

Endoneurium

The endoneurium is:

- The innermost layer that surrounds individual nerve fibers, offers little mechanical support

- A loose collagenous matrix that is an exten-sion of the blood–brain barrier.

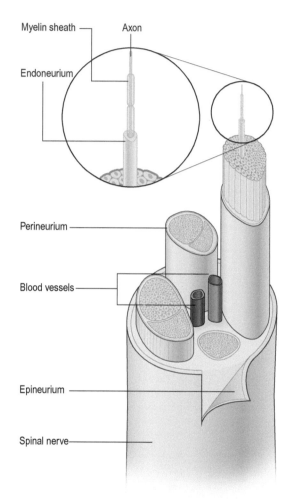

Myelin sheath — Axon
Endoneurium
Perineurium —
Blood vessels —
Epineurium —
Spinal nerve —

Figure 4.9

Neurofascial envelopes.

Clinical Consideration

The space between the distinct neurofascial cover-ings comprises a delicate, areolar CT much like that seen in the sliding layers associated with muscle and fascia. This layer is presumed to provide a similar slid-ing function and present with similar consequences when impacted by injury and trauma.

Peripheral nerves – wrapped in their neuro-fascial envelopes – travel throughout the body within fascial clefts or cleavage planes that function as 'neutral motion corridors'. These protective corridors help safeguard the nerve from compression and over extension. As the nerve and its protective coverings are connected via investing fibers, whatever impacts the various layers of the neurofascial corridor has great potential to impact the enveloped nerve.

Pathophysiological Consideration

A nerve fiber remains undisturbed upon fascial traction/stretch only within certain limits – typically up to 1 cm or anywhere from 8–20% of its 'non-tractioned' length (Sommer 2010). When stretch of the neurofascia reaches its boundary of 'normal limit', intrafascial mechanoreceptors are activated. Mechanoreceptors monitor tensional changes and can initiate rapid relaxation in response to sudden over-load or a quick burst of movement. Rapid relaxation response occurs to reduce the potential that the fascia will be torn. This mechanism provides protection from injury (Stecco et al. 2007, Chaitow 1998).

Peripheral nerves are most commonly traumatized by pressure, traction, friction, anoxia or cutting but can also be impacted by thermal or electrical injury. Spinal nerve roots lack well-developed epi and perineurium, rendering them susceptible to compressive forces, tensile deformation, chemical irritants (e.g. heavy metals, alcohol) and metabolic disturbances (Magee 2008). Neural trauma and sequelae will be covered in more detail later in this chapter.

Nerves are supplied by extra and intraneural blood vessels and neurofascial coverings are innervated by small nerves (Bove & Light 1997,

Sauer et al. 1999, Bove 2008). This 'nerve of a nerve' is referred to as nervi nervorum. Nervi nervorum are nociceptive and also nocifensive, meaning that they are responsive to damaging stimuli by contributing to local inflammation, thus helping to defend and maintain the nerve's local environment (Lembeck 1983, Light 2004, Bove 2008). Research suggests that nervi nervorum and their associated plexus of nociceptors play a role in nerve trunk and dyesthetic pain.

Innervation of Skin and Fascia

Nerves fibers are found throughout the expanse of skin and fascia with some regions showing a higher condensation of fibers than others. Fiber condensation is related to the functional requirements of a particular region or specific segment of tissue.

Clinical Consideration

There is an extensive network of nerve fibers in the fascia surrounding the muscles in the low back region. Tissues in this region are required to perceive complex information and perform highly complex functions.

Clinical Consideration

Higher nerve fiber condensations are found near and around blood vessels in the deep layer of fascia. It is suggested that the higher condensations here are related to fascia's ability to adjust its viscosity in response to demand (Stecco el al. 2006). Fascial fluid dynamics involve the extrusion of plasma from blood vessels into the interstitial fluid matrix (Kruger 1987). In turn, changes in local fluid dynamics result in changes in the viscosity of the extracellular matrix.

Clinical Consideration

Diane Jacobs PT (2014) on neurodynamics:

Peripheral nerves come all the way out to supply skin, sooner or later, proximally or distally,
making them fairly easy to affect mechanically
regardless of where or how one makes contact
with skin.

Nerve Receptors

Nerve receptors provide a means by which our
CNS can keep informed as to what is happening in our external and internal environment.
Various types of receptors detect and transmit information from the periphery to the CNS
and interpretation of this information drives
response.

There are five general classifications of receptors: mechano, thermo, noci, chemo and photo.
Receptors are classified according to what it typically has the lowest threshold for or is most easily
stimulated by (e.g. chemo/chemical); however,
any given receptor can respond to more than one
type of stimuli.

In skin, superficial and deep fascia, mechano,
thermo and nociceptors are collectively called
somatosensory receptors. Given the relevance
of mechano and nociceptors to the focus of this
book, each of these receptor types is covered in
greater detail.

Mechanoreceptors

Mechanoreceptors are specialized sensory
receptors that respond to a variety of stimuli
(e.g. sound, touch, pressure, movement, tissue stretch and distortion). In skin and fascia
mechanoreceptor condensation varies widely
and within an expanse of tissue several types
of mechanoreceptors can be present, thus perception of various stimuli can occur simultaneously. Mechanoreceptors (this includes
proprioceptors – movement and positioning
detectors) provide skin and fascia with the ability to perceive tissue deformation (e.g. stretch,
shear, tensional load and pressure) and respond
to such stimuli.

Clinical Consideration

It appears that manual therapies employ mechanosensory afferents (group I–IV). Manual technique effectiveness is – in part – due to evocation
of neuronal activity of particular magnitude and in a
pattern not seen during 'normal' activity (Pickar et
al. 2007). Mechanical (manual) stimulation of intrafascial mechanoreceptors evokes cellular 'down-
stream' effects linked to fascial tonus changes
and healing (Langevin et al. 2002), as illustrated
in Figure 4.10.

There are several types of mechanoreceptors
and proprioceptive mechanoreceptors (e.g.
muscle spindles, Ruffini, Golgi, Pacini,
paciniform and interstitial receptors (IRs); see
Table 4.1).

Proprioceptive mechanoreceptors are found
throughout skin and fascia, showing that these
tissues play an important proprioceptive role
(Yahia et al. 1993). Proprioceptors are more
concentrated in transitional zones occurring
near the myotendinous junctions (MTJ), ten-
operiosteal junctions, in fascial connections
between muscle/ligaments and joint capsules,
retinaculum and in aponeuroses functioning as
a 'coupling unit'.

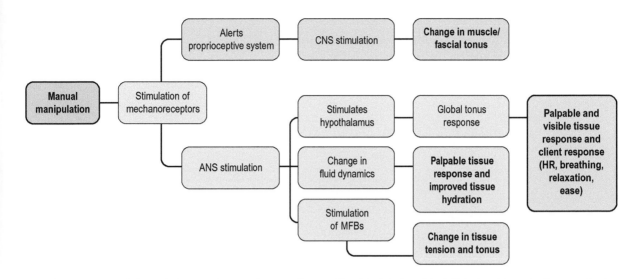

Figure 4.10

Mechanoreceptor mediated effects.

Clinical Consideration

Although muscle spindles (stretch receptors) have traditionally been associated with muscle tissue, more recent research indicates that these receptors are embedded in myofascial tissue. Muscle spindle response to detectable stretch can be altered if myofascia (e.g. endo or perimysium) is too rigid. In such cases, normal firing of the muscle spindles can be altered (Stecco 2004).

Clinical Consideration

Retinaculae in particular display a greater density of nerve receptors than that typically seen in muscle bellies or some other soft tissues (Stecco et al. 2010). It is suggested that fascia plays an integrating function as a proprioceptive organ and that it can coordinate the action of different muscles by acting as a common 'ectoskeleton'

Clinical consideration (Cont.)

(Jones 1944) or myokinetic linkage system (Stecco 2004). For example, such is seen in the thoracolumbar region during locomotion and load lifting (Jones 1944, Vleeming et al. 1995, Graceovetsky 2007).

Clinical Consideration

The form of stimulus to which a receptor responds and where they are found in higher concentrations factor into our ability to achieve desired effects/productive results.

Example 1

According to Cottingham (1985), Golgi receptors are stimulated during soft tissue manipulation, Hatha yoga postures and slow active stretching resulting in a lower firing rate of specific alpha-motor neurons,

Receptor type	Common location	Responsive to	Therapeutic outcome
Golgi receptors and Golgi tendon organs (GR/GTO)	Dense fascia, joint related tissues, and near myotendinous junctions	Contractile tension and active moderate, sustained stretch	Tonus decrease in related motor fibers
Large Pacini and paciniform corpuscles	Layers of deeper skin and deeper, dense fascia	Vibration, pressure changes and light, brief tangential loading	Enhanced proprioceptive feedback and motor control
Merkel cells	Superficial skin	Localized pressure, sustained loading and tissue displacement	May include certain neuromodulation and neuroendocrine responses
Ruffini organs	Below the skin in dense CT/fascia and joint related tissues	Slow, sustained, deeper pressure, slow deep strokes and lateral/tangential forces or stretch (Kruger 1987	Sedation of sympathetic activity
Interstitial receptors (IRs)	Plentiful in various presentations of fascia, including periosteum	Are multi-modal in their function as noci (pain), thermo, chemo and the majority as mechanoreceptors (e.g. intrafascial mechanoreceptors); in their role as mechanoreceptors, IRs respond to tension, pressure, tissue stretch and ultra-light touch	Ability to influence autonomic responses e.g. blood pressure changes and improved parasympathetic/sympathetic balance

Table 4.1

Summary of receptor typology and therapeutic outcomes. With manually applied techniques, the degree, direction and duration of application factor significantly into the desired therapeutic outcomes as each of these elements influence the various mechanoreceptors in a variety of ways (Kruger 1987, Schleip 2003b, Chaitow 2014).

Clinical consideration (Cont.)

which then translates into a decrease in myofascial tonicity and a decrease in striated muscle tonus.

Example 2

Ruffini stimulation results in lowering of SNS activity and increased local proprioceptive awareness (Kruger 1987). Slow deep pressure typically induces PSNS dominance, which tends to quiet SNS activity and, in turn, the more trophotropic anterior lobe of

Clinical consideration (Cont.)

the hypothalamus is activated resulting in decreased global muscular tonus (Fig. 4.10).

Example 3

IRs, found in abundance throughout skin, fascia and all aspects of connective tissue, are intimately linked to the ANS – as the ANS governs all manner of organ system functioning, IR stimulation can impact the various systems (Hammer 1998, Arbuckle 1994).

Significant neural-mediated mechanisms or neurobiological functions have been identified as potential catalysts for tissue changes that occur as a result of manual manipulation. Of particular interest is CT and fascia's ability to change its fluid ratio. A change in local fluid dynamics can result in a change in the viscosity of ground substance in the ECM. The shift involves the nervous and vascular systems and CT cells (e.g. myofibroblasts found in fascia). It has been determined that many of the IRs can apparently influence plasma extra-vasation (i.e. the movement of plasma from blood vessels into the ECM (Kruger 1987), see Figure 4.10 and Table 4.1.

With manually applied techniques, the degree, direction and duration of application factor significantly into the desired therapeutic outcomes as each of these elements influence the various mechanoreceptors in a variety of ways.

Golgi receptors and Golgi tendon organs

Golgi receptors and Golgi tendon organs (GR/GTO) are:

- Found in dense fascia, joint related tissues, and near myotendinous junctions
- Known, thus far, to respond to contractile tension and active moderate, sustained stretch – to what extent manually applied load can elicit Golgi responses remains unclear (Schleip 2003a, 2003b)
- Therapeutic outcome is a tonus decrease in related motor fibers.

Large Pacini and paciniform corpuscles

Large Pacini and paciniform corpuscles:

- Are found in layers of deeper skin and deeper, dense fascia

- Have an affinity for vibration, pressure changes and light, brief tangential loading
- Therapeutic outcome include enhanced proprioceptive feedback and motor control.

Merkel cells

Merkel cells:

- Are found in superficial skin
- Respond to localized pressure, sustained loading and tissue displacement
- Therapeutic outcomes may include certain neuromodulation and neuroendocrine responses.

Ruffini organs

Ruffini organs:

- Are found below the skin in dense CT/fascia and joint related tissues
- Are especially responsive to slow, sustained, deeper pressure, slow deep strokes and lateral/tangential forces or stretch (Kruger 1987)
- Therapeutic outcomes include sedation of sympathetic activity.

IRs

IRs:

- Are plentiful in various presentations of fascia, including periosteum
- Are multi-modal in their function as noci (pain), thermo, chemo, and the majority as mechanoreceptors (e.g. intrafascial mechanoreceptors)
- In their role as mechanoreceptors, respond to tension, pressure, tissue stretch and ultra-light touch
- Therapeutic outcomes include the ability to influence autonomic responses, e.g. blood

pressure changes and improved parasympa-thetic/sympathetic balance.

Nociceptors

A nociceptor is a receptor specialized in detecting stimuli that objectively can damage tissue and subjectively are perceived as painful.

Dommerholt (RMTBC Pain Conference 2014)

Nociceptors, which are threat detectors, are responsive to various noxious stimuli (e.g. extreme hot, cold, swelling, tissue damage or prior tissue damage) (Winkelstein 2004, Jacobs 2014). Although there is a common tendency to identify nociceptors as pain receptors, not all nociceptive signals are interpreted as pain and not every pain sensation originates from a nociceptor. However, acute pain almost always originates from nociceptors in somatic or visceral tissue. Pain mechanisms and various types of pain will be discussed in greater detail later in this chapter.

As is the case with mechanoreceptors, nociceptor condensations vary from region to region; for example, the thoracolumbar fascia (aka lumbodorsal fascia) is densely innervated with nociceptors, and nociceptors in this region have a more extensive distribution in the spinal cord than is seen in other tissues (e.g. more so than what is seen in the gastroc/soleus). The higher nociceptor condensation and more extensive spinal cord distribution may explain why we see a higher prevalence of chronic low back pain (ChLBP) in comparison to chronic lower limb pain (Tesarz 2009, Tesarz et al. 2011).

NS Function

The primary functions of the NS include:

- Control and coordination of the body functions (e.g. those involved in maintaining homeostasis)

- Receiving sensory impulses/information

- Analyzing and interpreting information and initiates responses

- Storing previous stimuli as the experiences or memory which can then guide or influence future responses.

The NS mediates complex multisystem relationships. Together with the endocrine system it controls and integrates the activities of the various parts of the body. Like the connective tissue system, the NS is physically connected to and communicates with all other systems of the body. Therefore any trauma or conversely any beneficial effect on the NS has far reaching, multisystem implications.

Proprioception, Interoception and Nociception

Proprioception

Although proprioception, the ability to sense bodywide and body part position, location, orientation and movement, has been classically viewed as a muscle and joint-related-tissue activity, current research supports that both skin and fascia play an important role in proprioception as well.

Clinical Consideration

According to Yahia et al. (1993):

High concentrations of mechanoreceptors in superficial fascia play a proprioceptive role and receptors in and near the skin are more active in detecting and regulating movement than joint ligament receptors – therefore, even superficial scars and burns could potentially impact proprioception and subsequently movement and stability.

Fascia plays a particularly significant role in dynamic proprioception, and fascia researchers now suggest that the majority of proprioception occurs in fascia/myofascia (Stecco et al. 2006, Chaitow & DeLaney 2008, van der Wal 2009). The presence of Ruffini organs and Pacini receptors in deep fascia suggests that fascia participates in perception of posture, motion, tension and position (Stecco et al. 2007).

Interoception

Interoception, or sensing the state of one's well-being, is mediated by IRs that are known to influence the autonomic system.

Interoception includes a wide range of physiological sensations including muscular effort, ticking, pain, hunger, thirst, warmth, cold, organ-distension, sensual and pleasant touch (Richards 2012, Schleip & Jäger 2012). The interoceptive pathway terminates in the insular cortex, which participates in consciousness, emotional state and control of homeostasis. Insular cortex

Clinical Consideration

Mechanoreceptors in skin gather and relay any external (touch) information being provided. In addition to this information being relayed to the brain, the skin can communicate globally across its own expanse and deeply as it is contiguous with the various layers of fascia, and all that the fascia is connected to (Abu-Hijleh & Harris 2007, Chaitow 2014). The ECM within the hypodermis or superficial fascia sends out projections towards the surface of the skin providing a communication route between the deeper layers of fascia and the surface. Therefore movement, touch or other forms of stimuli can be communicated across all layers, from superficial to deep, and from the subterranean to the surface (Paoletti 2006). This connection pathway provides a plausible mechanism

Clinical Consideration (Cont.)

for various manual therapy approaches to achieve the 'tissue release' or tonus changes we feel beneath our hands during treatment. Release can be mediated by the nervous system (responding to mechanoreceptor stimulation) or via the mechanotransduction pathway, as discussed in Chapter 2 (Schleip 2003a, 2003b, Langevin 2006).

Pathophysiological Consideration

Trauma, mechanoreceptors and proprioceptive disinformation

Trauma, including pathophysiological scars, can result in aberrant mechanoreceptor function. Fibrosis and adhesions that occur with pathological scars can lead to innocuous mechanical stimuli being perceived as noxious, resulting in the subsequent relay of incoherent or misinformation to local, regional, or central nerve centers (i.e. proprioceptive disinformation). Under- or overestimation of the mechanical stimuli received results in inappropriate muscular reactions, such as interference with recruitment and timing of recruitment, which endangers equilibrium, coordination and stability. Consequently, proprioceptive disinformation can adversely impact the rehabilitative process or increase the incidence of comorbid injuries (e.g. falling with subsequent sprains or fracture).

functions include perception, motor control, self-awareness and cognition, and subsequently dysfunction can impact perception of afferent information.

The interoceptive system, considered the substrate of recognition of self, plays a fundamental role in the relationship between one's subjective state of well-being and physiological health.

Volitional cortical control in humans can directly modify homeostatic integration (Petrovic et al. 2002, Craig 2003, Critchley et al. 2002, Damasio et al. 2000, Derbyshire et al. 2003). This supports that how we feel about *how we feel* can influence how we function, right down to the physiological level.

Clinical Consideration

In addition to the ability to respond to pain and thermal stimuli, interoceptors found in hairy skin sense changes in mechanical stimuli in the form of light touch, pressure and stretch, establishing a plausible mechanism for the effects of gentle manual techniques. The anatomical communication route that exists between skin and deeper structures (e.g. bone), noted previously also supports a plausible mechanism for deeper changes or effects following treatment (Schleip & Jäger 2012, Chaitow 2014).

Nociception

Nociception, tissue threatening stimuli, is activated by varying thresholds not activated during typical functional movement. In addition to sensitivity to tissue deformation, nociceptive afferent receptors are sensitive to endogenous chemicals (e.g. bradykinin, serotonin, prostaglandin E2, adenosine triphosphate and histamine) released as a result of disrupted tissue or by inflammatory cells. These nociceptive stimulants can have long-lasting effects and often potentiate one another (Mense 1993, Reinert et al. 1998, Graven-Nielsen & Mense 2001, Mense 2003, Mense 2009, Waters-Banker et al. 2014). Muscle

Clinical Consideration

In addition to sense of well-being, it is also known that nurturing touch plays an important role in promotion of physical growth during infant/child development.

Clinical Consideration (Cont.)

This *well-being* touch, linked to interception in adults, suggests a plausible mechanism for growth factor mediated CT/fascial changes initiated by gentle touch. Growth factor plays an important role in collagen remodelling in response to injury and demand (Van den Berg 2012, Chaitow 2014).

Clinical Consideration

Manual techniques targeting interoceptors can influence ANS mediated changes such as an increase in local blood flow and ECM hydration. In addition to physiological effects, interoceptive mediated psychoemotional benefits can also be derived (Schleip 2003a, 2003b).

fibers contain no afferent receptors within the confines of their cell membranes. Instead, afferents are located in the perimysium, adjacent to the vasculature that serves as the entry point for various immune cells (Reinert et al. 1998) – thus giving further credence to fascia nociception and fasciagenic pain.

Pain

The nervous system includes the patient from skin cell to sense of self. It might be a tiny thing, at only 2% of the whole body, but it's what keeps us alive, and creates a pain for us to feel somewhere.

Diane Jacobs PT (2014)

Pain is described as an 'unpleasant sensory and emotional experience associated with actual or potential tissue damage, or described in terms

Clinical Consideration

Massage immunomodulation

According to Waters-Banker et al. (2014), the influence of massage on apoptotic signaling may be one explanation for its physiologic benefits. Apoptotic signaling of neutrophils has been shown to influence a phenotype change in the macrophage population (Fadok et al. 2001). This further suggests that, via influencing macrophage phenotype change, additional benefits from this would include prompting transition into the repair and regeneration phase of healing, thereby preventing the exacerbation of a toxic environment and subsequent decrease in endogenous chemical availability and potential nerve sensitization. Massage may provide an important utility in its ability to prevent transient and more detrimental plastic changes in afferent nerve density in the periphery and spinal cord. Attenuating the inflammatory and subsequent NS response supports the viability of utilizing MT to treat, manage and prevent acute and chronic pain syndromes as well as inflammatory presentations. By altering signaling pathways involved with the inflammatory process, massage may decrease secondary injury, nerve sensitization and collateral sprouting, resulting in increased recovery from damage and reduction or prevention of pain.

of such damage' (Mersky & Bogduk 1994; see Table 4.2).

The actual concept of pain is one that involves numerous factors that are processed at several higher centers of the brain, including the linkage of an emotional response. The somatoemotional aspects of trauma and pain and associated comorbidities will be covered in greater detail in Chapter 7.

Neurons transmit pain and other sensory information via electrical signals. In response to a stimulus, ions travelling through channels in neuron membranes actuate a change in the electrical potential of the membrane. When this change is large enough, a voltage spike is produced and the signal is ultimately transmitted to the brain. When certain neurons fire too easily or too often hyperexcitablility can arise (Ratté et al. 2014).

Injury-induced hyperexcitability is not limited to nociceptors. Hyperexcitability also develops in myelinated afferents that normally convey innocuous information (e.g. normal movement and touch) and under neuropathic conditions, mechanical allodynia can occur (Campbell et al. 1988, Koltzenburg et al. 1994, Devor 2009, King et al. 2011, Ratté et al. 2014).

Hyperexcitability can make something perceived as painful feel even worse (hyperalgesia), or it can make things hurt that should not (allodynia). According to Ratté et al. (2014), increasing the flow of ions through the cell membrane can eventually result in a 'tipping point' to be crossed, which triggers a change in the voltage spiking pattern (i.e. lowering of threshold and increase in firing rate – see Fig. 4.11). However, as several different types of ion channels contribute to the current, there are several different ways in which the tipping point can be crossed. This ability to produce the same result by multiple means is a common feature of complex systems. It makes systems more robust, as a given result can still be achieved if one particular attempt to achieve this result fails. The work of Ratté and colleagues helps to explain why drugs that target just one type of ion channel may fail to relieve neuropathic pain as maladaptive changes in any one of several other ion channels may circumvent the therapeutic effect (Ratté et al. 2014).

Neuropathic pain is notoriously difficult to treat as it does not respond well to common painkillers. Ratté and colleagues suggest that a paradigm shift will be needed to effectively treat neuropathic pain - recommending that

Term	Definition, mechanism, characteristics and other important information
Allodynia	Pain due to a stimulus that does not normally provoke pain – an unexpected pain response associated with different types of somatosensory stimuli applied to different tissues. A consequence of neural hyperexcitation
Fasciagenic Pain	Because fascia has been largely overlooked as a potential pain generator and because scarring impacts fascia, specific consideration is given here. Fascia contains type C nociceptors and some of the free nerve endings in fascia are substance P-containing receptors, commonly assumed to be nociceptive and rendering fascia a potential pain generator (Tesarz 2009). And, as previously noted, neurofascial coverings are innervated by nervi nervorum **Pathophysiological consideration** Elevated concentrations of biochemical substances associated with pain, inflammation and intercellular signaling are found at active MTrP locations (e.g. inflammatory mediators, neuropeptides, catecholamines, pro-inflammatory cytokines, pain modulators). Increased levels of pain modulators, such as Substance P and bradykinins, are plausible explanations for the occurrence of pain associated with active MTrPs (Shah et al. 2005). **Pathophysiological consideration** Under normal circumstances an axon is not mechanically sensitive – otherwise every time we moved we would collapse in pain. However, inflammation of a neurofascial envelope can render the associated nociceptors mechanically hypersensitive (Bove 2008).
Hyperalgesia	Heightened pain sensation from a stimulus that normally provokes pain, a consequence of hyperexcitation involving peripheral or central sensitization or both • Primary hyperalgesia: occurs at the site of injury, associated with increased sensitivity of peripheral receptors (e.g. local nocis activated by substances released as a result of injured tissue) • Secondary hyperalgesia: occurs in tissue outside the site of injury, associated with central sensitization (e.g. changes in spinal cord glial and satellite cells and voltage spiking pattern changes) • Opioid-induced hyperalgesia: sensitization associated with long-term use of exogenous opioids (e.g. heroine, oxycodone)
Neuropathic pain	Pain that arises as a consequence of injury or disease affecting the somatosensory NS (Treede et al. 2008, Correa-Illanes et al. 2010). Neuropathic pain may occur as a manifestation of various conditions that cause nerve damage, such as viral infections (postherpetic neuralgia), metabolic disorders (diabetes mellitus), drug-induced toxicity, inflammation, cancer, trauma, and postsurgical complications. Hyperalgesia to light touch that can occur with neuropathic pain is comparable to secondary hyperalgesia and thought to be associated with central sensitization. Treede (2008) suggests that neuropathic pain be viewed as a clinical description not a diagnosis.
Neuropathy	Disturbance of function or pathological change in a nerve
Nociception	Detection of (noxious) stimuli that are capable of producing tissue injury. Consequences of encoding may be autonomic (e.g. elevation of blood pressure) or behavioral (e.g. withdrawal reflex)
Nociceptive pain	Pain that arises from actual or threatened damage to non-neural tissue
Radicular or radiating pain/ sensation	Usually perceived as lancinating, sharp, shooting pain or paresthesia felt in a dermatome, myotome or sclerotome because of direct involvement of a spinal nerve or nerve root. It is distinguished from nociception as the axons are stimulated along their course rather than at the terminal-end receptors. Stimulation may occur as a result of mechanical deformation of a dorsal root ganglion, mechanical stimulation of previously damaged nerve roots, inflammation of a dorsal root ganglion and, possibly, by ischemic damage to dorsal root ganglia (Howe et al. 1977, Murphy 1977, Howe 1979). Radicular pain differs from referred pain in several respects. While pain can also be perceived deeply, radicular pain displays a cutaneous quality (perceived in the skin as well as deeply) whereas referred pain lacks any cutaneous quality (IASP 2014)

Term	Definition, mechanism, characteristics and other important information
Referred pain	Pain perceived at a location other than the site of the painful stimulus/origin (e.g. referred pain associated with MTrPs). Referred pain may thus occur in a region that is either remote from or directly contiguous with the source of pain, but the two locations are distinguishable on the basis of their different nerve supply. Pain can be referred into the corresponding myotome, dermatome or sclerotome from any somatic or visceral tissue innervated by a nerve root, but, confusingly, sometimes it is not referred according to the commonly known pattern. Referred pain is a common occurrence in problems associated with the musculoskeletal system. Pain quality is usually described as deep and aching and although its central locus is recognizable and constant, its margins are hard to define (Kellgren 1938, 1939, Feinstein et al. 1954, Magee 2008, IASP 2014)
Sensitization	Changes in the PNS or CNS (adaptive or pathologic) that lead to heightened nociceptive responses and/or lower thresholds, i.e. a lower intensity stimuli results in increased responsiveness. Clinically, sensitization may only be inferred indirectly from presenting phenomena such as hyperalgesia or allodynia, and may include dysfunction of endogenous pain control systems: • Central sensitization: increased responsiveness of nociceptive neurons in the CNS • Peripheral sensitization: increased responsiveness of nociceptive neurons in the periphery

Table 4.2

Important pain terms. Various terms are used to describe pain mechanisms (e.g. nociceptive) and characteristics (e.g. allodynia) (www.iasp-pain.org)

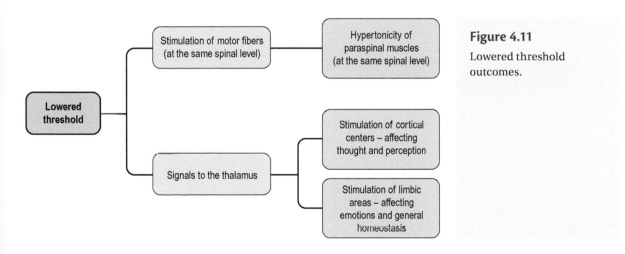

Figure 4.11

Lowered threshold outcomes.

treatments aimed at restoring normal regulation of excitability, rather than targeting ion channels themselves, may present the best course of action (Ratté et al. 2014).

Allodynia: pain due to a stimulus that does not normally provoke pain – an unexpected pain response associated with different types of somatosensory stimuli applied to different tissues. A consequence of neural hyperexcitation. See also Table 4.2.

Clinical Consideration

According to Jacobs (2014):

> Skin is well supplied with exteroceptive receptors and fibers that transmit information to the brain using fast dorsal column pathways and non-nociceptive slow spinothalamic pathways, to centers in both the internal regulation system and the primary sensory cortex of the brain. As long as manual therapy is mostly non-nociceptive, treatment will be physically safe for most pain presentations. Ruffini endings are particularly capable of transducing lateral stretch to skin. It is slow adapting, which means it will actively fire the entire time a skin stretch is held, allowing the nervous system time and providing stimulation that will alter the motor output and pain output at spinal cord and more rostral levels.

Clinical Consideration

Acute and chronic or persistent pain present as different clinical entities. Acute pain, provoked by a specific disease or injury, serves a useful biologic purpose and is self-limited, lasting less than 6 months. The therapy of acute pain is aimed at treating the underlying cause and interrupting the nociceptive signals. The therapy of chronic pain must rely on a multidisciplinary approach and should involve more than one therapeutic modality (Grichnik & Ferrante 1991).

Fasciagenic pain: because fascia has been largely overlooked as a potential pain generator and because scarring impacts fascia, specific consideration is given here. Fascia contains type C nociceptors and some of the free nerve endings in fascia are substance P-containing receptors, commonly assumed to be nociceptive and rendering fascia a potential pain generator (Tesarz 2009). And, as previously noted, neurofascial coverings are innervated by nervi nervorum.

Hyperalgesia: heightened pain sensation from a stimulus that normally provokes pain, a consequence of hyperexcitation involving peripheral or central sensitization or both.

- Primary hyperalgesia: occurs at the site of injury, associated with increased sensitivity of peripheral receptors (e.g. local nocis activated by substances released as a result of injured tissue).

- Secondary hyperalgesia: occurs in tissue outside the site of injury, associated with central sensitization (e.g. changes in spinal cord glial and satellite cells and voltage spiking pattern changes).

- Opioid-induced hyperalgesia: sensitization associated with long-term use of exogenous opioids (e.g. heroin, oxycodone).

Neuropathic pain: pain that arises as a consequence of injury or disease affecting the somatosensory NS (Treede et al. 2008, Correa-Illanes et al. 2010). Neuropathic pain may occur as a manifestation of various conditions that cause nerve damage, such as viral infections (postherpetic neuralgia), metabolic disorders (diabetes mellitus), drug-induced toxicity, inflammation, cancer, trauma, and postsurgical complications. Hyperalgesia to light touch that can occur with neuropathic pain is comparable to secondary hyperalgesia and is thought to be associated with central sensitization. Treede and colleagues (2008) suggest that neuropathic pain is viewed as a clinical description not a diagnosis.

Neuropathy: a disturbance of function or pathological change in a nerve.

Nociception: detection of (noxious) stimuli that are capable of producing tissue injury. Consequences of encoding may be autonomic (e.g. elevation of blood pressure) or behavioral (e.g. withdrawal reflex).

Nociceptive pain: pain that arises from actual or threatened damage to non-neural tissue.

Radicular or radiating pain/sensation: usually perceived as lancinating, sharp, shooting pain or paresthesia felt in a dermatome, myotome or sclerotome because of direct involvement of a spinal nerve or nerve root. It is distinguished from nociception as the axons are stimulated along their course rather than at the terminal-end receptors. Stimulation may occur as a result of mechanical deformation of a dorsal root ganglion, mechanical stimulation of previously damaged nerve roots, inflammation of a dorsal root ganglion and, possibly, by ischemic damage to dorsal root ganglia. Radicular pain differs from referred pain in several respects. While pain can also be perceived deeply, radicular pain displays a cutaneous quality (perceived in the skin as well as deeply) whereas referred pain lacks any cutaneous quality (Bogduk 2009, Lin et al. 2013, IASP 2014).

Referred pain: pain perceived at a location other than the site of the painful stimulus or origin (e.g. referred pain associated with MTrPs). Referred pain may thus occur in a region that is either remote from or directly contiguous with the source of pain, but the two locations are distinguishable on the basis of their different nerve supply. Pain can be referred into the corresponding myotome, dermatome, or sclerotome from any somatic or visceral tissue innervated by a nerve root, but, confusingly, it sometimes is not referred according to the commonly known pattern. Referred pain is a common occurrence in problems associated with the musculoskeletal system. Pain quality is usually described as deep and aching and although its central locus is recognizable and constant, its margins are hard to define (Magee 2008, Bogduk 2009, IASP 2014).

Sensitization: changes in the PNS or CNS (adaptive or pathologic) that lead to heightened nociceptive responses and/or lower thresholds; i.e. a lower intensity stimuli results in increased responsiveness. Clinically, sensitization may only be inferred indirectly from presenting phenomena, such as hyperalgesia or allodynia, and may include dysfunction of endogenous pain control systems.

- Central sensitization: increased responsiveness of nociceptive neurons in the CNS.

- Peripheral sensitization: increased responsiveness of nociceptive neurons in the periphery.

Neuroplasticity

As noted, neurons communicate with each other via electrical signals and synapses. Our brains learn and form memories by strengthening synapses that are frequently used and weakens those that are used less often.

Neuroplasticity, an intrinsic adaptation trait of the NS, enables modification of function and structure in response to demands via the strengthening, weakening, pruning, or adding of synaptic connections and by promoting neurogenesis. Contrary to common belief, neurogenesis in the adult brain can persist into the elder years (Rakic 2002); therefore, the brain does not remain static but instead, throughout life, continues to change its physical structure and functional organization in response to each sensory input, motor act, association, reward signal, action plan and awareness (Pascual-Leone et al. 2005). So, not only can an 'old dog learn new tricks', new cells and streamlined synaptic connections will support the ability to expertly master *said-tricks* well into the elder years.

Neuroplasticity occurs on a variety of levels, ranging from cellular changes in response to learning, to large-scale changes involved in cortical remapping in response to injury.

Neuroplastic adaptation can occur as positive or negative: recovery post-stroke to normal levels of performance is a case of *positive* plasticity. For example when a region of tissue or body part is immobilized, brain regions devoted to sensing, initiating and controlling movement will change as a result of lack of neuronal activity or stimulation. In turn this results in re-allocation of these nerves to other functions (e.g. nociception) and/or actual shrinkage of gray matter within the associated brain region – denoting *negative* plasticity. Other forms of negative plasticity include an excessive release of neurotransmitters in response to injury, resulting in nerve cell apoptosis and chronic pain (Doidge 2007).

Clinical Consideration

A key principle of neuroplasticity is that brain activity promotes brain reorganization. Even relatively simple brain exercises, such as new intellectual challenges, interacting in social situations, or getting involved in physical activities, will stimulate the formation of connections. Building on the principle that neuronal activity promotes new connections, rehabilitation therapy attempts to stimulate particular neurons that have been inactive, with the intended goal to promote self-repair and reorganization through specific motor activity. As an example, practicing a particular movement over and over enables your brain to form and strengthen the connections necessary for that movement (HOPES 2010).

Chronic/Persistent Pain

The brain mostly talks to itself, making up its own stories to enjoy – some of which may not be congruent with physical reality.

Diane Jacobs (RMTBC Pain Conference 2014)

Chronic or persistent pain is so pervasive and potentially incapacitating that the National Institutes of Health (NIH) identify it as a freestanding disorder, rather than as a complication of some underlying condition (NIH 2014).

When pain is chronic, pain signals persist for more than 6 months, often years. Although the original cause may be linked to a previous injury or infection, or an ongoing cause (e.g. arthritis, cancer or pathophysiological scar) some people suffer chronic pain in the absence of any past injury or evidence of body damage. Those with chronic pain disorders with known or unknown causes may have altered cerebral pain processing and loss of gray matter, leading to impaired function (Apkarian et al. 2004, Rodriguez-Raecke et al. 2009, Valet et al. 2009, Wrigley et al. 2009, Granert et al. 2011).

Central and peripheral sensitization

Chronic pain is associated with significant functional, structural and chemical changes in the brain – often termed sensitization, super or hypersensitization (Siddall & Cousins 2004, Tracey & Bushnell 2009). The process of sensitization involves noxious stimuli that results in prolonged pain or misinterpretation of non-noxious stimuli (secondary hyperalgesia and allodynia). These changes occur at the level of the brain cortex, peripheral nerves and/or receptors (Puretić & Demarin 2012). Sensitization explains how pain can exist in the absence of acute trauma or observable irritation of neuronal structures (Chaitow & DeLany 2008, Woolf 2011).

Neuropeptides, released from the nerve itself during the inflammatory response following tissue injury (e.g. surgical and nonsurgical wounds), include substance P and calcitonin gene-related peptide (CGRP). The influence of these vasodilators eventually leads to edema and subsequent sensitizing effects on nociceptors. The consequent decrease in the excitatory threshold to mechanical stimuli allows the nerve to become increasingly sensitive to stimuli that normally are classified as non-noxious (Mense 1993, 2003, 2009, Cady et al. 2011, Waters-Banker et al. 2014).

Prolonged activation of nociceptors and nociceptive input eventually can lead to neuroplastic changes in the peripheral and CNS and the development of various chronic pain syndromes (Krenz et al. 1999, Graven-Nielsen & Mense 2001, Mense 2003, Waters-Banker et al. 2014).

The unrestricted production of neurotrophic growth factors after the sensitization of afferent fibers eventually can lead to collateral sprouting of the afferents in the periphery and fibers within the lamina of the spinal cord. Sprouting of afferents amplifies their input to various pathways within the spinal cord. A potent neurotrophic growth factor, nerve growth factor (NGF), is a known neuronal sensitizing agent. NGF is released during injury and, when uncontrolled, can lead to debilitating chronic pain syndromes (Carew et al. 1979, Krenz et al. 1999, Krenz & Weaver 1998, Mense 2009, Waters-Banker et al. 2014).

In the presence of pain and via the support of various neuropeptides – afferent receptor sensitivity can change in such a way that normal physiological pressure changes often lead to strong and chronic firing of these receptors. Basically, the more the NS is subjected to nociceptive signaling, the more sensitive it becomes to non-injurious or *innocuous* stimuli. Additionally, over a certain

threshold, all mechanoreceptors can potentially become algoceptors (i.e. pain receptors) with consequent propagation of nociceptive signals.

Mitchinson and Rosenberg (2007) suggest that with the recent emphasis on assessing pain as the fifth vital sign tempered by renewed concerns for patient safety, it is time to reintegrate the use of effective and less dangerous approaches to relieve patient distress (Merboth & Barnason 2000, Taylor et al. 2005). If MT's greatest effect is related to modulating the perception of the unpleasantness of pain (Piotrowski et al. 2003), then it is no giant leap to consider MT's utility in the treatment of acute pain and the prevention and treatment of chronic pain. In the world of pain management, research supports that, *hands-down* (pun perhaps intended), multi-modal approaches derive better patient outcomes than singular interventions.

Clinical Consideration

Following persistent inflammation in skeletal muscle, an increase in free nerve-ending fiber density in the perimysium can occur within 12 days. The mechanism proposed suggests NGF as the contributing factor to the increase in substance P production in the dorsal root ganglion. This illustrates the rapidity with which the PNS can become 'efficient' at pain transmission and supports the importance of timely modulation of the early immune response (Reinert et al. 1998, Waters-Banker et al. 2014).

Clinical Consideration

A hypersensitive nerve – and whatever it supplies – tends to 'overreact' in response to many forms of stimulation, including *innocuous* stretch, movement and pressure (Sharpless 1975).

Clinical Consideration (Cont.)

Example

Hypersensitive nerves (associated with muscle) are prone to spontaneous electrical impulses that trigger false pain signals or provoke involuntary muscular activity such as increased tone or tension (Culp & Ochoa 1982). In turn, this increase in tone/tension can subsequently increase the risk of secondary injury (e.g. sprain/strain, tendinopathies, MTrPs).

Clinical Consideration

Hypersensitive afferents can display other forms of aberrant behavior.

Example 1

Hypersensitized nerve fibers become receptive to chemical transmitters all along their length rather than just at their receptor endings (Thesleff & Sellin 1980).

Example 2

Hypersensitized nerves are prone to accept contacts from other types of nerves including autonomic and sensory nerve fibers (Thesleff & Sellin 1980). Impaired communication between sensory and autonomic nerves may contribute to complex regional pain syndrome.

Clinical Consideration

It is suggested that local twitch response (associated with MTrPs) may be due to altered sensory spinal processing resulting from hypersensitized peripheral mechanical nociceptors (Mense et al. 2001).

Pathophysiological Consideration

Pain experts suggest that pain due to peripheral or central neural damage or aberration (neuropathic pain) may differ in clinical features and responsiveness to pharmacological therapy, from pain caused by activation of primary afferents in somatic or visceral tissues (nociceptive pain).

Clinical Consideration

Neuropathic pain may be resistant or less responsive to opioid therapy, suggesting the necessity of using alternative analgesics to achieve pain relief in patients with neuropathic pain (Wilkie et al. 2001). Additionally, there is growing concern over the detrimental side effects, including opioid-induced hyperalgesia. Although this family of drugs provides analgesic and antihyperalgesic effects initially, subsequently they are associated with the expression of hyperalgesia, suggesting that opioids can activate both pain inhibitory and pain facilitatory systems. Paradoxically, opioid therapy aiming at alleviating pain may render patients more sensitive to pain and potentially may aggravate their pre-existing pain (Angst & Clark 2006).

Clinical Consideration

MT has been found to be an effective and safe adjuvant therapy for the relief of acute postoperative pain in patients undergoing major operations. Patients reported markedly less intense and less unpleasant pain and less anxiety than patients who received standard pain medication or individual attention but no MT. The day after surgery, some patients reported that massage delivered about as much pain relief as a dose from a morphine drip. It is suggested that MT works by creating

Wound Healing

The NS plays an important role in mediating normal wound healing via the involvement of various neuropeptides and growth factors. Noxious stimuli causes nerves to release neuropeptides such as substance P and CGRP and certain growth factors (e.g. NGF). And, along with healthy scar formation, in order to re-establish normal functioning post-injury, innervation of the injured tissue must also be re-established.

Wounds initially display hyperinnervation, similar to hypervascularization seen in early wound healing. With normal wound healing, nerve density will normalize with scar maturation. Although densities may return to normal, normal responsiveness is not always re-established, as nerve end organs cannot regenerate and therefore sensory deficit or aberrancies may occur. In spite of the clinical significance of abnormal innervation in scars, the NS has been largely ignored in the pathophysiology of scars.

The role of the NS in wound healing, normal and abnormal, is covered in greater detail in Chapter 5.

Impact of Trauma and Pathophysiological Scars on the NS

As nerves traverse throughout the body they track between and pass through various tissues and structures. The greater proportion of our larger nerves track in the superficial fascia and smaller nerves in the clefts created between perimysial bundles.

Irritation or compression at any point along the complex network of the NS can evoke changes not only locally but also in distant regions and can elicit autonomic disturbances.

Excessive scarring in the layers of tissue a nerve is travelling through can impede all manner of NS functioning (e.g. nerve and electromagnetic conduction, local and systemic responsiveness, sensitization, intraneural blood and nerve supply).

Additionally, injured or distressed somatic tissues adjacent to nerve structures release inflammatory substances that can chemically irritate neural elements. This suggests that a nerve does not have to be entrapped in scar tissue, it can also be impacted by scarring in neighboring tissue.

Pressure and compression constitute the most common forms of nerve injury as complete severance is rare. While nerve injury grading classification systems, such as Seddon (1943) and Sunderland (1952), describe the severity of neural injury (neuropraxia, axonotmesis, neurotmesis) and consider negative symptomology (e.g. numbness and weakness), they do not include considerations for positive symptomology like neuropathic pain.

Clinical Consideration

According to Jacobs:

> Nociceptors signal high threshold stimuli – propagated from chemical, thermal or mechanical messages. If a nerve can't access oxygen and glucose or if the nerve is 'backed-up' with deoxygenated blood that can't escape (i.e. hypoxia and ischemia, due to tensional compression and diminished lymphatic drainage) then that nerve will complain via its mechanoreceptors, chemoreceptors and nociceptors.

Therefore, if MT can productively affect tensional compression and lymphatic flow with resultant impact on hypoxia and ischemia, the chain of events will culminate in less cranky nerves.

Compression Syndromes

Although peripheral nerves are fairly robust and capable of withstanding a hefty amount of distortion, under certain circumstances even a relatively small amount of pressure may trigger a cascade of immune-inflammatory responses leading to peripheral neuropathy. Certain neural parts are less protected and more vulnerable to compression or pressure injury; for example, at nerve roots and where a nerve travels through confined spaces such as structured tunnels (Coppieters & Nee 2012, Schmid et al. 2013).

Additionally, peripheral nerves can become entrapped in dense, fibrosed tissue or compressed by dense, fibrosed neurofascia. Peripheral neuropathies may exist where there is altered nerve conduction in the absence of severe enough compression to be graded as neuropraxia. Sunderland (1978) referred to such presentations as *irritative lesion*. This suggests that a nerve irritated at a *low-level* state,

something other than observable *squish* or full-rage inflammation, can be the source of neuropathic pain. Pathophysiological scars may constitute such irritative lesions.

Pathophysiological Consideration

Compression of type C nociceptors can contribute to the pain associated with entrapment syndromes (Hammer 1998). Pain can be local or referred.

Pathophysiological Consideration

If a neural sheath is twisted, impinged or shortened, by excessive scarring or dense, fibrosed tissue, the nerve and what it supplies will be impacted (Shacklock 2005).

Pathophysiological Consideration

Endoneurial fluid increases when a nerve is compressed, irritated or injured. In such cases MR neurography can detect nerve injury and irritation (Cudlip et al. 2002).

Pathophysiological Consideration

Unimpeded nerve conduction is essential to trophic effect (i.e. control and maintenance of cellular function). When conduction is impeded or blocked, innervated structures become atrophic. Atrophic structures can become highly irritable and develop hypersensitivity (Cannon & Rosenblueth 1949).

Double-crush injury

With double-crush injury, an axon compressed in one region can become susceptible to injury at another site (e.g. development of a cervical radiculopathy in conjunction with carpal tunnel syndrome) (Upton & McComas 1973, Moghtaderi & Izadi 2008, Coppieters & Nee 2012). Mechanisms similar to those associated with sensitization are implicated.

Clinical Consideration

With double-crush injuries, failure to treat at multiple levels will result in failure to relieve the patient's symptoms (Mackinnon 2002). This supports the importance of local and global treatment considerations (e.g. along the nerve path, corresponding myofascial meridians/myokinetic chains and neighboring tissue).

Clinical Consideration

As is the case with other tissues, neural tissue functions best when free of restriction or compression. Neural compression is linked to various neuropathies (e.g. carpal tunnel, sciatica, thoracic outlet). Neural sensitivity to compression ought to be taken into consideration during manual therapies. It is important to approach distressed neural tissues gently and from angles that avoid compressing the nerve further. Additionally, distressed nerves do not tolerate much stretch – treatment considerations are covered in more detail in Chapter 9.

Proprioceptive Disinformation

Densification, adhesions, fibrosis or excessive scarring can impact proprioception (Stecco et al. 2006, Stecco et al. 2010, Fourie 2012). Binding may occur among layers that should stretch and slide/glide on each other, distorting myofascial relationships which, in turn, can alter muscle motor function and proprioception (Fourie 2009, Stecco & Stecco 2009).

Recall from Chapter 2, when challenged by stretch or movement, dense and/or restricted fascia may alter proprioceptive afferent signals that lead to eventual abnormal biomechanics, aberrant movement patterns, muscle compensation, joint distress and pain (Bouffard et al. 2008, Stecco et al. 2010).

Normal tissue viscoelasticity is essential for proper neurological functioning, including proprioception (Stecco 2004, Stecco et al. 2010). In the absence of normal physiological elasticity, receptors embedded within the fascia may also be in an active state, even at rest. Any further stretching – even that produced by normal muscular contraction – could cause excessive stimulation with consequent propagation of nociceptive afferents. Further, over a certain threshold (i.e. consistent stimulus over time), all receptors can potentially become algoceptors (pain receptors) in response to consequent propagation of nociceptive signals (Ryan 2011).

Pathophysiological Consideration

Fascial restrictions (i.e. altered elasticity due to pathophysiological scarring) can exert an adverse effect on free nerve endings (functioning as mechanoreceptors), resulting in changes in tissue viscosity. This is particularly evident when the restricted fascia is challenged. Stretch or tensioning of restricted or dense fascia appears to trigger *incoherent* afferent signaling which in turn leads to aberrant firing sequences (i.e. muscle incoordination) along the myokinetic chain. Incoordination can lead to abnormal biomechanics, eventual abnormal muscle compensation and pain. 'Normal' fascial elasticity is essential for sound biomechanical and neurological functioning (Schleip 2003a, 2003b).

Impaired mechanoreceptors (e.g. receptors entrapped in dense, fibrosed tissue) react to mechanical forces by disinforming local, regional, or central nerve centers. Under or overestimation of the mechanical stimuli may occur. This proprioceptive disinformation causes inappropriate muscular reactions which endanger the patient's general equilibrium and can lead to alterations in contraction force, mistiming of myofascial contraction activation or muscular incoordination. Proprioceptive disinformation can also lead to subsequent secondary injuries such as tendinopathies, sprains, strains, falling and fractures.

References

Abu-Hijleh MF, Harris PF (2007) Deep fascia on the dorsum of the ankle and foot: extensor retinacula revisited. Clinical Anatomy 20: 186–195.

Angevine Jr, JB (2002) Organization of the nervous system. In: Ramachandran VS (ed) Encyclopedia of the Human Brain, Vol 3. Waltham, MA: Academic Press, p 313.

Angst MS, Clark JD (2006) Opioid-induced hyperalgesia. A qualitative systematic review. Anesthesiology 104: 570–87.

Apkarian AV, Sosa Y, Krauss BR et al (2004) Chronic pain patients are impaired on an emotional decision-making task. Pain 108: 129–36.

Arbuckle BE (1994) The selected writings of Beryl E. Arbuckle, DO. Indianapolis, IN: American Academy of Osteopathy.

Bhowmick S, Singh A, Flavell RA et al (2009) The sympathetic nervous system modulates CD4(+)FoxP3(+) regulatory T cells via a TGF-beta-dependent mechanism. Journal of Leukocyte Biology 86: 1275–1283.

Bogduk N (2009) On the definitions and physiology of back pain, referred pain, and radicular pain. Pain 147: 17–19.

Bouffard NA, Cutroneo KR, Badger GJ et al (2008) Tissue stretch decreases soluble TGF-beta1 and type-1 procollagen in mouse subcutaneous connective tissue: evidence from ex vivo and in vivo models. Journal of Cell Physiology 214: 389–395.

Bove G (2008) Epi-perineurial anatomy, innervation, and axonal nociceptive mechanisms. Journal of Bodywork and Movement Therapies 12(3): 185–190. doi:10.1016/ j.jbmt.2008.03.004.

Bove GM, Light AR (1997) The nervi nervorum: missing link for neuropathic pain? Pain Forum 6(3): 181–190.

Cady RJ, Glenn JR, Smith KM, Durham PL (2011) Calcitonin gene-related peptide promotes cellular changes in trigeminal neurons and glia implicated in peripheral and central sensitization. Molecular Pain 7:94.

Campbell JN, Raja SN, Meyer RA, Mackinnon SE (1988) Myelinated afferents signal the hyperalgesia associated with nerve injury. Pain 32: 89–94. doi: 10.1016/ 0304-3959(88)90027-9.

Cannon WB, Rosenblueth A (1949) The supersensitivity of denervated structures, a law of denervation. New York: Macmillan.

Carew T, Castellucci VF, Kandel ER (1979) Sensitization in Aplysia: restoration of transmission in synapses inactivated by long-term habituation. Science 205(4404): 417–419.

Chaitow L (1998) Positional release techniques in the treatment of muscle and joint dysfunction. Clinical Bulletin of Myofascial Therapy, 3(1): 25–35.

Chaitow L (2007) Soft tissue manipulation: diagnostic and therapeutic potential. Available at: www.leonchaitow.com [Accessed 10 March 2007].

Chaitow L (2014) Fascial dysfunction – manual therapy approaches. Pencaitland, UK: Handspring Publishing.

Chaitow L, DeLany J (2008) Clinical application of neuromuscular techniques: the upper body vol. 1, 2e. Edinburgh: Churchill Livingstone Elsevier.

Coppieters M, Nee R (2012) Neurodynamics: movement for neuropathic pain states. In: Schleip R, Findley TW, Chaitow L, Huijing P, eds. Fascia: the tensional network of the human body. Edinburgh: Churchill Livingstone Elsevier, Ch 7.19, pp 425–432.

Correa-Illanes G, Calderón W, Roa R, Piñeros J L, Medina D (2010) Treatment of localized post-traumatic neuropathic pain in scars with 5% lidocaine medicated plaster. Local and Regional Anesthesia 3: 77.

Cottingham JT (1985) Healing through touch – a history and a review of the physiological evidence. Boulder, CO: Rolf Institute Publications.

Craig AD (2003) Interoception: the sense of the physiological condition of the body. Current Opinion in Neurobiology 13(4): 500–505.

Critchley HD, Melmed RN, Featherstone E, Mathias CJ, Dolan RJ (2002) Volitional control of autonomic arousal: a functional magnetic resonance study. NeuroImage 16: 909–919.

Cudlip SA, Howe FA, Clifton A et al (2002) Magnetic resonance neurography studies of the median nerve before and after carpal tunnel decompression. Journal of Neurosurgery 96(6): 1046–1051.

Culp WJ, Ochoa JL (Eds) (1982). Abnormal Nerves and Muscles as Impulse Generators. New York: Oxford University Press.

Damasio AR, Grabowski TJ, Bechara A et al (2000) Subcortical and cortical brain activity during the feeling of self-generated emotions. Nature Neuroscience 3:1049–1056.

Derbyshire S, Whalley M, Oakley D (2003) Subjects hallucinating pain in the absence of a stimulus activate anterior cingulate, anterior insula, prefrontal and parietal cortices. Journal of Pain 4:39.

Devor M (2009) Ectopic discharge in Abeta afferents as a source of neuropathic pain. Experimental Brain Research 196: 115–128. doi: 10.1007/s00221-009-1724-6.

Doidge N (2007) The brain that changes itself: stories of personal triumph from the frontiers of brain science. New York: Viking.

Dommerholt J (2014) Science and trigger points, does it matter? Lecture notes from the Registered Massage Therapists' Association of British Columbia (RMTBC) Pain Management Conference, Vancouver, March 28–29.

Dorko BL (2003) The analgesia of movement: ideomotor activity and manual care. International Journal of Osteopathic Medicine 6(2): 93–95.

Fadok VA, Bratton DL, Guthrie L, Henson PM (2001) Differential effects of apoptotic versus lysed cells on macrophage production of cytokines: role of proteases. Journal of Immunology 166(11): 6847–6854.

Feinstein B, Langton JN, Jameson RM, Schiller F (1954). Experiments on pain referred from deep somatic tissues. The Journal of Bone and Joint Surgery, 36(5): 981–997.

Fourie W (2009) The fascia lata of the thigh – more than a "stocking": a magnetic resonance imaging, ultrasonography and dissection study. In: Fascia Research II: Basic Science and Implications for Conventional and Complementary Health Care. Huijing P, Hollander P, Findley T, Schleip R, eds. Munich: Elsevier, p 93.

Fourie W (2012) In: Schleip R et al. Fascia: the tensional network of the human body. Edinburgh, Churchill Livingstone Elsevier, Ch 7.17, pp 410–419.

Frymann VM (1988) Why does the orthodontist need osteopathy in the cranial field. The Cranial Letter 41: 4.

Goodman CC, Fuller KS (2012) Pathology for the physical therapist assistant. St Louis: Elsevier Saunders, p 717.

Graceovetsky S (2007) Is the lumbodorsal fascia necessary? Fascia Anatomy and Biomechanics Panel. Lecture notes from The 1st International Fascia Research Congress, Boston October 3–5.

Granert O, Peller M, Gaser C et al (2011) Manual activity shapes structure and function in contralateral human motor hand area. NeuroImage 54(1): 32–41.

Graven-Nielsen T, Mense S (2001) The peripheral apparatus of muscle pain: evidence from animal and human studies. The Clinical Journal of Pain 17(1): 2–10.

Grichnik KP, Ferrante FM (1991) The difference between acute and chronic pain. Mount Sinai Journal of Medicine 58(3): 217–20.

Hammer W (1998) The fascial connection. Dynamic Chiropractic, Dec 14 16:26.

Hammer WI (2008) The effect of mechanical load on degenerated soft tissue. Journal of Bodywork and Movement Therapies 12(3): 246–256.

HOPES (2010) Huntington's Outreach Project for Education at Standford. Neuroplasticity. Available at: http://web. stanford.edu/group/hopes/cgi-bin/wordpress/2010/06/neuroplasticity/ [Accessed 6 October 2014].

Howe JF, Loeser JD, Calvin WH (1977) Mechanosensitivity of dorsal root ganglia and chronically injured axons: a physiological basis for the radicular pain of nerve root compression. Pain 3: 25–41.

Howe JF (1979) A neurophysiological basis for the radicular pain of nerve root compression. Advances in pain research and therapy. 3: 647–57.

International Association for the Study of Pain (2014) IASP Taxonomy. Pain terms. Available at: http://www.iasp-pain.org/Taxonomy?navItemNumber=576.

Jacobs D (2014) Making connections; pain science, therapeutic context, manual therapy, nervous system and skin. Lecture notes from the Registered Massage Therapists' Association of British Columbia (RMTBC) Pain Management Conference, Vancouver March 28–29.

Jones FW (1944) Structure and function as seen in the foot. London: Baillière, Tindall and Cox.

Kandel ER, Schwartz JH, Jessell TM (2000) Principles of neural science. New York: McGraw-Hill.

Kellgren JH (1938) Referred pains from muscle. British Medical Journal, 1(4023):325.

Kellgren JH (1939) On the distribution of pain arising from deep somatic structures with charts of segmental pain areas. Clinical Science 4(35):5.

King T, Qu C, Okun A et al (2011) Contribution of afferent pathways to nerve injury-induced spontaneous pain and evoked hypersensitivity. Pain 152: 1997–2005. doi: 10.1016/j. pain. 2011.04.020.

Koltzenburg M, Torebjork HE, Wahren LK (1994) Nociceptor modulated central sensitization causes mechanical hyperalgesia in acute chemogenic and chronic neuropathic pain. Brain 117: 579–591. doi: 10.1093/brain/117.3.579.

Krenz NR, Meakin SO, Krassioukov AV, Weaver LC (1999) Neutralizing intraspinal nerve growth factor blocks autonomic dysreflexia caused by spinal cord injury. The Journal of Neuroscience, 19(17): 7405–7414.

Krenz NR, Weaver LC (1998) Sprouting of primary afferent fibers after spinal cord transection in the rat. Neuroscience 85(2): 443–458.

Kruger L (1987) Cutaneous sensory system. In: Adelman G (ed) Encyclopedia of Neuroscience (1): 293–294.

Langevin HM (2006) Connective tissue: a body-wide signaling network? Medical Hypotheses 66(6): 1074e1077.

Langevin HM, Churchill DL, Wu J et al (2002) Evidence of connective tissue involvement in acupuncture. The FASEB Journal 16: 872–874.

Lee MWL, McPhee RW, Stringer MD (2013) An evidence-based approach to human dermatomes. Australasian Musculoskeletal Medicine (online), 18 (1) Jun 2013: 14–22. Availability: <http://search.informit.com.au/documentSummary;dn=354755695799746;res=IELHEA> ISSN: 1324–5627 [cited 19 Aug 15].

Lembeck F (1983) Sir Thomas Lewis's nocifensor system, histamine and substance-P- containing primary afferent nerves. Trends in Neurosciences 6: 106–108.

Light AR (2004) 'Nocifensor' system re-revisited. Focus on 'Two types of C nociceptor in human skin and their behavior in areas of capsaicin-induced secondary hyperalgesia'.[comment]. Journal of Neurophysiology 91: 2401–2403. [PubMed: 15136601].

Lin CW, Verwoerd AJH, Maher CG et al (2014) How is radiating leg pain defined in randomized controlled trials of conservative treatments in primary care? A systematic review. European Journal of Pain 18(4): 455–464.

Mackinnon SE (2002) Pathophysiology of nerve compression. Hand Clinics 18(2): 989–997.

Magee DJ (2008) Orthopedic physical assessment, 5th edn. St Louis: Elsevier Saunders.

Mense S (1993) Nociception from skeletal muscle in relation to clinical muscle pain. Pain 54(3): 241–289.

Mense S, Simons DG, Russell IJ (2001) Muscle pain: understanding its nature, diagnosis, and treatment. Baltimore: Lippincott Williams & Wilkins.

Mense S (2003) The pathogenesis of muscle pain. Current Pain and Headache Reports 7(6): 419–425.

Mense S (2009) Algesic agents exciting muscle nociceptors. Experimental Brain Research 196(1): 89–100.

Merboth MK, Barnason S (2000) Managing pain: the fifth vital sign. Nursing Clinics of North America 35(2): 375–383.

Mersky H, Bogduk N (1994) ISAP Subcommittee on taxonomy, classification of chronic pain. Pain 1994: SI–5236.

Minasny B (2009) Understanding the process of fascial unwinding. International Journal of Therapeutic Massage and Bodywork 2(3): 10–17.

Mitchinson AR, Kim H, Rosenberg JM et al (2007) Acute postoperative pain management using massage as an adjuvant therapy: a randomized trial. Archives of Surgery 142(12): 1158–1167. doi:10.1001/archsurg.142.12.1158.

Moghtaderi A, Izadi S (2008) Double crush syndrome: an analysis of age gender and body mass index. Clinical Neurology and Neurosurgery 110(1): 225–29.

Murphy RW (1977) Nerve roots and spinal nerves in degenerative disk disease. Clinical Orthopaedics and Related Research, 129: 46–60.

National Institutes of Health, NIH (2014) [online] Available at: http://www.ninds.nih.gov/disorders/chronic_pain/chronic_pain.htm [Accessed September 19 2014].

Paoletti S (2006) The fasciae: anatomy, dysfunction and treatment. Seattle: Eastland Press.

Pascual-Leone A, Amedi A, Fregni F, Merabet LB (2005) The plastic human brain cortex. Annual Review of Neuroscience 28: 377–401. doi:10.1146/annurev.neuro.27.070203.144216.

Petrovic P, Kalso E, Petersson KM, Ingvar M (2002) Placebo and opioid analgesia – imaging a shared neuronal network. Science 295: 1737–1740.

Pickar JG, Sung PS, Kang YM, Ge W (2007) Response of lumbar paraspinal muscles spindles is greater to spinal manipulative loading compared with slower loading under length control. The Spine Journal 7(5): 583–595.

Piotrowski MM, Paterson C, Mitchinson A (2003) Massage as adjuvant therapy in the management of acute postoperative pain: a preliminary study in men. Journal of the American College of Surgeons 197(6): 1037–1046.

Puretić M, Demarin V (2012) Neuroplasticity mechanisms in the pathophysiology of chronic pain. Acta Clinica Croatica 51(3): 425–429. Available at: http://hrcak.srce.hr/index.php?show=clanak&id_clanak_jezik=158033 [Accessed 10 November 2014].

Rakic P (2002) Neurogenesis in adult primate neocortex: an evaluation of the evidence. Nature Reviews Neuroscience 3(1): 65–71. doi:10.1038/nrn700.

Ratté S, Zhu Y, Yeop-Lee K, Prescott S (2014) Criticality and degeneracy in injury-induced changes in primary afferent excitability and the implications for neuropathic pain. eLife 3:e02370. doi: 10.7554/eLife.02370.

Reinert A, Kaske A, Mense S (1998) Inflammation-induced increase in the density of neuropeptide-immunoreactive nerve endings in rat skeletal muscle. Experimental Brain Research 121(2): 174–180.

Richards S (2012) Pleasant to the touch. The Scientist. Available at: http://www.the-scientist.com/?articles.view/articleNo/32487/title/Pleasant-to-the-Touch/ [Accessed 10 November 2014].

Rodriguez-Raecke R, Niemeier A, Ihle K et al (2009) Brain gray matter decreases in chronic pain is the consequence and not the cause of pain. Journal of Neuroscience 29: 13746–50.

Ryan C (2011) The story of fascia – Interview with Julie Day. Massage Matters Canada Magazine, Summer Issue.

Sauer SK et al (1999) Rat peripheral nerve components release calcitonin gene-related peptide and prostaglandin E-2 in response to noxious stimuli: Evidence that nervi nervorum are nociceptors. Neuroscience 92: 319–325.

Schleip R (2003a) Fascial plasticity – a new neurobiological explanation: Part 1. Journal of Bodywork and Movement Therapies 7(1): 11–19.

Schleip R (2003b) Fascial plasticity–a new neurobiological explanation Part 2. Journal of Bodywork and Movement Therapies 7(2): 104–116.

Schleip R, Jäger H (2012) Interoception: a new correlate for intricate connections between fascial receptors, emotion and self recognition. In: Schleip R, Findley TW, Chaitow L, Huijing P, eds. Fascia: the tensional network of the human body. Edinburgh: Churchill Livingstone Elsevier, pp 89–94.

Schleip R, Naylor IL, Ursu D et al (2006) Passive muscle stiffness may be influenced by active contractility of intramuscular connective tissue. Medical Hypotheses 66(1): 66–71.

Schmid AB, Nee RJ, Coppieters MW (2013) Reappraising entrapment neuropathies –mechanisms, diagnosis and management. Manual Therapy, 18(6): 449–457.

Schuman E (2013) The remarkable neuron: Erin Schuman at TEDxCaltech. Available at: https://www.youtube.com/watch?v=yr6kh_QOk0s [Accessed 10 September 2014].

Seddon HJ (1943) Three types of nerve injury. Brain 66(4): 237–288.

Shacklock M (2005) Clinical neurodynamics: a new system of musculoskeletal treatment. Oxford, Butterworth Heinemann.

Shah I, Phillips T, Danoff J et al (2005) An in vivo microanalytical technique for measuring the local biochemical milieu of human skeletal muscle. Journal of Applied Physiology 99: 1977–1984.

Sharpless SK (1975) Supersensitivity-like phenomena in the central nervous system. Federation Proceedings 34: 1990–1997.

Siddall PJ, Cousins MJ (2004) Persistent pain as a disease entity: implications for clinical management. Anesthesia and Analgesia 99: 510–20.

Simon DG, Mense S (2007) Understanding and measurement of muscle tonus as related to clinical muscle pain. In: Findley T, Schleip R, eds. Fascia research, basic science and implications for conventional and complementary health care. Munich: Elsevier.

Sommer C (2010) Practical considerations for structural integration, biased by the nervous system. Structural Integration June 2010.

Staubesand J, Li Y (1996) Zum Feinbau der Fascia cruris mit besonderer Berucksichtigung epi- und intrafaszialer Nerven. Manuelle Medizin 34: 196–200.

Stecco C, Gagey O, Belloni A, et al (2007) Anatomy of the deep fascia of the upper limb. Second part: study of innervation. Morphologie, 91(292): 38–43.

Stecco C, Porzionato A, Macchi V et al (2006) Histological characteristics of the deep fascia of the upper limb. Italian Journal of Anatomy and Embryology 111: 105–110.

Stecco C, Macchi V, Porzionato A et al (2010) The ankle retinacula: morphological evidence of the proprioceptive role of the fascial system. Cells Tissues Organs 192: 200–210.

Stecco L (2004) Fascial manipulation for musculoskeletal pain. Padova: Piccin, pp 123–130.

Stecco L, Stecco C (2009) Fascial manipulation for musculoskeletal pain and fascial manipulation: practical part. Padova: Piccin Nuova Libraries SpA.

Sunderland S (1952) A classification of peripheral nerve injuries producing loss of function. Brain (74): 491–516.

Sunderland S (1978) Nerves and nerve injuries, 2e. Edinburgh: Churchill Livingstone.

Sunderland S, Bradley KC (1949) The cross-sectional area of peripheral nerve trunks devoted to nerve fibres. Brain 72(3): 428–449.

Taylor S, Kirton OC, Staff I, Kozol RA (2005) Postoperative day one: a high risk period for respiratory events. American Journal of Surgery 190(5): 752–756.

Tesarz J (2009) The innervation of the fascia thoracolumbalis. In: Huijing PA, Hollander P, Findley TW, Schleip R (eds) Fascia research II – basic science and implications for conventional and complementary health care. Munich: Elsevier GmbH, p 37.

Tesarz J, Hoheisel U, Wiedenhofer B, Mense S (2011) Sensory innervation of the thoracolumbar fascia in rats and humans. Neuroscience 194: 302–308. doi:10.1016/j.neuroscience.2011.07.066.

Thesleff S, Sellin LC (1980) Denervation supersensitivity. Trends in Neurosciences 122–126.

Tracey I, Bushnell MC (2009) How neuroimaging studies have challenged us to rethink: is chronic pain a disease? Journal of Pain 10: 1113–20.

Treede RD, Jensen TS, Campbell JN et al (2008) Neuropathic pain: redefinition and a grading system for clinical and research purposes. Neurology 70(18): 1630–1635.

Upledger JE (1987) Craniosacral therapy II: beyond the dura. Seattle: Eastland Press, pp 115–130.

Upton A, McComas AJ (1973) The double crush in nerve entrapment syndromes. Lancet 2 (7825): 35–362.

Valet M, Gündel H, Sprenger T et al (2009) Patients with pain disorder show gray matter loss in pain processing structures: a voxel based morphometric study. Psychosomatic Medicine 71: 49–56.

Van den Berg (2012) The physiology of fascia: an introduction. In: Schleip R, Findley TW, Chaitow L, Huijing P, eds. Fascia: the tensional network of the human body. Edinburgh: Churchill Livingstone Elsevier, pp 149–155.

Van der Wal J (2009) The architecture of the connective tissue in the musculoskeletal system – an often overlooked functional parameter as to proprioception in the locomotor apparatus. International Journal of Therapeutic Massage and Bodywork: Research, Education and Practice 2(4): 9–23.

Vleeming A, Pool-Goudzwaard AL, Stoeckart R, van Wingerden JP, Snijders CJ (1995) The posterior layer of the thoracolumbar fascia]. Its function in load transfer from spine to legs. Spine 20(7): 753–758.

Resources and further reading

Doidge N (2007) The Brain that Changes Itself: Stories of Personal Triumph from the Frontiers of Brain Science. New York: Viking.

Jacobs D, PT – Dermoneuromodulation: http://www.dermoneuromodulation.com/.

Ward RS, Tuckett RP, English KB et al (2004) Substance P axons and sensory threshold increase in burn-graft human skin. Journal of Surgical Research 118: 154–60.

Waters-Banker C, Dupont-Versteegden EE, Kitzman PH, Butterfield TA (2014) Investigating the mechanisms of massage efficacy:the role of mechanical immunomodulation. Journal of Athletic Training 49(2): 266–273 doi: 10.4085/1062-6050-49.2.25.

Wilkie DJ et al (2001) Nociceptive and neuropathic pain in patients with lung cancer: a comparison of pain quality descriptors. Journal of Pain and Symptom Management 22; 5: 899–910.

Winkelstein BA (2004) Mechanisms of central sensitization, neuroimmunology and injury biomechanics in persistent pain: implications for musculoskeletal disorders. Journal of Electromyography and Kinesiology 14(1): 87–93.

Woolf CJ (2011) Central sensitization: implications for the diagnosis and treatment of pain. Pain 152(3): S2–S15.

Wrigley PJ, Press SR, Gustin SM et al (2009). Neuropathic pain and primary somatosensory cortex reorganization following spinal cord injury. Pain 141: 52–9.

Yahia L, Pigeon P, DesRosiers E (1993) Viscoelastic properties of the human lumbodorsal fascia. J Biomed Eng 15(5): 425–429.

Zigmond MJ, Bloom FE, Landis SC, Roberts JL, Squire LR (1999) Fundamental Neuroscience, San Diego: Academic Press.

Neuroscience and Pain Science for Manual Therapists: https://www.facebook.com/pages/Neuroscience-and-Pain-Science-for-Manual-Physical-Therapists/114879238784?ref=nf.

CHAPTER 5

Wound healing and scars

Never be ashamed of a scar. It simply means you are stronger than whatever tried to hurt you

Unknown

Any wound that breaches the dermis results in some degree of scarring, no matter how the wound occurred (Fitch 2005). Scar formation – a natural biological process – is the body's means by which it protects itself from infection and re-establishes structural continuity by *knitting* itself back together following injury or trauma.

Although the 'replacement-tissue' that forms the scar differs from the original tissue, *normal* or healthy scarring is intended to restore or preserve tissue integrity and function. On the other hand, if any aspect of the process is faulty or mismanaged, pain and dysfunction can occur at debilitating levels. Both normal (physiological) and abnormal (pathophysiological) scars are covered in this chapter.

The aim of this chapter is to provide a solid base for understanding and working with tissue that is a little out of the ordinary. Although each client's physiology may differ from the next, there are enough similarities between individuals to inform treatment protocol and to effect positive changes. In some cases, treatment may not significantly impact scar aesthetics or scar tissue structural organization; however, there is evidence to support the claim that manual scar management techniques can impact pain, function and quality of life in positive and productive ways (DeNoon 2005, Josenhans 2007, Cherkin 2011, Bove & Chapelle 2012, Fourie 2008, 2009, 2012, Werner 2012, Rodriguez & del Rio 2013).

A massage therapist can play an active role in a client's healing and recovery. The benefits of MT (interventions which assist the healing process or which may be employed *after* scarring

has taken place), treatment protocols, contraindications and modifications will be explored in greater detail in subsequent chapters.

Wound Healing

Wound healing, a complex physiological response to injury, consists of four overlapping and precisely programmed stages: homeostasis, inflammation, proliferation and remodeling (Table 5.1). For a wound to heal successfully, all four stages must occur in the proper sequence and time frame.

Without the thorough completion of all four stages, homeostasis will not be restored and healing will not reach its maximum potential. Any interruptions, aberrancies or prolongation of the process can result in delayed, improper or impaired healing and complications. It is important to note that the healing process for viscera and fascia is the same as that observed in skin (Bond et al. 2008, Sarrazy et al. 2011, Bordoni & Zanier 2014).

Many factors influence and can interfere with one or more stages of this process. The appropriate levels of cytokines and growth factors ensure that cellular responses are mediated in a coordinated manner. The TGF-β family is of particular interest because they play a role in all four stages of wound healing and are thought to have the broadest spectrum of effects including: cell proliferation and differentiation, ECM matrix production and immune modulation. (Finnson et al. 2013).

Aberrant TGF-β signaling has been implicated in pathological skin disorders, including chronic wounds, excessive scarring and fibrosis, all of

Stage	Primary events, features and typical time frames
1: Homeostasis	Within seconds after injury, rupture of tissues/vessels results in blood-borne cells, proteins and platelets seeping into the periphery (ECM), initiating clot formation to slow/stop blood loss. Activated platelets adhere together creating a clot/ provisional matrix which provides structural support for cellular attachment and subsequent cellular proliferation within the wound. Once bleeding is relatively controlled, various signaling molecules stimulate chemotaxis
2: Inflammation	Neutrophils, mast cells and macrophages locally migrate to clean up potentially contaminating microorganisms, degrade surplus components and rid the area of waste material. Macrophage secreted chemotactic and growth factors, along with other inflammatory agents, mediate the typical cascade of events associated with inflammation response. As this stage subsides, inflammatory mediators and immune cell concentrations decrease at the wound site; however, the area may still be edematous and warm as the immune system remains active until the barrier is repaired. This stage typically lasts from 1 to 4 days
3: Proliferation	Within 48–72 hours after the initial injury (overlapping stage 2), epithelial proliferation and fibroblast migration toward the provisional matrix occur, constituting the first signs of scar formation – granulation tissue. This forms a structural framework to bridge the wound and allow vascular ingrowth in the form of fresh capillary beds. The wound gap begins to decrease as MFBs contract and physically draw the severed tissue fragments together. Eventually, collagenase is released to degrade the fine Type III collagen that helped form the provisional matrix as a stronger matrix replaces the provisional one to better support day-to-day function. Fibroblasts synthesize GAGs and Type I collagen and continued Type 1 collagen proliferation ensures the scar tissue becomes stronger. In some cases edema, elevated temperature around the wound and pain may still be present. This stage typically lasts 4–21 days but may last for up to 6 weeks
4: Remodeling	Regression of capillary hypervascularity commences prompting a return to normal vascular density. The wound continues to undergo MFB-mediated contraction, ensuring the formation of a mechanically sound scar. Adequate amounts of TGF-β1 and mechanical tension assure the restoration of normal/physiological ECM and tissue architecture. Normal scar tissue progresses from being red and prominent, to becoming thin and pale. As long as the scar appears redder than normal, remodeling is still under way. Normally, this stage should be relatively painless and yield an innocuous scar that exhibits normal coloration, is relevant in size and is mobile. There should be no significant degree of pain associated with a properly healing wound nor any residual pain experienced, once remodeling has completed. The remodeling stage can last from months to years

Table 5.1

Stages of wound healing

which can compromise normal tissue function (Finnson et al. 2013).

Pathophysiological Consideration

Understanding the mechanisms involved in regulating TGF-β signaling provides important insights into how to prevent or reduce aberrant wound healing and excessive scarring (Finnson et al. 2013)

Clinical Consideration

Because therapeutic agents that target the TGF-β signaling pathway have been shown to improve wound healing and reduce scarring (Finnson et al. 2013), targeting the TGF-β signaling pathway represents a viable strategy for improving wound healing and reducing pathological scarring (Finnson et al. 2013). Transforming growth factor beta-1 (TGF-β1) activation is – in part – influenced by tissue tension (Wipff & Hinz 2009, Meyer-ter-Vehn et al. 2011). It is suggested that the manual manipulation of fascia has the potential to change the cell-matrix tension state (i.e. restoration of tensional homeostasis) and possibly influence localized TGF-β1 activity (Grinell 2008).

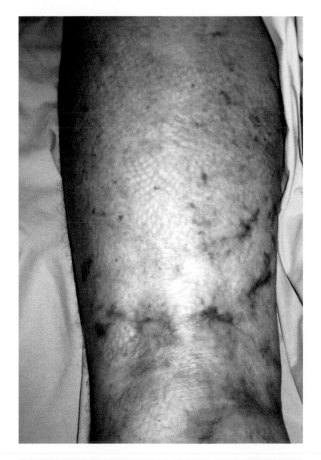

Figure 5.1

Hypertrophic scar example.

The Four Stages of Wound Healing (Marieb 2003; see Also Table 5.1)

Stage 1: Homeostasis

The healing process begins within seconds after injury when tissue and blood vessels are disrupted. Vessel wall rupture results in the release of blood-borne cells, proteins and platelets into the periphery (ECM). Platelets are activated upon coming into contact with collagen and other ECM constituents outside of the blood vessels. Activated platelets adhere together, forming an initial plug to slow or stop blood loss. The platelet coagulation cascade results in the production of a stable fibrin-reinforced clot and provisional matrix. A provisional matrix, comprising fibrin and Type III collagen, provides structural support for cellular attachment and subsequent cellular proliferation within the wound (Tredget et al. 1997). Once bleeding is controlled, various signaling molecules (e.g. pro-inflammatory cytokines and growth factors, such as TGF-β1; epidermal growth factor – EGF; insulin-like growth factor – IGF1; and platelet derived growth factor – PDGF), stimulate chemotaxis, the migration of inflammatory and reparative cells (e.g. neutrophils, macrophages, epithelial and endothelial cells, mast cells and fibroblasts) to the wound, initiating the next stage (Gauglitz et al. 2011, Guo & DiPietro 2010, Bordoni & Zanier 2014, Zhu et al. 2013).

Stage 2: Inflammation

In this stage, specific types of cells perform specific tasks. Neutrophils, mast cells and macrophages clean up potentially contaminating micro organisms, degrade surplus components and rid the area of waste material.

Macrophages also secrete a variety of chemotactic and growth factors (e.g. fibroblast growth factor (FGF), epidermal growth factor (EGF), TGF-β1 and interleukin-1 (IL-1). These and other inflammatory mediators (e.g. chemokines, cytokines and substance P) are responsible for the typical cascade of events associated with inflammation response.

As this *reactive* stage begins to subside, inflammatory mediators and the number of neutrophils and macrophages are reduced at the wound site. The scarred area may still be edematous, presenting as red in color with a noticeable rise in temperature from surrounding tissue. The immune system remains active until the barrier is repaired. Under normal circumstances this stage typically lasts from 1 to 4 days – with the overt signs of edema beginning to diminish.

Stage 3: Proliferation

Within 48–72 hours after the initial injury, the healing process moves into the proliferation stage. Endothelial cells and fibroblasts are the most prominent cell types present in this stage, which, generally overlapping with the inflammatory stage, is characterized by epithelial proliferation and fibroblast migration toward the provisional matrix (i.e. first signs of scar formation – granulation tissue) (Bordoni & Zanier 2014, Bran et al. 2012). Granulation tissue comprises procollagen, elastin, proteoglycans (PGs) hyaluronan (HA), forming a structural repair framework to bridge the wound and allow vascular ingrowth (Reinke & Sorg 2011).

In addition to their role in collagen proliferation, cytokines (e.g. TGF-β1) also stimulate the release of collagenase – intended to degrade the fine Type III collagen that helped form the provisional matrix (Slemp & Kirschner 2006).

At this point in the healing process a stronger matrix replaces the provisional one that was necessary to establish homeostasis. Fibroblasts stimulate Type I collagen proliferation as well as glycosaminoglycans (GAGs) and PGs forming a sturdier structural matrix – one that will better support day-to-day function.

If the wound is not too deep (i.e. has not damaged some or all of the nerve, muscle, lymph, hair and sebaceous glands), fresh capillary beds form thus constituting the hypervascularization seen in the early stages of wound healing. Increased vascularity assists the formation of granulation tissue that begins the process of restoring damaged tissue. Granulation tissue contains fibroblasts, which synthesize mucopolysaccharides and collagen fibers that are necessary for the development of new connective tissue.

This continues what began in Stage 1 – nutrition and waste exchange that accelerate collagen proliferation. Some effects from the inflammatory/ *reactive stage* may start to decrease; however, in some cases edema, elevated temperature around the wound and pain may still be present.

The alpha-smooth muscle actin within myofibroblasts (MFBs) becomes organized in filamentous bundles, called stress fibers, and the wound gap generally begins to decrease as MFBs contract and physically draw the severed tissue fragments together. Additionally, continued Type 1 collagen proliferation ensures the scar tissue becomes stronger. This stage typically lasts 4–21 days but may last for up to 6 weeks. Once the wound is closed, the immature scar can make the transition into the final maturation stage.

Clinical Consideration

During wound healing, continuous or cyclical loading (brief, light stretch or compression) of mechano-sensitive tissues stimulates resident fibroblasts to secrete collagenase (Tortora et al. 2007) reducing the potential of excess collagen formation (fibrosis and pathological cross-linking). Cyclical stretch and/ or compression – involving approximately 10% of available tissue elasticity – doubles collagenase production, whereas continuous stretching appears to be 50% less productive (Carano & Siciliani 1996, Langevin 2010).

Stage 4: Remodeling

In this stage, regression of capillary hypervascularity occurs, ensuring a return to normal vascular density and the wound continues to undergo contraction (mediated by MFBs), which contributes to the formation of a mechanically sound scar (Hinz et al. 2001, Hinz et al. 2012, Hinz 2013). Adequate amounts of TGF-β1 and mechanical tension (produced by MFBs) play an important role in assuring this stage culminates in the restoration of normal physiological (i.e. as close to pre-trauma) ECM and tissue architecture (Desmoulière et al. 2005). However, even physiological scars exhibit *slightly out of the ordinary* features (e.g. smaller Type I collagen than that seen in undamaged tissue and the fiber arrangement is less orderly or somewhat 'non-specific') (Bran et al. 2012, Profyris et al. 2012, Bordoni & Zanier 2014).

The increase in scar matrix strength can somewhat impact tissue elasticity; however, with healthy scars this will not result in pain or dysfunction. *Normal* scar tissue progresses from being weak and easily broken down, to being red and prominent, to finally becoming thin, pale and stable. The strength of the scar tissue increases gradually, and reaches a plateau about 7 weeks after wounding (Huang et al. 2013). As long as the scar appears redder than normal, remodeling is still under way.

If the wound is healing normally, this stage should be relatively painless and yield an innocuous scar that exhibits normal coloration, is relevant in size and mobile. There should be no significant degree of pain associated with a properly healing wound nor any residual pain experienced, once remodeling has completed. The remodeling stage can last from months to years (Bran et al. 2012, Profyris et al. 2012, Bordoni & Zanier 2014, Cho et al. 2014).

Clinical Consideration

Although the effect of massage on the remodeling stage of wound healing is unknown, it may shorten the time needed to form a healthy, mature scar (Cho et al. 2014).

Scar Chronology

The wound healing process begins at the time of the injury and may take up to 2 years to complete (Kania 2012). Subsequent chapters will cover how MT can assist in a long-term recovery plan for your client.

Scar chronology is broken down into immature and mature (Goel & Shrivastava 2010), with the identifiable presentations of each noted as follows:

Immature:

- <1 year old
- Thick and firm
- Elevated or raised in height
- Not easily pliable
- Red or pinkish in color
- Blanches with pressure.

Mature:

- >1 year old
- Soft
- Flat
- Pliable
- Displays normal vascularity (does not blanch).

Pathophysiological Scars

Pathophysiological scars are generally accepted to be the result of prolonged, aberrant wound healing that involves excessive fibroblast participation and collagen deposition (Huang et al. 2013) – see Figure 5.3. Regardless of etiology and size, pathophysiological scars will display characteristics that differ from normal skin, viscera and fascia in the following ways:

- Are thickened, dense

- Display textural variations (e.g. rough, lumpy, dimpled, puckered)

- Tend to exhibit compromised elasticity and mobility

- May display altered or abnormal neuro-functioning (hypersensitivity, hyposensitivity, increased electrical activity with movement) (Bordoni & Zanier 2014, Valouchová & Lewit 2009)

- Some mature scars may be pale due to limited blood supply or appear reddish due to hypervascularization that lasts beyond the 'normal' time frame (i.e. early stage of wound healing).

Types of Pathophysiological Scars

In order to assist with this next section, a few key terms are briefly described in Table 5.2.

The type of tissue damage and severity of the injury factor significantly in forming the proper protocol for long-term recovery

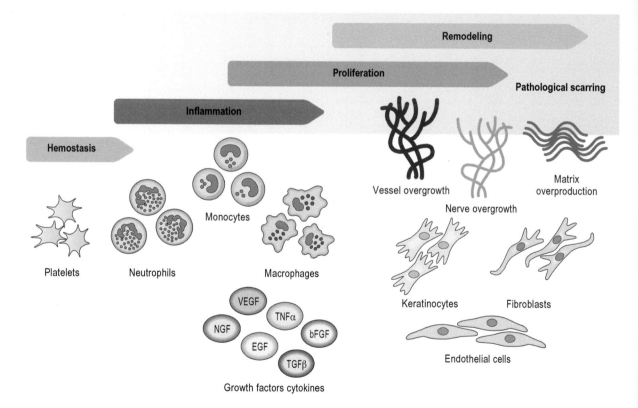

Figure 5.3

Adapted from Huang et al. (2013). Pathophysiological scar formation can begin in the inflammatory stage of wound healing and continue through the remodelling stage; characterized by prolonged and stronger inflammation stage with inappropriately released cytokines culminating in an aberrant healing response and abnormal scar.

and rehabilitation. Being able to identify the differences in the types of scar tissue will help to safely and effectively deliver care and develop more precise long-term protocols for clients.

Traumatic scars will be explored in greater detail in subsequent chapters where discussion will center around specifics on scarring from burns, surgery (e.g. mastectomy) and other types of traumatic events. Special consideration will be given to each type of scar presentation along with specific treatment protocols.

A few key terms and an overview of the various types of pathophysiological scars are briefly

Term	Definition and other information
Scar	Commonly used in reference to the 'normal' end product – describing a mark left in the skin, fascia, muscle (or other tissue) and organs as a result of healing of a wound, sore or injury
Adhesion	Commonly used to describe problematic areas of profuse or abnormal scarring occurring in organs and tissues. Adhesions can result in pain/dysfunction
Fibrosis	Replacement of the normal structural elements of tissue by excess accumulation of dysfunctional fibrotic tissue (Rodriguez & del Rio 2013). A process driven by excessive or sustained production of TGF-ß1 and consequent superfluous MFB activity (Smith et al. 2007, Karalaki et al. 2009, Fourie 2012). When used in reference to the myofascial/musculoskeletal system this term is commonly used to describe what occurs as a result of onerous tension or mechanical strain associated with poor remodeling following injury; culminating in superfluous, maladaptive, poorly constructed collagen (e.g. aberrant fiber/bundle arrangement, increased incidence of pathological cross-links and reduced elastic-malleability) (Henry & Garner 2003, Diegelmann & Evans 2004). It is a reasonable conclusion that prevention or resolution of fibrosis can diminish the occurrence of common sequelae and comorbidities
	Pathophysiological consideration It is reasonable to consider fascial tension/rigidity as an etiological factor in myofascial injuries and in pathophysiological scars (Gabbiani 2003, Solon et al. 2007, Grinell 2008, Chiquet et al. 2009, Hinz 2009, Heiderschelt et al. 2010, Rodriguiz & del Rio 2012). **Pathophysiological consideration** Fibrosis is commonly considered to be a by-product of an abnormal or chronic inflammatory response as a result of cumulative or overuse-type trauma, immobilization and **poor wound healing**. When not effectively managed, fibrosis can result in a milieu of functional deficits. The fall-out from fibrosis include the following and associated sequelae: increased risk of recurrent injury, muscle contraction dysfunction, altered force transmission, impaired tissue; slide/ glide and stretch, neural, circulatory and lymphatic compression, antalgia, pain and pain translation (i.e. shift from acute to chronic pain) (Simons, Travell & Simons 1999, Gabbiani 2003, Shah et al. 2005, 2008, Hinz 2007, Grinell 2008, Chiquet et al. 2009, Lowe 2009, Ciciliot & Schiaffino 2010). **Clinical consideration** Mechanical disruption of fibrotic tissue increases the pliability of scars (Bhadal et al. 2008, Chan et al. 2010, Cho et al. 2014).

Table 5.2

Important pathophysiological scar-related terms

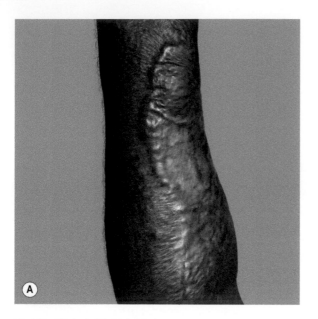
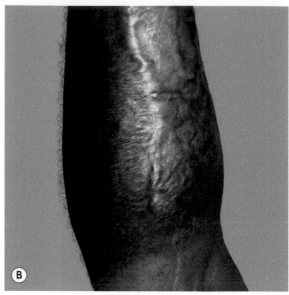

Figure 5.2

Keloid scar example.

described in Table 5.3. The various types of scars may occur individually or combined.

Pathophysiological Scar Formation – What can go Wrong

Multiple factors can contribute to impaired wound healing. To generalize, these factors can be categorized as local and systemic:

- Local: directly influence the characteristics of the wound itself, for example oxygenation, infection and the various aspects of the inflammatory cascade.

- Systemic: encompass the individual general state of health – in particular, factors which may affect his or her ability to heal. Some systemic factors include: genetic predisposition, age, stress levels, existing pathologies, neuro-inflammatory and neurogenic issues

(covered in greater detail in Chapter 4), medications, nutritional and lifestyle practices (e.g. sedentary tendencies, smoking and exposure to other pollutants). Research shows that smoking (nicotine) has a detrimental impact on all stages of wound healing resulting in delayed healing and a higher incidence of scar complications. Smoking cessation reverses some but not all of the mechanisms involved as many of the pathologic processes induced by smoking appear to be prolonged or even irreversible despite abstinence from smoking (Avery & Bailey 2008, Sorenson 2012).

Essentially the primary presentation seen with pathological scars is excessive collagen proliferation. Normally, the body stops collagen production when adequate strength of the scar is obtained. When collagen production does not shut down, pathological scars will form (Box 5.1).

Scar type/term	Description and other important information
Cicatric	Generalized term used to describe a scar left by the formation of new connective tissue over a healing sore or wound. This type of scar may have considerable contraction. It may be necessary to divide the scar and then graft on new skin, as is done for burns
Contracture	Common post-burn injury crossing joints or skin creases at right angles. Contractures are often disabling or result in dysfunction as they prevent or limit normal mobility. Contracture occurs before the scar fully matures and often presents as hypertrophic According to Klingler (2012): *... painful contractures resulting in limited/reduced range of motion are often associated with rigid collagenous tissue within and surrounding skeletal muscle, as well as other CTs involved in force transmission (e.g. retinaculae, thoracolumbar fascia, tendon).*
Hypertrophic scar	An elevated, excessive scar that is limited to the original boundaries of the incision or wound (Bordoni & Zanier 2014, Zhu et al. 2013). Common features include raised, thickened, red and sometimes ropelike scarring. Hypertrophic scars can lead to deformity, disfigurement and loss of function and can take weeks to form. Scars formed at the fringe of skin grafts are prone to hypertrophy (e.g. those associated with deep second-degree burns and other scars requiring grafts). Both hypertrophic and keloid scars occur more commonly in the regions of the anterior chest, shoulder/periscapular, lower abdomen and ear lobes (Ogawa 2008, Bordoni & Zanier 2014) (see Fig. 5.1)
Keloid scar	An abnormal scar that forms at the site of an injury or an incision and spreads beyond the borders of the original lesion. The scar is made up of a swirling mass of collagen fibers and fibroblasts. Keloid scars reach out like little fingers and extend well beyond the original injured area. Common features include thickened, raised, itchy clusters of scar tissue that grow beyond the edges of the wound or incision and are often red or darker in color than surrounding skin. Keloids occur when the body continues to produce the tough, fibrous collagen after a wound has healed. Keloids most commonly appear over the sternum, ears and shoulders and occur more in dark-skinned people. The tendency to develop keloid scars lessons with age. Some scars may start as hypertrophic and eventually develop into keloid (see Fig. 5.2)
Atrophic scar	Common presentation is a fibrotic, cutaneous depression displaying a sunken or pitted appearance (Weiss et al. 2010)
Widespread scar	Can appear when the fine lines of surgical scars gradually become stretched and widened. These typically flat, pale, soft, symptomless scars are more common following knee or shoulder surgery (Rudolph 1987). Stretch marks (abdominal striae) are variants of widespread scars involving injury to the dermis and subcutaneous tissues without breaching the epidermis. There is no elevation, thickening, or nodularity in mature widespread scars, which distinguishes them from hypertrophic scars (Bayat et al. 2003) **Clinical Consideration** As discussed previously; if tensional homeostasis can be achieved/restored, thereby mediating superfluous collagen proliferation, it seems plausible that the risk of pathophysiological scarring can be reduced

Table 5.3

Scar types and related terms

Box 5.1

Factors that drive excessive collagen proliferation

During the remodeling stage, premature or anomalous mechanical strain/tensional loading can exaggerate scar tissue formation (Akaishi et al. 2008, Wolfram et al. 2009, Bordoni & Zanier 2014).

Rubbing or friction, for example, due to a wound dressing or bandage being too tight, can also result in an over-stimulation of inflammatory response and subsequent pathological scar formation (Akaishi et al. 2008).

According to Bordoni & Zanier (2014) the direction of the lesion may also be a consideration as those that lie horizontal to a body segment (e.g. calf) induce three times greater tensional pull (i.e. mechanical strain) on the developing scar (Miyamoto et al. 2009). Although it seems plausible, it has not been confirmed whether lesion direction predisposes one to a higher incidence of pathophysiological scar formation or has an effect on the scar once the healing process has concluded.

Pathophysiological scars can perpetuate aberrant signaling (e.g. neuro-inflammatory and neurogenic signaling). This in turn can create a viscous cycle of persistent presence of pro-inflammatory and pain agents (e.g. substance P, calcitonin, cytokines and growth factors) further driving excessive/pathological scar formation.

Inflammatory mediated disruption in the balance of fibrin-forming and fibrin-dissolving capacities, favoring un-checked fibrin deposition (Chapelle & Bove 2013).

Breathing patterns, acidic pH and anxiety have also been identified as other potential contributing factors (Chaitow 2014).

CT and fascia's response to the internal (inflammatory mediators and growth factors) and external (mechanical strain) stresses applied will determine how the scar matures. The scar can become either dense and unyielding or pliable and mobile. Remodelling is not (necessarily) restricted to the injured area. Neighboring, non-injured tissue also changes its collagen production rate in response to inflammation.

Fourie 2012

Pathophysiological Consideration

In his exploration of the tendon sliding system, Guimberteau noted, at the FRC III 2012, that when – certain – tendons move, the movement is barely discernible in neighboring tissues if no restrictions are present (e.g. adhesions, fibrosis). According to Guimberteau, variances in non-injured tissue and tissue during and after scar formation can be seen endoscopically. Notably, with irregular or abnormal healing (even though the surface tissue looks normal) below the surface undifferentiated tissue can be present for several months (e.g. thick/dense and devoid of loose sliding tissue). Additionally, the hypervasculization typically seen in the early stages of normal healing will persist far longer with abnormal or irregular healing. When reconstructive hardware is used (e.g. screws, plates, and synthetic joint parts) normal scar formation does not occur.

Generally speaking, the greater the damage, the more extensive the scarring and the more extensive the abnormal scarring, greater is the potential for functional loss or abnormal functioning (e.g. dermal scars are less resistant to ultraviolet radiation, hair follicles do not grow back within scar tissue and extensive cardiac muscle scarring can lead to heart failure). Altered or abnormal healing increases the likelihood of excessive scarring (adherences), which in turn can impact the functioning of various tissues and systems.

Pathological scars in skin and fascia alter not only the structure and functioning of these tissues but also impacts the individual and their body's capacity to interact with his/her internal and external environment.

Prolonged Inflammation and Immobilization

Inflammatory response is our body's natural/normal process of repair following injury. If all goes well, undue damage does not typically occur and the event culminates in a positive resolution (e.g. tissue healing, normal repair/remodeling and recovery of pain-free function). However, the fall-out from excessive or prolonged inflammation and immobilization constitutes some of the most prevailing issues we may deal with in our practice.

Prolonged Inflammation

Inflammation will persist as long as debris is present at the wound site. Ineffective 'clean-up' during the inflammatory stage may prolong healing. Both bacteria and endotoxins can lead to the prolonged elevation of pro-inflammatory cytokines (e.g. interleukin-1 (IL-1)) extending this stage beyond its normal length of time. Consequently this can result in the wound transitioning into chronic state with failure to heal. In vitro evidence suggests that the presence of macrophages delays wound contraction, therefore the withdrawal of macrophages from the wound site may be essential for subsequent stages to occur in normal sequence and timing. Prolonged inflammation can lead to an increased level of matrix proteases (e.g. collagenase) that are known to degrade the ECM or conversely the excessive/prolonged presence of cytokines that stimulate excessive collagen production – resulting in pathophysiological scars (Edwards & Harding 2004, Menke et al. 2007).

Clinical Consideration

Drainage of excess fluid from interstitial spaces reduces the concentration of pro-inflammatory cytokines (Fryer & Fossum 2009).

Immobilization

The impact of immobilization or restricted movement can potentially complicate the healing process and health and well-being in general.

In immobilized tissue, cross-links form between the pre-existing or original collagen fibers as well as newly forming fibers. Pathological collagen cross-links can impact slide/glide potential between the tissue layers.

Immobilization diminishes the ability of the various ground substance (GS) hydrophilic compounds to up-take water, resulting in a higher concentration of particulate to solute (i.e. gel-like state of the GS). A reduction in hydration also impacts the distance between the collagen fibers. When collagen fibers are in closer proximity to one another and in a bath of more gel-like fluid, cross-links appear to form more readily (Fig. 5.4).

Clinical Consideration

Fascia hydrodynamically responds to mechanically applied strain (e.g. compression, stretch) via its sponge-like squeeze and refill mechanism in the bioarchitecture of hydrophilic compounds (e.g. GAGs and PGs). This suggests that some of the effects of manual therapy (e.g. changes in tissue pliability, decreased stiffness, ease of movement, changes in the state of under-hydrated tissues and reduced edema) can be attributed to changes in fluid concentration and content (Klingler et al. 2004).

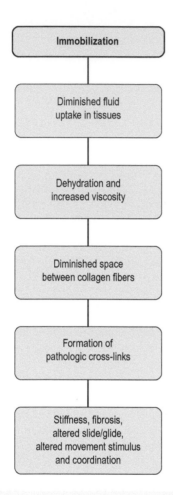

Figure 5.4

The fall-out associated with immobilization.

As noted by Barbe at the FRC III in 2012, immobilization may result in correlating grey matter shrinkage and subsequently there is a diminished or lost ability for movement stimulus and/or coordination. Nerve regions that were originally devoted to sensing, initiating and controlling movement lack activity/stimulation when the region is immobilized, resulting in re-allocation of these nerves to other functions and/or actual shrinkage of grey matter (Granert et al. 2011).

The Nervous System: Wound Healing And Pathophysiological Scars

As noted in Chapter 4, the NS plays an important role in wound healing. Noxious stimuli triggers the release of neuropeptides such as substance P and calcitonin gene-related peptide (CGRP) and certain growth factors such as NGF. Neuropeptides are released from nerve terminals and also are stimulated by cellular and chemical components involved in inflammation. (Lawman et al. 1985, Quinlan et al. 1998, Gibran et al. 2002, Muangman et al. 2004, Scott et al. 2007, Hanna & Katz 2011, Ogawa 2011, Chéret et al. 2013).

When all goes well, all is well, but multiple factors can contribute to impaired wound healing, including neural mediated ones.

Neuropeptides

Under physiological and pathophysiological conditions, neuropeptides released during wound healing modulate a number of important aspects of the process such as cell proliferation, cytokine and growth factor production, antigen presentation, mast cell degradation, increased vascular permeability and neovascularization (Lawman et al. 1985, Quinlan et al. 1998, Gibran et al. 2002, Muangman et al. 2004, Scott et al. 2007, Hanna & Katz 2011, Chéret et al. 2013).

Altered neuropeptide levels are implicated in pathophysiological scar formation, pruritus and chronic pain (Henderson et al. 2006, Scott et al. 2007, Almarestani et al. 2008, Cheng et al. 2011, Widgerow 2013, Xiao et al. 2013).

Substance P

During wound healing there is early release of substance P in the local milieu of the epidermis and ECM. In addition to its role in pain signaling, substance P is also known to induce inflammation and mediate angiogenesis, keratinocyte proliferation and fibrogenesis. Altered levels of substance P can instigate excessive inflammation and subsequent sequelae (Quinlan et al. 1998, Quinlan et al. 1999, Broome & Miyan 2000, Scott et al. 2007).

Substance P concentration has been found to be significantly greater in hypertrophic scars than in normal uninjured skin and the proliferative effect of substance P on fibroblasts is thought to contribute to keloid formation (Crowe et al. 1994, Scott et al. 2007, Jing et al. 2010).

When stimulated by substance P, mast cells in hypertrophic scars were found to release more histamine than those found in normal skin. Additionally, mast cells are capable of promoting proliferation of fibroblasts. Therefore mast cells are thought to play a role in fibroblast mediated hypertrophic scar formation and pruritus mediated by the release of excess histamine (Scott et al. 2007, Cheng et al. 2011, Widgerow 2013).

In addition to acute pain signaling, substance P is implicated in mediating certain chronic pain related symptoms, such as hyperalgesia and allodynia, seen with mature hypertrophic scars (Henderson et al. 2006, 2012).

Pathophysiological Consideration

According to Scott and colleagues (Scott et al. 2007), hypertrophic scars exhibit excessive neuropeptide activity. Altered substance P levels may contribute to impaired cutaneous healing responses associated with hypertrophic scar formation.

Pathophysiological Consideration

Neuroinflammation may play a role in the formation of hypertrophic scars, as a result of increased cellular proliferation, cytokine and growth factor stimulation and excess ECM deposition (Scott et al. 2007).

Pathophysiological Consideration

Neuropeptides have a direct fibroblastic effect and undue mechanical stretching of skin can lead to significant increase in neuropeptides (Scott et al. 2007, Cheng et al. 2011, Widgerow 2013).

CGRP

Pruritic hypertrophic scars show elevated levels of CGRP in comparison to normal skin (Crowe et al. 1994, Anderson et al. 2010). It is suggested that CGRP levels contribute to pain and pruritus during wound healing (Henderson et al. 2006, 2012).

CGRP is known to associate with nociceptive fibers and elevated levels are linked to sensory symptoms (e.g. itch and pain) associated with healing and chronic inflammation (Henderson et al. 2006, Almarestani et al. 2008, Hamed et al. 2011).

There is a significant increase in nerve fibers responsive to CGRP found in patients with chronic pain. This increase is observed both at the site of the scar and in distal/uninjured sites, suggesting a change occurs in the systemic response to injury in those with chronic pain. This supports that chronic pain is not a simple, local response but rather a systemic response that is aberrant (Hamed et al. 2011).

However, it is not yet clear how CGRP elevation could lead or contribute to chronic pain. Its presence is known but mechanism is still a mystery. One suggested possibility is that the increased density of CPRG responsive fibers leads to inappropriate cross-stimulation of fibers due to the close-packed proximity and that this leads to more central plasticity and subsequent chronic pain. What is evident is that reducing cutaneous CGRP concentrations and CGRP responsive fibers may play a role in the pathogenesis and the prevention of chronic pain associated with pathophysiological scars (Hamed et al. 2011).

Nerve growth factor (NGF)

The diverse biological effects of NGF include the process of wound repair and the development and survival of certain sympathetic and sensory neurons in both the central nervous system (CNS) and PNS. NGF is secreted and synthesized by a variety of cells, such as inflammatory and repair cells, including fibroblasts.

NGF plays a key role in the initiation and maintenance of inflammation in various organs. Thus it has been suggested that NGF is also involved in cutaneous wound repair. Exogenous NGF was shown to accelerate wound healing in normal and healing-impaired diabetic mice and to promote the healing of pressure ulcers in humans (Li et al. 1980, Lewin & Mendell 1993, Matsuda et al. 1998, Bernabei et al. 1999, Werner & Grose 2003).

Etiological considerations thought to underlie human hypertrophic scar formation include mechanical tension, nerve factors, inflammation, and foreign-body reactions. Undue mechanical tension appears to be the most significant causative factor. It is hypothesized that NGF is one of the mediators connecting mechanical tension with pathophysiological scarring (Ramos et al. 2008, Moore et al. 2009, Gabriel 2011, Schouten et al. 2012, Xiao 2013).

Mechanical tension stimulates mechanosensitive nociceptors and in turn, stimulated fibers induce the hyper-release of neuropeptides and NGF, even in the absence of mechanical tension, once the malignant cycle has begun.

Excess neuropeptides and NGF are implicated in the over-expression of repair material, constituting pathophysiological scar formation (Xiao et al. 2013).

Clinical Consideration

As noted above, undue mechanical tension is considered the most significant causative factor associated with pathophysiological scar formation. Therefore it is suggested that stabilizing a scar during formation via the control of mechanotransduction-mediated mechanical tension – involving MFBs – appears to be a primary target to prevent or reduce the incidence of pathophysiological scars. Additionally, sedation of exposed nerve endings and attenuation of neurogenic inflammation are also important scar management considerations, as well as proper wound dressings to prevent infection and maintain proper wound hydration. A multimodal approach to attenuating scar tensional stress and undue sensory stimulation will likely yield the best possible outcomes (Widgerow 2013).

Clinical Consideration

Careful application of massage therapy during the repair process can decrease undue tissue tension. A decrease in mechanical tension can attenuate tension-driven responses. In addition to the influence of mechanoreceptors on pain (via both ascending and descending pathways), mechanical stretching of fibroblasts can alter interstitial osmotic pressure as well as increase blood flow, thereby reducing concentrations of pro-inflammatory cytokines and reduce sensitization of peripheral nociceptors, by diluting the concentration of sensitizing agents (Fryer & Fossum 2009).

Nerve density in pathophysiological scars

During wound healing, scar tissue becomes both vascularized and innervated (Bove & Chapelle 2012). Under, over or aberrant innervation can potentially be problematic.

Example 1: as sensory nerves play a role in modulating immune response, denervated skin exhibits reduced leukocyte infiltration leading to impaired first line of defence, constituting a kind of *no one minding the store* predicament (Galkowska et al. 2006, Sibbald & Woo 2008).

Example 2: it is suggested that increased density of substance P and CGRP responsive fibers is associated with chronic pain and pruritus (Henderson et al. 2006, Scott et al. 2007, Almarestani et al. 2008, Cheng et al. 2011, Hamed et al. 2011, Widgerow 2013).

In healing wounds, it appears that regeneration of nerve fibers correlates with epithelialization during healing. Immediately following injury, the wound bed is devoid of nerves. Gradually, nerve fibers localize to the edges and later to the center of the wound beds. By 14 days post-injury, burn wounds display excessive numbers of nerve fibers (hyperinnervation) below the advancing epithelium. In normal wound healing, these numbers normalize with time and after 4 weeks, the distribution of nerve fibers in re-epithelialized areas is similar to that of normal skin (Dunnick et al 1996, Scott et al. 2007).

Innervation density is not the exclusive consideration in terms of restoration of normal neural responsiveness. It has been suggested that loss of sensory function in pathophysiological scars is not so much due to diminished re-innervation but more to do with aberrancies in nerve function within the scar or from changes in the perception of stimuli (e.g. sensitization and plasticity changes). It has also been suggested that a change in tissue structure (e.g. decrease in pliability in the tissues around, near or associated with the nerve) results in sensory deficits (Anderson et al. 2010).

Hypertrophic scars

Hypertrophy of a scar is accompanied by hypertrophy of noci-responsive nerves within the scar. Hypertrophic scars exhibiting a greater number of noci-responsive fibers, presented with more serious pathologies (Derderian et al. 2005).

Aberrations in the *re-innervation* of scars may either cause aberrant wound healing or neural hypertrophy may be a result of disturbed interplay in wound healing mechanisms such as excessive concentrations of NGF and undue mechanical tension, as noted previously (Zhang & Laato 2001, Xiao et al. 2013).

Pruritus associated with hypertrophic scars involves a complex interaction between the CNS, PNS and skin. Pruritus not only accompanies hypertrophic scars but is also thought to contribute to the development of hypertrophic scars.

In addition to itch being caused by histamine, neurokinin, tachykinins, bradykinin and neuropeptides, peripheral nerve damage may be central to the burn injury itch syndrome and may be a central component contributing to hypertrophic scar development. Various neuropeptides are released in response to injury activate mast cells, which release kinins, histamine and other agents, which in turn excite nociresponsive-fibers leading to exaggerated neurogenic inflammation. Fourteen days post-injury, a rebound increase in substance P responsive nerve fibers

is observed in pathophysiological scars. It is suggested that this exaggerated re-innervation is associated with pruritus and the development of hypertrophic scars. Therefore, attenuating pruritus not only alleviates patient discomfort but also may halt cellular/molecular processes that contribute to the development of pathophysiological scars (Scott et al. 2007, Xiao et al. 2013).

Keloid scars

Sensations of itch and pain are common in keloids. Itch occurs more frequently at the periphery of keloids whereas pain occurs more in the center.

As is the case with hypertrophic scars, histamine release by mast cells has been implicated in contributing to itch; however, antihistamines are shown to be largely ineffective. This suggests other factors may contribute to pruritogenesis. Sensory testing in symptomatic keloids show abnormal findings, suggesting the presence of small nerve fiber neuropathy possibly related to exaggerated neurogenic inflammation (Lee et al. 2004, Tey et al. 2012).

There appears to be no correlation between innervation density and intensity of itch or pain, suggesting that such sensations are not exclusively related to neuronal density, but that there are other factors at play (Tey et al. 2012).

Pruritic keloids tend to display a lower than normal epidermal neural density. Tey and co-workers suggest a possible hypothesis; chronic stimulation of itch-transmitting nerve fibers results in a self-regulated hypoplasia in an attempt to modulate the intensity and persistence of sensory input (neuroplasticity *pruning* at work) (Tey et al. 2012). Reduced nerve density in the epidermis, where itch-conducting fibers terminate, may therefore be a consequence of chronic pruritus. Although there is reduced neural density in the epidermis, neuronal density is shown to be elevated in the dermis. Fibers appear longer and thinner, possibly due to compression from thickened or dense collagen fibers and the extensive deposition of ECM in deeper tissue. An alternate hypothesis suggests that the compressive effect in the keloidal dermis may contribute to the reduced epidermal nerve density (Hochman et al. 2008, Tey et al. 2012). According to Bove, regenerating nerves cannot push through dense fibrous tissue.

Clinical Consideration

In the treatment of pathophysiological scars, the focus inevitably shifts from ensuring survival to the inclusion of quality of life considerations such as improved aesthetic and functional aspects of the scar. An aspect of wound healing that has not been investigated as extensively as others is the restoration of sensory function and the consequences of changes in neuroanatomy and function. There is strong evidence for local and systemic sensory function deficits, such as

Clinical Consideration (Cont.)

pruritus, paresthesia and a high incidence of chronic pain in pathophysiological scars (Hamed et al. 2011). These considerations warrant due diligence. In addition to sensory protection provided by proper wound bandaging in the early stages of healing, successful management of pathophysiological scars ought to include manual therapy measures aimed at sensory disturbance prevention and attenuation of mechano-receptor stimulation.

Mechanotransduction: Wound Healing and Pathophysiological Scars

Like the nervous system, the mechanotransduction pathway is an important cell communication system that plays a role in wound healing and pathophysiological scar formation. The mechanophysiological conditions of injured tissue greatly influence the degree of scar formation, scar contracture, and pathophysiological scar progression/generation (e.g. keloids and hypertrophic scars) (Ogawa 2011).

Mechano-biology involves the multiple interactions among cells, the ECM, and cytokines. Cell surface integrins interface with both extracellular and intracellular scaffolding proteins. Alterations in the mechanical environment can therefore be immediately sensed by the cell and converted into a biochemical signal that can be conveyed throughout the broader expanse of the biotensegrity system (Ingber 1997, Garg et al. 2012).

The interrelated mechanosensory functions of ion channels, integrins, and scaffolding proteins play a role in complex signaling cascades initiated by alterations in the mechanical environment, including alterations seen during wound healing (Ingber 1997, Wynn 2004, Ogawa 2011, Garg et al. 2012).

It is well established that undue mechanical forces on a wound impairs healing and is considered by many the most significant factor in pathophysiological scar formation (Krammer et al. 1999, Yu & Stamenkovic 2000, Yano et al. 2004, Distler et al. 2006, Reichelt 2007, Akaishi et al. 2008, Ogawa 2008, 2011, Chin et al. 2009, Cheng et al. 2011, Wong et al. 2011, Garg et al. 2012, Widgerow 2013).

As noted in Chapter 2, MFBs play an important role in; inflammation, remodeling, excess scarring and fibrosis. MFBs mediate wound closure/contraction – covered in greater detail in Chapter 5. During wound healing the differentiation of fibroblasts into MFBs occurs in the wound by day 5. If the wound contraction cycle is repeated intermittently and sufficient times, subsequent consequences can include excess scarring and fibrotic conditions (Akaishi et al. 2008; Garg et al. 2012).

Ravi et al. (2012) found that when traction (mechanical tension) was applied along the edges of an incision in a mouse model, the wound recapitulated nearly all the features of human hypertrophic scars. Conversely, stress-shielding of high tension wounds resulted in a decrease in pro-fibrotic TGFβ1 signaling, diminished cellular and vascular density, reduced scarring and restoration of near normal skin architecture. This supports that wounds under elevated stress develop increased fibrosis and mechanical forces alone could significantly alter wound characteristics (Gurtner et al. 2011; Garg et al. 2012).

The common view is that keloids and hypertrophic scars arise from the dermis and therefore it is theorized that modulating mechanical forces on the dermis could reduce the risk of pathophysiological scar formation after surgery (Akaishi et al. 2010; Ogawa et al. 2012). The work of Guimberteau supports that aberrant scar presentations occur below the skin as well, implying that mechanical force tension in deeper tissues should also be considered.

An improved understanding of how mechano sensory pathways influence remodeling and how manual methods can influence mechanosensory pathways will likely yield improved wound healing outcomes.

Clinical Consideration

Off-loading wound tension, and resultant responses via the mechanotransduction pathway, can mitigate hypertrophic scarring and promote healthy tissue regeneration (Garg et al. 2012). The extent to which mechanotransduction effects can be influenced by manual methods remains speculative. However, there is evidence that alteration of local tissue tension can influence post-traumatic healing via mechanotransduction-mediated changes in collagenase and TGFβ1 production (Langevin 2006, Tortora et al. 2007, Wipff & Hinz 2009, Chaitow 2014).

Clinical Consideration

Mechanical forces such as stretching tension, shear force, compression, hydrostatic pressure and osmotic pressure can be perceived by two general classes of receptors: sensory nerve receptors and receptors associated with the mechanotransduction signaling system; such as integrins and mechanosensitive ion channel and cytoskeleton receptors (Ogawa 2011). Therefore clinical approaches aimed at attenuating mechanical forces and influencing such receptors ought to propel better outcomes in the prevention and treatment of scars.

Degrees, Severity and Extent of Traumatic Scars

The depth, severity, extent of the injury/trauma all factor significantly in the designing of safe and effective treatment protocols. Pre-existing health issues can impair wound healing. Issues such as diabetes, immune suppressing conditions, heart disease and liver or kidney issues should be considered when evaluating scar management protocol.

The normal sequencing of the stages of wound healing, the time taken to full maturation and the quality of the end product (i.e. scar) depend on several factors (Kania 2012):

- Depth of damage
- Area of damage
- Amount of tissue loss
- Previous medical condition(s)

- Genetic factors.

With burn trauma in particular, there are four standard measurements of wound depth thereby giving the healthcare professional a better understanding of muscles, tendons, ligaments, nerves and a host of other considerations that may have been involved in the injury. The four measurements, expressed in degrees, are covered in greater detail in Chapter 6. As burn trauma often impacts larger surface areas, Chapter 6 will also discuss area of damage and amount of tissue loss considerations in greater detail.

NP/CM	Impact	Outcome
Substance P	Elevated levels linked to excessive inflammation and subsequent sequelae; including fibroblasts proliferation and increased histamine release by mast cells	Increased incidence of: • pathophysiological scars • pruritus and other sensory disturbances (e.g. hyperalgesia and allodynia) • heightened pain sensation
CGRP	Elevated levels linked to sensory symptoms associated with wound healing and chronic inflammation	Increased incidence of: • pruritus • heightened pain sensation • pain translation/development of chronic/persistent pain
NGF	Altered levels linked to disruption of normal wound healing processes	Adverse impact on: • neuron development/survival • inflammatory processes Increased incidence of: • pathophysiological scars • aberrant re-innervation/nerve density
Various NPs, histamine and kinins	Elevated levels linked to exaggeration of neurogenic inflammation, increased receptor hypersensitivity and aberrant re-innervation; including, density aberrancies and increased concentration of receptors sensitive to certain stimulants, such as Substance P and CGRP, that drive various outcomes	Increased incidence of: • pathophysiological scars • pruritus and other sensory disturbances • pain translation/development of chronic/persistent pain • small nerve fiber neuropathy

Table 5.4

Role of neuropeptides (NP) and other chemical mediators (CM) in pathophysiological scars and associated sequelae

References

Akaishi S, Ogawa R, Hyakusoku H (2008) Keloid and hypertrophic scar: neurogenic inflammation hypotheses. Medical Hypotheses 71: 32–8.

Akaishi S, Ogawa R, Hyakusoku H (2010). Visual and pathologic analyses of keloid growth patterns. Annals of Plastic Surgery 64(1): 80–82.

Almarestani L, Longo G, Ribeiro-da-Silva A (2008) Autonomic fiber sprouting in the skin in chronic inflammation. Molecular Pain 4(1): 56.

Anderson JR, Zorbas JS, Phillips JK, Harrison JL, Dawson LF, Bolt SE, Fear MW (2010) Systemic decreases in cutaneous innervation after burn injury. Journal of Investigative Dermatology 130:1948–1951; doi:10.1038/jid.2010.47.

Avery NC, Bailey AJ (2008) Restraining cross-links responsible for the mechanical properties of collagen fibers: natural and artificial. In Fratzl P Collagen Structure and Mechanics, pp 81–110. New York: Springer.

Barbe M (2012) Changes in fascia related to repetitive motion disorders – Opening Keynote. Lecture notes from The 3rd International Fascia Research Congress, Vancouver March 28–30 2012.

Bayat A. McGrouther DA, Ferguson MWJ (2003) Skin scarring. British Medical Journal 326 (7380): 88.

Bernabei R, Landi F, Bonini S et al (1999) Effect of topical application of nerve-growth factor on pressure ulcers. Lancet 354: 307.

Bhadal N, Wall IB, Porter SR, et al (2008) The effect of mechanical strain on protease production by keratinocytes. British Journal of Dermatology 158(2): 396–8.

Bond JS, Duncan JA, Mason T et al (2008) Scar redness in humans: how long does it persist after incisional and excisional wounding? Plastic and Reconstructive Surgery 121(2): 487–496.

Bordoni B, Zanier E (2014) Skin, fascias, and scars: symptoms and systemic connections. Journal of Multidisciplinary Healthcare 7: 11.

Bouffard NA, Cutroneo KR, Badger GJ et al (2008) Tissue stretch decreases soluble TGF-β and type I procollagen in mouse subcutaneous connective tissue: Evidence from ex vivo and in vivo models. Journal of Cellular Physiology 214: 389–395.

Bove GM, Chapelle SL (2012) Visceral mobilization can lyse and prevent peritoneal adhesions in a rat model. Journal of Bodywork and Movement Therapies 16(1): 76–82.

Bran GM, Brom J, Hormann K, Stuck BA (2012) Auricular keloids: combined therapy with a new pressure device. Archives of Facial Plastic Surgery 14(1): 20–26.

Broome CS, Miyan JA (2000) Neuropeptide control of bone marrow neutrophil production. A key axis for neuroimmunomodulation. Annals of the New York Academy of Sciences 917: 424–34.

Carano A, Siciliani G (1996) Effects of continuous and intermittent forces on human fibroblasts in vitro. European Journal of Orthodontics 18(1): 19–26.

Chaitow L (2014) Fascial dysfunction – manual therapy approaches. Pencaitland, UK: Handspring Publishing.

Chan MW, Hinz B, McCulloch CA (2010) Mechanical induction of gene expression in connective tissue cells. Methods in Cell Biology 98: 178–205.

Chapelle SL & Bove GM (2013) Visceral massage reduces postoperative ileus in a rat model. Journal of Bodywork and Movement Therapies 17(1): 83–88.

Cheng B, Liu H-W, Fu X-B (2011) Update on pruritic mechanisms of hypertrophic scars in postburn patients: the potential role of opioids and their receptors. Journal of Burn Care and Research 32: e118–e125.

Chéret J, Lebonvallet N, Carré JL et al (2013).Role of neuropeptides, neurotrophins, and neurohormones in skin wound healing. Wound Repair and Regeneration 21(6): 772–788.

Cherkin DC, Sherman KJ, Kahn J et al (2011) A comparison of the effects of 2 types of massage and usual care on chronic low back pain: a randomized, controlled trial. Annals of Internal Medicine 155(1): 1–9.

Chin MS, Lancerotto L, Helm DL et al (2009) Analysis of neuropeptides in stretched skin. Plastic and Reconstructive Surgery 124: 102–113.

Chiquet M, Gelman L, Lutz R, Maier S (2009) From mechanotransduction to extracellular matrix gene expression in fibroblasts. Biochimica et Biophysica Acta 1793(5): 911–920.

Cho YS, Jeon JH, Hong A et al (2014) The effect of burn rehabilitation massage therapy on hypertrophic scar after burn: a randomized controlled trial. Burns 40(8): 1513–1520.

Ciciliot S, Schiaffino S (2010) Regeneration of mammalian skeletal muscle. Basic mechanisms and clinical implications. Current Pharmaceutical Design 16(8): 906–914.

Crowe R, Parkhouse N, McGrouther D et al (1994) Neuropeptide-containing nerves in painful hypertrophic human scar tissue. British Journal of Dermatology; 130: 444–452.

DeNoon DJ (2005) Need Pain Relief? Massage gets high marks. Available at: http://www.webmd.com/pain-management/news/20051026/need-pain-relief-massage-gets-high-marks [Accessed 1 June 2014].

Derderian CA, Bastidas N, Lerman OZ et al (2005) Mechanical strain alters gene expression in an in vitro model of hypertrophic scarring. Annals of Plastic Surgery 55(1): 69–75.

Desmouliere A, Chaponnier C, Gabbiani G (2005) Tissue repair, contraction, and the myofibroblast. Wound Repair and Regeneration 13(1): 7–12.

Diegelmann R F, Evans MC. (2004). Wound healing: an overview of acute, fibrotic and delayed healing. Frontiers in Bioscience 9(1): 283–289.

Distler JH, Jungel A, Caretto D et al (2006) Monocyte chemoattractant protein 1 released from glycosaminoglycans mediates its profibrotic effects in systemic sclerosis via the release of interleukin-4 from T cells. Arthritis and Rheumatology 54(1): 214–25.

Dunnick CA, Gibran NS, Heimbach DM (1996) Substance P has a role in neurogenic mediation of human burn wound healing. Journal of Burn Care and Rehabilitation 17: 390–6.

Edwards R, Harding KG (2004). Bacteria and wound healing. Current Opinion in Infectious Diseases 17: 91–96.

Finnson KW, McLean S, Di Guglielmo GM, Philip A (2013) Dynamics of transforming growth factor beta signaling in wound healing and scarring. Advances in Wound Care 2(5): 195–214.

Fitch P (2005) Scars of life. Journal of Soft Tissue Manipulation. 12(4): 3–6.

Fourie W (2008) Lymphatic scarring and secondary lymphoedema post breast cancer treatment. Text of invited presentation given at the British Lymphology Society Annual Conference. Belfast, October.

Fourie W (2009) The fascia lata of the thigh – more than a 'stocking': a magnetic resonance imaging, ultrasonography and dissection study. In: Fascia research II: Basic science and implications for conventional and complementary health care. Munich: Elsevier Urban and Fischer.

Fourie W (2012) Surgery and scarring. In: Schleip R et al (eds) Fascia: the tensional network of the human body. Ch 7.17, pp 411–420. Edinburgh: Churchill Livingstone Elsevier.

Fryer G, Fossum C (2009) Therapeutic mechanisms underlying muscle energy approaches. Physical therapy for tension type and cervicogenic headache: physical examination, muscle and joint management. Boston: Jones and Bartlett.

Gabbiani G (2003) The myofibroblast in wound healing and fibrocontractive diseases. Journal of Pathology 200: 500–503.

Gabriel V (2011) Hypertrophic scar. Physical Medicine and Rehabilitation Clinics of North America 22(2): 301–310.

Galkowska H, Olszewski WL, Wojewodzka U et al (2006) Neurogenic factors in the impaired healing of diabetic foot ulcers. Journal of Surgical Research 134: 252–258.

Garg RK, Wong VW, Gurtner, GC (2012) Of mice and men. Mechanical signaling and scar formation across species. Journal of Wound Technology. Jan, 15: 24–25.

Gauglitz GG, Korting HC, Pavicic T et al (2011) Hypertrophic scarring and keloids: pathomechanisms and current and emerging treatment strategies. Molecular Medicine 17(1–2): 113.

Gibran NS, Jang YC, Isik FF et al (2002) Diminished neuropeptide levels contribute to the impaired cutaneous healing response associated with diabetes mellitus. Journal of Surgical Research 108: 122–8.

Goel A, Shrivastava P (2010) Post-burn scars and scar contractures. Indian Journal of Plastic Surgery: official publication of the Association of Plastic Surgeons of India 43(Suppl): S63.

Granert O, Peller M, Gaser C et al (2011) Manual activity shapes structure and function in contralateral human motor hand area. Neuroimage 54(1): 32–41.

Graven-Nielsen T, Mense S (2001) The peripheral apparatus of muscle pain: evidence from animal and human studies. The Clinical Journal of Pain 17(1): 2–10.

Grinnell F 2008 Fibroblast mechanics in three-dimensional collagen matrices. Journal of Bodywork and Movement Therapies 12(3): 191–193.

Guimberteau (2012) Scars and Adhesion Panel. Lecture notes from The 3rd International Fascia Research Congress, Vancouver, 28–30 March.

Guo S, DiPietro LA (2010). Factors affecting wound healing. Journal of Dental Research 89(3): 219–229.

Gurtner GC, Dauskardt RH, Wong VW et al (2011) Improving cutaneous scar formation by controlling the mechanical environment: large animal and phase I studies. Annals of Surgery 254(2): 217–225.

Hamed K, Giles N, Anderson J et al (2011) Changes in cutaneous innervation in patients with chronic pain after burns. Burns 37(4): 631–637.

Hanna KR, Katz AJ (2011) An update on wound healing and the nervous system. Annals of Plastic Surgery 67: 49–52.

Heiderscheit B, Sherry M, Silder A, et al (2010) Hamstring strain injuries: recommendations for diagnosis, rehabilitation and injury prevention. Journal of Orthopaedic and Sports Physical Therapy 40(2): 67–81.

Henderson J, Terenghi G, McGrouther DA, Ferguson MW (2006) The reinnervation pattern of wounds and scars may explain their sensory symptoms. Journal of Plastic Reconstructive and Aesthetic Surgery 59(9): 942–50.

Henderson J, Ferguson MW, Terenghi G (2012). The feeling of healing. Plastic and Reconstructive Surgery 129 (1): 223e–224e.

Henry G, Garner, WL (2003) Inflammatory mediators in wound healing. Surgical Clinics of North America 83: 483–507.

Hinz B (2007) Formation and function of the myofibroblast during tissue repair. Journal of Investigative Dermatology 127: 526–537.

Hinz, B (2009) Tissue stiffness, latent TGF-beta1 activation, and mechanical signal transduction: implications for the pathogenesis and treatment of fibrosis. Current Rheumatology Reports 11(2): 120–126.

Hinz B, Celetta G, Tomasek JJ et al (2001) Alpha-smooth muscle actin expression upregulates fibroblast contractile activity. Molecular Biology of the Cell 12: 2730–41.

Hinz B, Phan SH, Thannickal VJ et al (2012) Recent developments in myofibroblast biology: paradigms for connective tissue remodeling. American Journal of Pathology 180 (4): 1340–1355.

Hinz B (2013) It has to be the [alpha] v: myofibroblast integrins activate latent TGF-[beta] 1. Nature Medicine 19(12): 1567–1568.

Hochman B, Nahas FX, Sobral CS et al (2008) Nerve fibres: a possible role in keloid pathogenesis. British Journal of Dermatology 158: 651–652.

Huang C, Murphy GF, Akaish S, Ogawa R (2013) Keloids and hypertrophic scars: update and future directions. Plastic and Reconstructive Surgery Global Open 1(4).

Ingber DE (1997) Tensegrity: the architectural basis of cellular mechanotransduction. Annual Review of Physiology 59(1): 575–599.

Jing C, Jia-Han W, Hong-Xing Z (2010) Double-edged effects of neuropeptide substance P on repair of cutaneous trauma. Wound Repair Regeneration 18: 319–324.

Josenhans E (2007) Physiotherapeutic treatment for axillary cord formation following breast cancer surgery. ZVK Science Prize.

Kania A (2012) Scars. In: Dryden T, Moyer C (eds) Massage therapy: Integrating research and practice. Human Kinetics Ch 15, pp 173–184.

Karalaki M, Fili S, Philippou, A, Koutsilieris, M. (2009). Muscle regeneration: cellular and molecular events. In vivo, 23(5): 779–796.

Klingler W, Jurkat-Rott K, Lehmann-Horn F, Schleip R (2012) The role of fibrosis in Duchenne muscular dystrophy. Acta Myologica 31(3): 184–95.

Klingler W, Schleip R, Zorn A (2004) European Fascia Research Project Report. 5th World Congress Low Back and Pelvic Pain, Melbourne.

Kobesova A et al (2007) Twenty-year-old pathogenic 'active' postsurgical scar: a case study of a patient with persistent right lower quadrant pain. Journal of Manipulative and Physiological Therapeutics 30(3): 234–238.

Krammer A, Lu H, Isralewitz B et al (1999) Forced unfolding of the fibronectin type III module reveals a tensile molecular recognition switch. Proceedings of the National Academy of Sciences in USA Feb 16; 96(4): 1351–6.

Langevin HM (2006) Connective tissue: a body-wide signaling network? Med Hypotheses 66: 1074–1077.

Langevin H (2010) Presentation: Ultrasound Imaging of Connective Tissue Pathology Associated with Chronic Low Back Pain. 7th Interdisciplinary Congress on Low Back and Pelvic Pain, Los Angeles.

Lawman MJ, Boyle MD, Gee AP, Young M (1985) Nerve growth factor accelerates the early cellular events associated with wound healing. Experimental and Molecular Pathology 43(2): 274–281.

Lee SS, Yosipovitch G, Chan YH, Goh CL (2004) Pruritus, pain, and small nerve fiber function in keloids: a controlled study. Journal of the American Academy of Dermatology 51: 1002–1006.

Lewin GR, Mendell LM. (1993) Nerve growth factor and nociception. Trends in Neuroscience 16: 353–359.

Li AK, Koroly MJ, Schattenkerk ME et al (1980) Nerve growth factor: acceleration of the rate of wound healing in mice. Proceedings of the National Academy of Sciences in USA 77: 4379–81.

Lowe JC (2009) Factors that induce fibrosis of fascial tissues. [accessed April 10, 2009 from HYPERLINK "http://www.drlowe.com" www.drlowe.com.]

Marieb EN (2003) Human anatomy and physiology, 5th edn. Redwood City, CA: Benjamin Cummings Publishing, 5.

Matsuda H, Koyama H, Sato H et al (1998) Role of nerve growth factor in cutaneous wound healing: accelerating effects in normal and healing-impaired diabetic mice. Journal of Experimental Medicine 187: 297–306.

Menke NB, Ward KR, Witten TM et al (2007). Impaired wound healing. Clinics in Dermatology 25: 19–25.

Meyer-ter-Vehn T, Han H, Grehn F, Schlunck G (2011) Extracellular matrix elasticity modulates TGF-β–induced p38 activation and myofibroblast transdifferentiation in human tenon fibroblasts. Investigative Ophthalmology and Visual Science 52(12): 9149–9155.

Miyamoto J, Nagasao T, Miyamoto S et al (2009) Biomechanical analysis of stresses occurring in vertical and transverse scars on the lower leg. Plastic Reconstructive Surgery 124(6): 1974–1979.

Moore ML, Dewey WS, Richard RL (2009) Rehabilitation of the burned hand. Hand Clinics 25(4): 529–541.

Muangman P, Muffley LA, Anthony JP et al (2004) Nerve growth factor accelerates wound healing in diabetic mice. Wound Repair and Regeneration 12: 44–52.

Ogawa R (2008) Keloid and hypertrophic scarring may result from a mechanoreceptor or mechanosensitive nociceptor disorder. Medical Hypotheses 71(4): 493–500.

Ogawa R (2011) Mechanobiology of scarring. Wound Repair and Regeneration 19(s1), s2–s9.

Ogawa R, Okai K, Tokumura F, Mori K et al (2012). The relationship between skin stretching/contraction and pathologic scarring: the important role of mechanical forces in keloid generation. Wound Repair and Regeneration, 20(2): 149–157.

Profyris C, Tziotzios C, DoVale I (2012) Cutaneous scarring: pathophysiology, molecular mechanisms, and scar reduction therapeutics Part I. The molecular basis of scar formation. Journal of the American Academy of Dermatology 66: 1–10.

Quinlan KL, Song IS, Bunnett NW et al (1998) Neuropeptide regulation of human dermal microvascular endothelial cell ICAM-1 expression and function. American Journal of Physiology 275: C1580–90.

Quinlan KL, Naik SM, Cannon G et al. (1999) Substance P activates coincident NF-AT- and NF-kappa B-dependent adhesion molecule gene expression in microvascular endothelial cells through intracellular calcium mobilization. Journal of Immunology 163(10): 5656–65.

Ramos ML, Gragnani A, Ferreira LM (2008) Is there an ideal animal model to study hypertrophic scarring? Journal of Burn Care and Research 29(2): 363–368.

Reichelt J (2007) Mechanotransduction of keratinocytes in culture and in the epidermis. European Journal of Cell Biology 86 (11-12): 807–16.

Reinke JM, Sorg H (2011) Wound repair and regeneration. European surgical research. Europaische chirurgische Forschung. Recherches Chirurgicales Europeennes 49(1): 35–43.

Rodríguez RM, del Río FG (2013) Mechanistic basis of manual therapy in myofascial injuries. Sonoelastographic evolution control. Journal of Bodywork and Movement Therapies 17(2): 221–234.

Sarrazy V, Billet F, Micallef L et al (2011) Mechanisms of pathological scarring: role of myofibroblasts and current developments. Wound Repair and Regeneration 19(s1), s10–s15.

Schleip R, Klingler W, Lehmann-Horn F (2005) Active fascial contractility: fascia may be able to contract in a smooth muscle-like manner and thereby influence musculoskeletal dynamics. Medical Hypotheses 65(2): 273–277.

Schouten HJ, Nieuwenhuis MK, van Zuijlen PP (2012) A review on static splinting therapy to prevent burn scar contracture: do clinical and experimental data warrant its clinical application? Burns 38(1): 19–25.

Scott JR, Muangman P, Gibran NS (2007) Making sense of hypertrophic scar: a role for nerves. Wound Repair and Regeneration (Suppl. 1): S27–31.

Shah JP, Danoff JV, Deshai MJ et al (2008) Biochemicals associated with pain and inflammation are elevated in sites near to, and remote from active myofascial trigger points. Archives of Physical Medicine and Rehabilitation 89: 16–23.

Shah J, Phillips T, Danoff J et al (2005) An in vivo microanalytical technique for measuring the local biochemical milieu of human skeletal muscle. Journal of Applied Physiology 99: 1977–1984.

Sibbald RG, Woo KY (2008) The biology of chronic foot ulcers in persons with diabetes. Diabetes Metabolism Research Reviews 24 (Suppl 1): 25–30.

Simons DG, Travell JG, Simons LS (1999). Travell & Simons' Myofascial Pain and Dysfunction: Upper Half of Body (Vol 1). Philadelphia:Lippincott Williams & Wilkins.

Slemp AE, Kirschner RE (2006) Keloids and scars: a review of keloids and scars, their pathogenesis, risk factors, and management. Current Opinions in Pediatrics 18(4): 396–402.

Smith CA, Stauber F, Waters C et al (2007). Transforming growth factor-ß following skeletal muscle strain injury in rats. Journal of Applied Physiology, 102(2): 755–761.

Solon J, Levental L, Sengupt K, Georges P, (2007) Fibroblast adaptation and stiffness matching to soft. Elastic Substrates 93 (12): 4453–4461.

Sorensen LT (2012) Wound healing and infection in surgery: the pathophysiological impact of smoking, smoking cessation, and nicotine replacement therapy: a systematic review. Annals of Surgery 255(6): 1069–1079.

Tey HL, Maddison B, Wang H et al (2012) Cutaneous innervation and itch in keloids. Acta Dermato-Venereologica 92(5): 529–531.

Tortora GJ, Funke BR, Case CL (2007) Introduction to Microbiology. San Francisco: Pearson Benjamin Cummings.

Tredget EE, Nedelec B, Scott PG, Ghahary A (1997) Hypertrophic scars, keloids, and contractures. The cellular and molecular basis for therapy. Surgical Clinics of North America 77(3): 701–730.

Valouchová P, Lewit K (2009) Surface electromyography of abdominal and back muscles in patients with active scars. Journal of Bodywork and Movement Therapies 13(3): 262–267.

Werner R (2012) Scar tissue: when a solution becomes a problem. Massage & Body Work Magazine (July/August).

Werner S, Grose R (2003) Regulation of wound healing by growth factors and cytokines. Physiological reviews 83(3): 835–870.

Widgerow AD (2013) Hypertrophic burn scar evolution and management: review. Wound Healing Southern Africa 6(2): 79–86.

Williams PE, Goldspink G (1984) Connective tissue changes in immobilised muscle. Journal of Anatomy 138(Pt 2): 343.

Wipff PJ, Hinz B (2009) Myofibroblasts work best under stress. Journal of Bodywork and Movement Therapies 13: 121–127.

Wolfram D, Tzankov A, Pülzl P, Piza-Katzer H (2009) Hypertrophic scars and keloids—a review of their pathophysiology, risk factors, and therapeutic management. Dermatologic Surgery 35(2): 171–181.

Wong VW, Akaishi S, Longaker MT, Gurtner GC (2011) Pushing back: wound mechanotransduction in repair and regeneration. Journal of Investigative Dermatology 131: 2186–2196.

Wynn TA (2004) Fibrotic disease and the T(H)1/T(H)2 paradigm. Nature Reviews Immunology 4(8): 583–594.

Xiao H, Wang D, Huo R et al (2013). Mechanical tension promotes skin nerve regeneration by upregulating nerve growth factor expression. Neural Regeneration Research 8(17): 1576.

Yano S, Komine M, Fujimoto M et al (2004) Mechanical stretching in vitro regulates signal transduction pathways and cellular proliferation in human epidermal keratinocytes. Journal of Investigative Dermatology 122: 783–790.

Yu Q, Stamenkovic I (2000) Cell surface-localized matrix metalloproteinase-9 proteolytically activates TGF-b and promotes tumor invasion and angiogenesis. Genes & Development14: 163.

Zhang LQ, Laato M (2001) Innervation of normal and hypertrophic human scars and experimental wounds in the rat. Ann Chir Gynaecol 90(Suppl 215): 29–32.

Zhu Z, Ding J, Shankowsky HA, Tredget EE (2013) The molecular mechanism of hypertrophic scar. Journal of Cell Communication and Signaling 7(4): 239–252.

Resource and Further Reading

The Wound Healing Society: http://woundheal.org/

Burns, mastectomies and other traumatic scars

Someone who has experienced trauma has gifts to offer all of us – in their depth, their knowledge of our universal vulnerability, and their experience of the power of compassion.

Sharon Salzberg (2015)

Burns, mastectomies and other traumatic injuries can involve significant penetration of the skin layers, sometimes penetrating deeper layers of tissue down to bone. Extensive tissue damage due to trauma (planned or unplanned) can compromise sensation, proprioception, circulation, lymphatic drainage, thermoregulation and dermal excretory capacities (Fitch 2005).

As discussed in previous chapters, scar tissue can affect the body in a variety of ways. Fibrotic scars and scars that are bound to the underlying tissues, organs or skeletal structures can restrict movement and organ motility (Fitch 2005, Bove & Chapelle 2012). In addition to physical disability and dysfunction, traumatic scars can also result in a spectrum of psychosocial sequelae, which will be covered in greater detail in Chapter 7.

The depth and extent of the scar strongly influence the consequent sequelae. Extensive tissue damage requires additional recovery time and increases the potential for complications, including excessive scarring and successive surgeries (Kania 2012).

The aim of this chapter is to provide more in-depth understanding of the types of pathophysiological scars and scars seen in conjunction with specific types of trauma.

Excessive Scarring

Excessive scarring was first described in the Smith papyrus around 1700 BC (Berman & Bieley 1995). A few millennia later, Mancini & Quaife (1962) and Peacock et al. (1970) differentiated excessive scarring into hypertrophic and keloid scar formation and defined their distinguishing characteristics: both scar types rise above skin level, but while hypertrophic scars do not extend beyond the initial site of injury, keloids typically project beyond the original wound margins (Gauglitz et al. 2011).

Excessive or pathophysiological scars form as a result of prolongations or aberrations of physiologic wound healing and may develop following any injury to the deep dermis, including burn injury, lacerations, abrasions, surgery, piercings and vaccinations. Wound healing in pathophysiological scars is characterized by a prolonged and stronger inflammation phase with inappropriately released cytokines followed by a subsequent delay in the healing response (Huang et al. 2013). Excessive scarring resulting in pain, pruritus, adherences and contractures can affect quality of life, physically, physiologically and psychologically (Gauglitz et al. 2011). Scar depth can have a negative impact on the healing process and, subsequently, impact the functions of the dermal layer and deeper layers of tissue (e.g. muscle, fascia).

Each year in industrialized nations, 100 million people develop scars as a result of 55 million elective operations and 25 million operations due to trauma (Gauglitz et al. 2011). From 55% to 100% of surgical patients will experience post-surgical scar/adhesion complications that may not become evident until months or years later (Diamond 2012).

Although there is extensive research on the pathophysiologic process of wound healing and scar formation, there is still no consensus on the best treatment strategy for preventing and reducing the issues associated with pathophysiological scars (Van der Veer et al. 2009, Cho et al. 2014).

A Deeper Look at Hypertrophic and Keloid Scars

Chapter 5 provided a brief overview of the various types of pathophysiological scars and how scars form. To further the understanding of the healing process and the impact of traumatic scars, this next section will provide a more in-depth look at hypertrophic and keloid scars – see Table. 6.1 for a comparative summary of hypertrophic and keloid scars.

Wound healing is an intricate biological process involving overlapping phases. When this process is disrupted or altered, abnormalities in scarring appear. Both hypertrophic and keloid scars are a result of disruption in the fundamental processes of wound healing. Race, age, genetic predisposition, hormone levels, atopy/hypersensitivity and immunologic responses, type of injury, wound size/depth, anatomic region, and local mechanical tension all factor into wound healing process and subsequent nature of the scar (Niessen et al. 1999, Cho et al. 2014).

Multiple studies on hypertrophic and keloid scar formation have been conducted over several decades, leading to many therapeutic strategies to prevent or attenuate excessive scar formation. Most therapeutic approaches remain clinically unsatisfactory, however, with an agreement that there is a meager understanding of the complex mechanisms underlying the processes of scarring and wound contraction and fibroproliferative disorders in general (Gauglitz et al. 2011, Rabello et al. 2014).

Scar pathogenesis involves cellular and extracellular matrix (ECM) components in both the epidermal and dermal layers that are regulated by a wide array of interfering factors in the inflammation, proliferation, and remodeling stages of healing (Huang et al. 2013).

Hypertrophic scarring after deep or partial-thickness wounds is common. A review of the literature on the prevalence of hypertrophic scarring found that females, children, young adults, and people with darker, more pigmented skin are particularly at risk and, in this subpopulation, the prevalence is up to 75% (Engrav et al. 2007). Hypertrophic scars are morphologically characterized by (Linares 1996, Cho et al. 2014):

• Abnormal collagen

• Reduced elastin

- Persistent cellularity
- Alterations in proteoglycan composition and amount

- Prolonged inflammatory reaction resulting in persistent hypervascularity and excess deposition of ground matrix.

Feature	Hypertrophic scar (HS)	Keloid scar (KS)	Both
Demographic prevalence		Pigmented skin	Age 10–30, rare in elderly
Regional prevalence	Across areas of high stress/tension (e.g. joints)	Anterior chest, shoulders, earlobes, upper arms and cheeks	
Risk factors	Common complication following burn injury, bacterial colonization and wound infection		
Etiology/ pathophysiology	Increased, altered phenotype, fibroblasts, which exhibit a higher expression of TGF-β1 than normal fibroblasts Increased or prolonged TGF-β1 activity Increased MFBs – contributing to increased ECM/collagen synthesis and tissue contraction MFBs in HSs are less sensitive to apoptotic signals, which can prolong collagen deposition and result in fibrosis Acidic mucopolysaccharides Alterations in PG composition and amount Persistent hypervascularity Persistent &/or hypercellularity Usually develops within 1–3 months following trauma or infection Rapid growth phase for up to 6 months, tend to spontaneously regress Will eventually enter the final stage of wound healing	Increased infiltration of immune cells – supporting KS formation is driven by T cell-keratinocyte/ fibroblast interactions Possibly increased/excessive MFBs May develop anywhere from a year up to several years after minor injuries and may even form spontaneously on the mid-chest in the absence of any known injury More sustained and aggressive than HSs Do not regress spontaneously, tend to reoccur following excision Failure to enter the final stage of wound healing	Persistent/pathological wound-healing signals or improper regulation of wound healing cells Prolonged inflammatory response Overproduction of fibroblast proteins Overabundant collagen deposition resulting in ECM, dermal and epidermal fibrosis. Failed release of collagenase in proper amount/ timing contributes to lower degradation of and excessive proliferation/deposition of collagen Aberrant epidermal regulation of dermal remodeling – epidermal keratinocytes intercommunicate with underlying fibroblasts, this intercommunication plays an important role in pathophysiological scar formation – keratinocytes induce fibroblasts to secrete CT growth factor, a cofactor/ downstream mediator of TGF-β driven fibrosis Aberrant activation of keratinocytes prolongs epidermal inflammation leading to abnormal epidermal interactions, suggesting that fibroblast mediated collagen production is not adequately regulated by keratinocytes – leading to excess collagen deposition

Table 6.1 (Continued)

Feature	Hypertrophic scar (HS)	Keloid scar (KS)	Both
Histopathological characteristics	Abnormal/overabundant ECM/collagen, primarily, larger than usual Type III collagen with abundant whorl-like nodules containing MFBs, reduced elastin Flattened epidermis Expanded dermis comprises flatter and less clearly demarcated, loosely arrayed wavy collagen bundles that are somewhat fragmented and shortened and display prominent vertically oriented blood vessels	Thick/hyalinized ('*keloidal collagen'), irregularly branched, disorganized Type I and III collagen bundles without nodules. Non-flattened epidermis. Randomly oriented collagen swirls and whorls that vary in length Numerous, thickened fibrocollagenous fascicles Horizontal fibrous bands in the upper reticular dermis and the presence of prominent fascia-like bands	Increased a-smooth muscle actin (a-SMA) More fibronectin than in normal skin Randomly oriented excessive collagen fibers Expanded dermis
Clinical presentation	Hard, usually linear, slightly-raised scar with well demarcated epidermal borders (do not extend beyond the general geographic wound margins) Appears red or pink in color Commonly pruritic	Firm, mildly tender, bosselated & more raised than HSs, with a shiny surface & occasional telangiectasia, infiltrates the surrounding tissue, well demarcated, irregular borders Thinned epithelium is prone to ulceration, hyperpigmentation and discoloration (pink/purple – initially erythematous, turning brownish, may pale as the scar ages) Scar margins tend to exhibit considerable peripheral tension whereas center of the scar less so Can cause significant pain and hyperesthesia	Raised above skin surface Discoloration Pain, pruritus, adherences and contractures can affect quality of life: physically, physiologically and psychologically Disfigurements present biopsychosocial considerations

*Keloidal collagen is not always detectable in KSs.

Table 6.1

Comparison of scars (Ogawa 2008, Bordoni & Zanier 2013, Bordoni & Zanier 2013, Zhu et al. 2013, Rabello et al. 2014)

Hypertrophic scarring can result in disfigurement and scarring that affects quality of life which, in turn, can lead to lowered self-esteem, social isolation, prejudicial societal reactions and job discrimination. Scarring also has profound rehabilitation consequences, including loss of function, impairment, disability, and difficulties pursuing recreational and vocational pursuits (Engrav et al. 2007).

Bacterial colonization and wound infection tend to promote the formation of hypertrophic scars (Niessen et al. 2004, Chan et al. 2005, Baker et al. 2007, Berman et al. 2007, Cho et al. 2014). Hypertrophic scarring usually develops within 1–3 months following wound infection, wound closure with excess tension or other traumatic skin injury (Brissett & Sherris 2001, Cho et al. 2014). Hypertrophic scarring exhibits a rapid growth phase for up to 6 months, and then gradually regresses over a period of a few years.

Keloids seem to be a more sustained and aggressive fibrotic disorder than hypertrophic scars (Brown & Bayat 2009). Research to date strongly suggests a more prolonged inflammatory period, with immune cell infiltrate present with keloids (Slemp & Kirschner 2006).

Precise etiologic factors associated with keloid formation are elusive. Keloids may develop anywhere from a year up to several years after minor injuries and may even form spontaneously on the mid-chest in the absence of any known injury (Brissett & Sherris 2001, Cho et al. 2014). Keloids are persistent and do not regress spontaneously.

Keloids appear as firm, mildly tender, bosselated (small knob-like projections) tumors with a shiny surface and sometimes telangiectasia (small, widened blood vessels on the skin which are usually meaningless, but may be associated with several diseases) (NIH 2015). The epithelium is thinned and there may be focal areas of ulceration.

Keloids are typically pink to purple in color and may be accompanied by hyperpigmentation. The borders of the keloid are well demarcated but irregular in outline. A hypertrophic scar has a similar appearance but is usually linear, if following a surgical scar, or papular or nodular if following inflammatory and ulcerating lesions. Both lesions are commonly pruritic, but keloids may be the source of significant pain and hyperesthesia (excessive physical sensitivity, especially of the skin) (Gauglitz et al. 2011).

In most cases, hypertrophic scarring develops in wounds at anatomic locations with high tension (joints), such as shoulders, neck, knees and ankles, whereas anterior chest, shoulders, earlobes, upper arms and cheeks have a higher predilection for keloid formation. Eyelids, cornea, palms, mucous membranes, genitalia and soles are generally less affected. Keloids tend to recur following excision, whereas new hypertrophic scar formation is rare after excision of the original hypertrophic scar (Gauglitz et al. 2011).

Histologically, both hypertrophic and keloid scars contain an overabundance of dermal collagen. Hypertrophic scars comprise primarily Type III collagen that lie parallel to the epidermal surface with abundant nodules containing myofibroblasts (MFBs), large extracellular collagen filaments and plentiful (acidic) mucopolysaccharides (Slemp & Kirschner 2006). Keloid tissue, in comparison, primarily comprises disorganized Type I and III collagen, containing hypocellular collagen bundles with no nodules or excess MFBs (Slemp & Kirschner 2006).

Both scar types overproduce multiple fibroblast proteins, including fibronectin, suggesting either pathological determination of wound healing signals or a failure of the appropriate regulation of wound-healing cells (Gauglitz et al. 2011, Chapelle & Bove 2013).

Pathophysiological Consideration

According to Bove and Chapelle (2012):

Inflammation caused by peritoneal trauma (any etiology) leads to a disruption of the balance between the fibrin-forming and fibrin-dissolving capacities of the peritoneum, favoring the deposition of a fibrin-rich exudate on the damaged area. If the fibrin is not resolved by the fibrinolytic system within days, adhesions form. Persistent adhesions can prevent the normal sliding of the viscera during peristalsis and movements of the body, such as respiration.

Clinical Consideration

The margins of keloid scars tend to pull outward (i.e. exhibit considerable peripheral tension) whereas the center of the scar is subjected to milder tension (Akaishi et al. 2008, Ogawa et al. 2011) Therefore, massage therapy (MT) treatment along the peripheral margins may be most helpful in terms of attenuating tissue tension.

Burns

A burn injury to the skin or other organic tissue is primarily caused by heat or due to radiation, radioactivity, electricity, friction or contact with chemicals. Skin injuries due to ultraviolet radiation and respiratory damage resulting from smoke inhalation are also considered to be burns.

Burn trauma is a worldwide public health problem. In 2004 nearly 11 million people were burned severely enough to require medical attention (WHO 2015).

Every year in the USA alone, approximately 9000 individuals experience burns that cover 20% or more of their total body surface area (TBSA). Non-fatal burn injuries leaves millions inflicted with lifelong disabilities and disfigurements. Additionally, burns are among the leading causes of disability-adjusted life-years (DALYs).

The degree of injury factors into subsequent complications, sequelae and treatment protocol. Treatment protocol will be covered in greater detail in Chapter 9.

Degree of Injury

Burn injuries are categorized as first degree, second degree, third degree and fourth degree, ranging from superficial to deep and involving part or all of the dermis (see Fig. 6.1). Even minor burns can result in complications (e.g. infection, dehydration).

First Degree

First degree trauma is limited to the epidermis. This type of injury to the first layer of skin rarely shows blistering or charring of skin. The first degree wound often heals in 3–7 days. The best example of a first degree burn injury is a sunburn or minor scald.

Second Degree

Second degree trauma is characterized as either superficial or deep. Tissue damage/destruction impacts the epidermis and may extend into the dermis (a.k.a. 'partial-thickness' injury or trauma).

In order to grasp the gravity of partial-thickness burn injuries one only need to consider the expanse and importance of the dermis. Considered the 'workhorse' of the integumentary system, the dermis constitutes an estimated 90% of the skin's thickness. An important fluid reservoir, it is estimated that the dermis comprises 80% water.

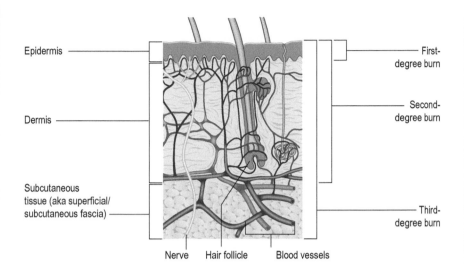

Epidermis

Dermis

Subcutaneous
tissue (aka superficial/
subcutaneous fascia)

Nerve   Hair follicle   Blood vessels

First-
degree burn

Second-
degree burn

Third-
degree burn

Figure 6.1

Depth of burn trauma
and structures
impacted.

Dermal water plays an important role in maintaining the physical properties of the skin (e.g. moisturizing and elasticity) (Nakagawa et al. 2010). Specialized cells in the dermis assist with regulating temperature and fighting infection. The dermis also houses vessels that supply blood and nutrients to the skin. Damage to the sweat glands, sebaceous glands, hair follicles, nerve receptors, blood vessels, lymph nodes/vessels, muscle and connective tissue may occur.

Partial-thickness burn injuries can be extremely painful, are often accompanied by blistering and edema/swelling, and may require debridement (removal of lacerated, weaken, debilitated or contaminated tissue) or skin grafting (transplanted tissue). Depending on the type of skin graft needed, the donor site may lose the epidermis and part or all of the dermis.

Third Degree

Third degree trauma involves destruction of all epidermal and dermal layers and is commonly referred to as a 'full-thickness' injury. Damage extends below hair follicles and sweat glands, into the subcutaneous tissue (i.e. connective tissue (CT) layer that is seeded with adipocytes).

With full-thickness trauma, there may be extensive edema and skin characteristics can change dramatically (e.g. charred, leathery appearance). Third degree injuries are usually not painful because of the destruction of nerve endings. Skin grafting or other replacement options are often required.

Fourth Degree

Fourth degree trauma involves destruction of epidermis, dermis, subcutaneous tissue, ligaments, tendons, nerves, blood vessels, possibly down to the level of bone. Fourth degree trauma often leads to amputation and significant functional impairment. Skin grafting and multistage reconstructive procedures are necessary.

Sequelae and Complications

A critical burn injury is a unique trauma that often is accompanied by significant metabolic disturbances as well as a change in the normal state of innate and adaptive immunity (Shankar et al. 2007). Human skin acts as a blockade against environmental insults and against colonization of pathogenic microbes, and is also an immune organ with significant surveillance and thermoregulatory functions. This knowledge helps us to understand that the loss of large portions of skin as the result of burns results in impaired immunity, metabolic compromises, fluid shifts, and heat loss (Shankar et al. 2007).

Burn injuries can cause severe muscle loss, muscle weakness, contractures, and traumatic scars, leading to lifelong physical impairments (Diego et al. 2013). Severe burns may require the removal of the dermal layer and subsequent skin graft procedure(s) (Ganio et al. 2013).

Burn injury sequelae can occur as a result of scarring associated with the burn trauma or graft proceedures.

Traumatic Scars

Hypertrophic scarring is the most common type of scar tissue formed after a burn injury. Hypertrophic scars are formed in 30–72% of burn survivors after injury. In addition to the above noted risk factors, hypertrophic scar development associated with burn injuries is mainly influenced by wound healing time (delayed 3 weeks or more), the depth (degree of injury), extent (size/surface area affected) and if multiple surgical or graft procedures are performed (Deitch et al. 1983, Cubison et al. 2006, Thompson et al. 2013, Cho et al. 2014). Unfortunately, most of the published information on post-burn scarring does not accurately define these factors and the body's whirlpool of physiological responses to burn injury continue to be studied and researched (Spurr & Shakespeare 1990, Bombaro et al. 2003, Cho et al. 2014).

What do we know? Fibroblasts play a key role in wound healing and scar formation as they:

- Actively release cytokines

- Stimulate ECM formation

- Regulate collagen synthesis and degradation.

A higher incidence of hypertrophic scarring may occur after injuries that affect the deeper layers of the dermis, which contains a larger number of reticular fibroblasts (Honardoust et al. 2012). Compared with the superficial layer of the skin, deep dermal fibroblasts demonstrate different cellular and molecular properties that influence their function during wound healing. As an example, deep dermal fibroblasts show a higher expression of transforming growth factor beta-1 (TGF-β1), CT growth factor, heat shock protein 47, α-SMA, and Type I collagen when compared with cells from superficial layers. Combined, these factors contribute to the increase in collagen synthesis, proliferation of denser collagen and greater contractile capabilities characteristic of hypertrophic scars.

Pathophysiological Consideration

Apoptosis (programmed cellular death) facilitates the decrease in cellularity (fibroblasts, MFBs and vascular cells) during the transition between granulation tissue and scar formation, suggesting a mechanism for granulation tissue evolution into the next stage of normal scar formation during wound healing (Honardoust et al. 2012). Interruption of apoptosis, resulting in the persistence of fibroblasts in the granulation tissue, has been linked to fibrotic conditions and pathological scar formation – as noted above, fibroblasts synthesize collagen and ECM. Decorin, a small leucine-rich proteoglycan, has been shown to influence apoptosis. Although not yet fully understood, it is known that decorin functions as a guardian in the context of constraining the activity of multiple growth factors and ECM components (e.g. TGFβ-1, collagen) (Neill et al. 2012).

Clinical Consideration

It has been identified that mechanical forces can induce changes in the expression of ECM proteins and proteases. In a study by Kanazawa et al. (2009), it was revealed that uniaxial, cyclical stretching of skin fibroblasts resulted in down-regulation of agents known to stimulate persistent collagen proliferation associated with fibrosis and abnormal scarring. In another in vitro model, human hypertrophic scar samples responded to mechanical loading by inducing apoptosis (Derderian et al. 2005). Although the exact mechanism remains to be determined, it is hypothesized that massage can impact cellular structural and signaling milieu, thereby inducing beneficial effects through the ability to affect fibroblast apoptosis and remodeling (Bhadal et al. 2008, Chan et al. 2010, Cho et al. 2014).

Clinical Consideration

Hypertrophy typically persists for 6–12 months and tends to regress over a period of 18–24 months (Oliveria et al. 2005). Pruritus is more likely to occur during active hypertrophy (i.e. early stages of maturation). It is prudent that the evolution of hypertrophic scars – whether the burn scar is in the early or late states of maturation – inform treatment protocol. Additionally, staging will impact short and long-term outcomes (Cho et al. 2014).

Clinical Consideration

MT may be a viable modality for attenuating post-burn hypertrophic scar pain, pruritus and scar characteristics such as thickness, melanin deposition, erythema, transdermal water loss and elasticity/tissue mobility (Cho et al. 2014).

Skin Grafts

As previously noted, the integument provides a protective barrier from external insults including trauma, radiation, harsh environmental conditions and infection. Our skin also serves an important aesthetic role. When damaged, restoration of an intact and functioning barrier is of utmost importance physiologically and psychologically.

Skin graft procedures are performed as a means of barrier and aesthetic restoration. Full-thickness skin grafts (FTSG) include the entire thickness of the dermis. While split-thickness skin grafts (STSG) include the epidermis and only a portion of the dermis.

Wound condition, location, thickness, size and aesthetic concerns are considerations in determining which procedure is appropriate (Ratner 1998).

STSGs serve a much broader range of application including resurfacing large wounds, mucosal deficits and muscle flaps, lining cavities and closing flap donor sites. STSGs are more fragile than FTSGs, typically not able to withstand radiation therapy, prone to mal-pigmentation in darker skinned individuals and can contract significantly during healing. Thinness, abnormal pigmentation, lack of hair growth and inconsistent texture render STSGs less aesthetic. Although both FTSG and STSG donor sites necessitate a second wound, the STSG donor site must re-epithelialize, often resulting in significant discomfort and posing a higher risk of infection (Ratner 1998).

Thermoregulation

Thermoregulation (through sweating, vasoconstriction or vasodilatation) and control of fluid loss are also essential functions performed by our skin. Although STSGs help restore a functional barrier, the blood vessels and sweat glands necessary for temperature regulation remain damaged.

When an individual is exposed to heat stress, cutaneous vasodilation and sweating in well-healed grafted skin is severely impaired compared with adjacent non-damaged skin. Likewise, grafted skin does not vasodilate or sweat appropriately upon exogenous administration of local vasodilators and sudorific drugs (i.e. sodium nitroprusside and acetylcholine), suggesting postsynaptic impairments, which are not resolved 4–8 years post-surgery (Lu & Fuchs 2014). These impairments in grafted skin become barriers to whole-body heat dissipation, especially when grafted skin represents a significant proportion of TBSA.

During physical activity, increases in metabolic heat production that are not properly compensated for by adequate heat loss responses (e.g. skin vasodilation and sweating) can lead to dangerous increases in core body temperature. Therefore, the ability of individuals with STSGs to safely participate in physical activity may be limited by their capacity to dissipate heat, especially when physical activity is performed in warm/hot temperature environments (Ganio et al. 2013).

Blood Flow

The control of skin blood flow occurs through two sympathetic neural pathways; one involves a sympathetic vasoconstrictor system and the other pathway modulates the skin blood flow through a non-adrenergic sympathetic active vasodilator system.

Interestingly, grafted skin is shown to preserve its vasoconstrictor ability. A study conducted on split-thickness grafted skin 5–9 months post-surgery showed that when exposed to cold stress (cold temperatures, high or cold wind, dampness and cold water) the grafted skin

demonstrated indicators of re-innervation and restoration of autonomic control of the cutaneous vasoconstrictor pathways. The same study showed that there were, however, impairments in cutaneous vasodilation and sweating during heat stress when compared to that of healthy, uninjured skin (Crandall & Davis 2010).

Increased skin blood flow and sweating are critical responses to correctly regulate internal temperature during exercise and/or hyperthermic exposure. The data indicates that diminished sweating responses in grafted skin are due to an absence of functional sweat glands. Weakened abilities to dissipate heat via cutaneous vasodilation and sweating from grafted skin do not recover for up to 4–8 years after graft surgery, raising the possibility that individuals with a significant amount of body surface area of grafted skin are at an increased risk of a heat-related injury. On the other hand, preserved vasoconstrictor responses to both indirect whole-body cooling and local cooling, regardless of graft maturity, suggest sustained capability to regulate internal temperature via cutaneous vasoconstriction during cold exposure (Crandall et al. 2009).

Inflammation and Edema

The inflammatory response in a critical burn injury is often unstable due to the global involvement of multiple tissue beds and their constituent immune and non-immune cells, placing significant metabolic and energy requirements on the repair process; for example, the extent of inflammation and energy requirements is directly proportional to the severity of injury sustained by the patient (Shankar et al. 2007).

The spectrum of inflammation runs from a mild elevation in cytokines associated with inflammation that largely go unnoticed clinically to a system-wide severe inflammatory response that eventually leads to microcirculatory failure of capillaries supplying individual vital organs, acute respiratory syndrome, severe coagulopathy, and the development of multiple organ failure sometimes seen in the initial treatment of a burn injury.

Exaggerated inflammation in burn injury wounds, which healed after 21 days, had a high rate of hypertrophic scarring formation (Tredget 2008). Edema, which occurs after a significant burn, is assumed to be a non-reversible process (Demling 2005).

Lymphatic Flow

As noted in Chapter 3, lymph is composed of interstitial fluid, which is collected from the tissues and taken up by the lymphatic system. The rate of lymph flow from burn-injured tissue directly correlates with the amount of fluid crossing the capillary membrane into the interstitial space during the edema process. The fluid is protein-rich, as evidenced by the high content of lymph albumin and globulin relative to the plasma protein value. The continued increase in lymph flow for more than 36 hours after burn injury indicates that the increased capillary permeability to protein persists for several days (Shankar et al. 2007).

Lymph flow rate and lymph protein content have been used frequently to monitor microvascular fluid filtration rate and protein permeability characteristics. Lymph flow rate reflects the degree of either fluid fluctuation or transport across the capillary at any given moment, as the lymph channels open very close to the capillary interstitium.

Several researchers have used various lymph preparations for the study of burn edema. The concentration of large molecules in lymph, such as protein or dextrans, has been used to determine the permeability characteristics of the microcirculation. Because lymph is derived from interstitial fluid, various vasoactive substances released from the burn may appear in high concentration in the regional lymph areas that are injured (Demling 2005).

Lymph flow appears to be a valid means of accurately monitoring partial-thickness burns, or non-burned tissue, where capillaries and lymphatics remain intact.

With deeper burns, capillary or microvascular occlusion decreases the perfusion (delivery of blood) to the burn tissue. Therefore, less fluid is likely to enter the interstitium and local lymphatics. In addition, subsequent lymphatic damage decreases the efficiency of the lymphatic network.

The concentration of larger molecules in the lymph fluid, such as proteins, has been used to study the permeability of microcirculation. The microcirculation is highly responsive to, and a vital participant in, the inflammatory response. Because a burn patient receives high volumes of fluid in the early stages of injury, the measured lymph flow rate in deep burns is likely to underestimate the actual degree of injury and the actual edema formation in deeper burns (Demling 2005).

Neuropathic Pain and Pruritus

As noted in Chapter 4, neuropathic pain is defined as pain initiated or caused by a primary lesion or dysfunction in the peripheral or central nervous system. Neuropathic-like pain symptoms consisting of a 'pins and needles', burning, stabbing, shooting or electric sensation is a common occurrence in burn injuries after the open wound has healed (Schneider et al. 2006). Researchers have documented neuropathy in up to 29% of patients with burn injuries.

Neuropathy is a common complication of a severe burn injury in the older survivor, the critically ill, an injury caused by electricity, or in those with a history of alcohol abuse. Peripheral neuropathy is a well-known disabling complication after major burn injury.

Determining why this occurs proves difficult due to the complex metabolic nature of burn trauma; the high incidence of sepsis; the use of neurotoxic antibiotics and potential iatrogenic (inadvertent medically induced) causes of neuropathy. However, some studies have shown the presence of neuropathy correlates with the TBSA that has been injured, the percentage of full-thickness burn and other severe illnesses (Kowalske & Holavanahalli 2001).

Pruritus

In addition to pain, burn trauma can also result in pruritus (itching) as a result of the burn trauma or as part of the wound healing process. As well as itching, scars have also been reported to exhibit burning and crawling sensations (Crandall et al. 2009).

Pruritus during wound healing is typically a short-lived, non-invasive presentation that decreases in frequency and intensity as the scar forms. However, with some pathophysiological scars, pruritus can be persistent and present as 'unbearable'.

In a Texas study (Ganio et al. 2013), 87% of post-burn patients reported daily episodes of pruritus. Fifty-two per cent reported experiencing itch for up to 30 minutes, some experiencing a single episode while others experiencing multiple episodes daily.

Management is particularly challenging due to elusive etiology. The exact mechanism and pathophysiology remain unclear and therefore effective treatment strategies are difficult to establish. Patel and Yosipovitch (2010) cite that there is no universally accepted treatment protocol for pruritus and management is to be tailored based on an individualistic approach.

Recent findings suggest that itching associated with inflammatory dermatosis can be reduced by antihistamines (Cheng et al. 2011). However, antihistamines are not effective for all presentations of pruritus associated with hypertrophic scars in post-burn patients. Opioid receptors in skin – when activated – can also provoke itching (Cheng et al. 2011).

Persistent or frequently intense bouts of pruritus can impact quality of life as disturbances in sleep, concentration and social interactions can occur (Yosipovitch et al. 2000, 2002a, 2002b).

Clinical Consideration

Burn rehabilitation MT has been shown to be effective in improving pain, pruritus, depression and scar characteristics in hypertrophic scars in post-burn patients (Roh et al. 2007, Cho et al. 2014).

Clinical Consideration

Skin rolling manipulations (targeting the adherences between the skin and superficial fascia (SF) can be a productive technique for addressing undue post-surgical scarring and scarring associated with burns (Kobesova et al. 2007).

Breast Cancer

The breast is made up of fatty, connective and lymphatic tissues. Breast cancer begins in the lobules (glands for milk production) and the ducts that connect to the lobules to the nipple.

According to the Canadian Cancer Society (CCS), breast cancer rates in women rose through the early 1990s and then decreased in the early 2000s. It is suggested that the increase related to improved detection and the increased use of hormone replacement therapy (HRT) during the preceding decades. HRT has been linked to increased breast cancer risk in post-menopausal women and it appears that the decrease in the early 2000s coincided with a large drop in the use of HRT when the risk relationship was publicized (CCS 2014).

According to Schmitz and colleagues (2012) in 2010, 1.5 million people were diagnosed with breast cancer worldwide.

Sequelae and Complications

Advances in diagnostic and treatment approaches have resulted in improved survival rates. It is estimated that there are 2.5 million breast cancer survivors alive in the US, and millions more worldwide (American Cancer Society 2010, Rosedale & Fu 2010, Schmitz et al. 2012).

While survival is obviously desirable, sequelae and complications are not. In addtion to the impact of the cancer itself, curative treatment approaches such as surgery (mastectomy), radiotherapy and chemotherapy, can also be the source of ongoing pain and dysfunction.

> *The incidence and prevalence of persistent adverse effects and the extent to which women's lives remain affected by breast cancer treatment is poorly understood.*
>
> (Schmitz et al. 2012)

According to Schmitz and colleagues, at 6 years post-diagnosis more than 60% of women experienced one or more side-effects amenable to rehabilitative intervention (Schmitz et al. 2012). For example:

- Postsurgical issues: infection, axillary web syndrome/cording, seroma, hematoma

- Skin/tissue reaction to radiotherapy: burns

- Upper body symptoms and functional issues: lymphedema, swelling, pain, numbness, tingling, muscle weakness, stiffness and range of movement (ROM) issues

- Fatigue.

Side-effects were reported to be 'severe to extreme, a bit to very much'.

Box 6.1

Early detection

Breast cancer is typically detected during a screening examination, prior to symptoms developing or after symptoms have established, including when a lump is found. Most masses discovered by a mammogram and most breast lumps are benign (non-cancerous).

As is the case with most cancers, early detection can factor significantly into prognosis and survival rate. Prognosis and survival considerations include: disease stage, lymph node status, hormone receptor status, tumor type, size and grade, degree of lymph and vascular invasion, age, recurrence and metastasis.

Many countries around the world provide screening programs as a means of early detection in women between the ages of 50–69 and for other identified risk groups (e.g. familial history, gene mutations – *BRCA1* or 2, history of breast cancer or atypical hyperplasia, dense breast tissue and history of regional radiation treatment).

Screening can include: mammography starting at a younger age; more frequent mammography; ultrasound; MRI; clinical breast exams. Additionally, the value of self-examination cannot be emphasized enough as many individuals are the first to notice changes in the look and feel of their own breasts.

Since the mid 1980s breast cancer mortality has declined in women in every age group, likely due to increased awareness, implemented screening measures and improvements in treatment.

Other available post-treatment sequelae statistics (Peuckmann et al. 2009):

- Chronic/persistent pain – 29%
- Paresthesia – 47%
- Arm/shoulder swelling – 25%
- Phantom sensations – 19%
- Allodynia – 15%.

Chronic pain related to breast cancer was significantly associated with poorer health-related quality of life (HRQOL) and higher medicine consumption. Chronic pain is 42% more prevalent in breast cancer survivors than in the general population. Other sequelae prevalence factors include age (<70 years), short education, being single (divorced, widowed, separated), radiotherapy, and time since operation <10 years. Radiotherapy and younger age were significantly associated with most sequelae (Peuckmann et al. 2009).

Although sequelae appears common, there remains a sizeable gap between patient need and measures taken to provide or refer for appropriate rehabilitative services (Cheville et al. 2008, 2009, Schmitz et al. 2012). It is established that the likelihood of referral is lower among minorities and the socioeconomically disadvantaged – a noted access to care disparity among not only cancer survivors but in the population at large.

There is a growing body of evidence which supports that rehabilitative and exercise intervention result in better outcomes when adverse treatment effects are identified and treated early on (Box et al. 2002, Stout Gergich et al. 2008, Torres Lacomba et al. 2010, Springer et al. 2010, Schmitz et al. 2010, Gerber et al. 2011).

Further, the 60% side-effect incidence (Schmitz et al. 2012) is likely an underestimate, given that several common sequelae of particular relevance to manual therapies were not measured

in the study, such as bone health, arthralgias and chemotherapy-induced peripheral neuropathy (Schmitz et al. 2012). If impairments are commonly observable and if cost-effective rehabilitative treatment has been shown to reduce morbidity and comorbidities, then it is reasonable that the service provision, referral and accessibility gaps are satisfactorily addressed.

Schmitz et al. (2012) note the broad spectrum term – rehabilitation; although MT is not specifically identified, when we scan the list of sequelae, with the exception of infection, every single issue noted falls squarely within our scope of practice. Clinical experience and supportive evidence affirms that MT can effectively prevent or reduce unnecessary pain and suffering for the many women and men who are breast cancer survivors. What is needed is improved access to care.

Mastectomy

As a result of early detection and the increase in breast cancer diagnosis, service providers around the world have reported an increase in mastectomy surgery. As an example, the English NHS had an increase in the number of operations performed from 24 684 to 33 814 over the period 1997–2006, a 37% increase (National Mastectomy Breast Reconstruction Audit 2008).

Surgical treatment for breast cancer is generally divided into two categories: breast-conserving therapy (BCT) and mastectomy.

BCT involves removing the least possible amount of breast tissue when removing the malignant tumor, and usually includes additional therapy after surgery, most often radiotherapy (Johns Hopkins Medicine 2014).

Mastectomy is removal of all breast tissue and may be performed as prevention/prophylactic or as treatment. There are various types of mastectomies – see Table 6.2 (Johns Hopkins Medicine 2014). Certain risk groups (those with gene

Mastectomy type	Description
Total simple	Removal of all the breast tissue, nipple and areola. No lymph nodes from the axillae are taken. General recovery from this procedure, if no reconstruction is done at the same time, is usually 1–2 weeks. Hospitalization varies; for some it may be an outpatient procedure and other patients may require an overnight stay
Modified radical	Removal of the breast, nipple and areola as well as axillary node dissection. General recovery, when surgery is done without reconstruction, is usually 2–3 weeks
Skin sparing	Removal of the breast, nipple and areola, keeping the outer skin of the breast intact. A tissue expander may also be placed as a space holder for later reconstruction. Tissue expansion is a procedure that enables the body to 'grow' extra skin for use in reconstruction. A silicone balloon expander is inserted under the skin near the area to be repaired and then gradually filled with salt water over time, causing the skin to stretch and grow. It is most commonly used for breast reconstruction following breast removal, but also to repair skin damaged by birth defects, accidents or surgery, and in certain cosmetic procedures (American Society of Plastic Surgeons)
Nipple sparing or subcutaneous	A newer (controversial) technique reserved for a smaller number of women with tumors that are not near the nipple areola area. An incision is made on the lateral side of the breast or around the edge of the areola. The breast tissue is *hollowed out*, and the areola removed – leaving the nipple intact. This method is used in conjunction with reconstruction. Sometimes the completed reconstruction is done at the same time and, in other cases, a tissue expander is inserted as a space holder for later reconstruction
Nipple and areola sparing	Similar to the nipple sparing procedure but leaving both the areola and nipple intact. And, similarly, reconstruction is done at the same time or an expander is inserted
Scar sparing	A fairly new procedure. The affected breast is hollowed out and whether done as skin sparing, nipple sparing, areola sparing or a combination, one goal of this surgery is to minimize the surgical incisions that are visible. It is not uncommon for an entire mastectomy procedure to be performed through an opening that is less than 2 inches in length
Preventive/ prophylactic	A procedure in which one or both breasts are removed in order to dramatically reduce the risk of developing breast cancer. Women who test positive for certain genetic mutations, such as *BRCA1* and *BRCA2*, or who have a strong family history of breast cancer, may elect for this kind of surgery. They may also elect to have their ovaries removed at the same time. When this type of mastectomy is performed, no lymph nodes are removed because there is no evidence of cancer

Table 6.2

Types of mastectomies

mutations) may opt for a mastectomy to reduce the risk of developing breast cancer whereas others will have a mastectomy upon diagnosis of malignancy. Mastectomy can sometimes be combined with chemo, radio, hormone and other targeted therapies.

As mastectomy is considered more invasive, it is important to understand the surgical procedures to get a clearer picture of what systems and structures can be effected and how MT treatment can best assist the healing process and address issues related to postsurgical scarring. Although common in the past, radical mastectomy is now rarely performed because in most cases, modified radical mastectomy has proven to be just as effective, while less invasive and disfiguring.

Traumatic Scars

Breast and axillary scar tightness are one of the most common impairments reported after a mastectomy (Fourie 2008). Scarring can vary widely depending upon the type of mastectomy and reconstructive considerations. Additionally, as with any surgery, skillful incisions and suturing are known to minimize the spectrum of sequelae and complications (e.g. poor wound closure, wound rupture, ischemia, necrosis, enhanced inflammatory response that may retard healing, wide-spread and hypertrophic scars) (Khan et al. 2002). There is some evidence to support that certain types of suture material may result in smaller, less reactive scars and a lower tendency toward hypertrophic scar development (Niessen et al. 1997). As previously noted, anatomical location can also factor into the tendency toward pathophysiological scarring.

Radiation scarring

Scar tissue as a result of a mastectomy or radiation can result in several side-effects (BreastCancer.org 2015a):

- Pain, paresthesia or anesthesia if scar tissue entraps a nerve or nerve receptors

- Pathophysiological scar tissue that forms in the space where breast tissue is removed

- Pathophysiological, lumpy scar tissue that forms around a suture (i.e. suture granuloma)

- Changes in breast appearance, scar tissue and fluid retention can make breast tissue feel harder or appear rounder than before surgery and/or radiation.

Radiation therapy is a burn from the inside out. When radiation is delivered, it affects many cells – not only the cancer cells, but normal cells as well. Some cells that are particularly sensitive are those that line small blood vessels. When radiation is given, some of these very tiny blood vessels are damaged and, sometimes, destroyed. Some parts of tissue receive less blood supply and become fibrotic. And some of that tissue, therefore, is not as well-nourished and as viable as it was in its pre-treatment state. In that case, some of those tissues can scar. It is not uncommon for the radiation site to remain warm to the touch for up to 6 months after treatment.

The total number of patients who suffer from late effects of radiation therapy has not decreased because of the increased total number of patients and better survival rates. Late adverse effects, occurring more than a few months after irradiation, include the extension and collapse of capillaries, thickening of the basement membrane, and scar tissue due to loss of peripheral vessels. The main causes of these late effects are the loss of stromal cells and vascular injury (Karasawa 2014).

Implants

Capsular contracture

Capsular contracture is a complex inflammatory response to the presence of a biomedical device (e.g. silicone or saline implants, orthopedic prostheses). Diverse cell signaling followed by migration of fibroblasts to the implant surface will result in the eventual envelopment of the implant in a fibrous collagen capsule. The fibrous capsule will eventually incapacitate the device (e.g. pacemaker, artificial joint) or capsular contracture can result in compression or squeezing, distortion, migration, hardness and pain – as is seen with breast implants (DiEqidio et al. 2014).

Capsular contracture is the most common complication following the insertion of breast implants. Within a decade, following implantation approximately 50% of patients will develop capsular contracture, leading to significant morbidity and need for reoperation (Fernandes et al. 2014).

Capsular contracture is more common following infection, hematoma, seroma and rupture of the implant shell with subsequent leakage of contents. It is also more common with subglandular placement.

With breast implants capsular contracture is graded by the Baker scale (Table 6.3).

Current literature supports that steps taken to attenuate inflammatory response and subsequent fibroblast migration may be the favored approach to preventing or minimizing capsular contracture. Essentially, capsular contracture displays the common features associated with pathological scar formation: pathogenic collagen bundles (too much, too stiff, incoherent organization) and the presence of MFBs which are capable of smooth-muscle like contractions.

Implants and pain

Pain of fluctuating intensity and duration may occur and persist following breast implant surgery. In addition, improper size, placement, surgical technique or capsular contracture may result in pain associated with nerve entrapment or interference with mobility and joint ROM.

Implants and necrosis

Necrosis – the formation of dead tissue around the implant – may prevent wound healing and require surgical correction and/or implant removal. Permanent scar deformity may occur following necrosis. Factors associated with increased necrosis include infection, use of steroids in the surgical pocket, smoking, chemotherapy/radiation, and excessive heat or cold therapy.

Lymphedema

Breast cancer treatment often impacts upper body function. Dysfunction may be due to fibrosis, lack of muscle strength, lack of flexibility, lymphatic insufficicncy (lymphedema) and neural hypersensitivity (Fourie 2008).

Lymphedema is caused by an inefficiency in the lymphatic system. Hydrophilic protein becomes congested in the interstitial spaces of the extremities or trunk, which causes swelling in the area.

Incidence statistics of lymphedema range from 5% to 60%, with the onset of symptoms occurring immediately following surgery to up to 30 years

Grade I	Grade II	Grade III	Grade IV
Breast appearance is natural/normal, feel is of *normal* softness and the capsule is pliable/supple	Breast appearance is natural/normal but feels somewhat hard to the touch and pliability/suppleness is somewhat diminished	The breast feels hard, pliability/ suppleness is more noticeably diminished and some distortion is evident (e.g. presents as an atypical rounded shape, or the implant is generally tilted upwards)	Similar to grade III but with greater distortion and hardening of the capsule – pain/discomfort may accompany this grade of contracture

Table 6.3

Baker scale

post-surgery (Poage 2008). Statistics for development of lymphedema for breast cancer patients range from 2.4% to 56%. Once lymphedema is established it can be managed but not cured (Fourie 2008).

Cancer treatment is the leading cause of lymphedema in developed countries. Development and severity of lymphedema have a significant impact on comfort, psychological distress and overall quality of life. Development of lymphedema and at what point in a patient's recovery stage it may manifest are wide ranging. Some research studies indicate factors such as variations in anatomy, surgical procedures and radiotherapy may play a part in lymphedema development (Fourie 2008).

Quantitative lymphoscintigraphy – a method used to check the lymph system for disease (e.g. lymphoma, lymphedema) – reveals that lymph drainage is slowed in the subcutis (deeper part of the dermis), where most of the edema lies, and in the subfascial muscle compartment, which normally has much higher lymph flows than the subcutis.

Although the associated musculature does not swell significantly, the impaired drainage correlates with the severity of arm subfascial swelling, indicating an important role for muscle lymphatic function (Stanton et al. 2009). The far-reaching consequences of chronic lymph stasis is not completely understood; however, what is known is that the accumulation of the protein-rich interstitial fluid lends to early and progressive predisposition to tissue fibrosis. Components of the epidermal and dermal layers thicken significantly which, in turn, increases the thickness of the subcutaneous adipose layer (Rockson 2013).

Early indications of lymphedema include self-reported sensations of heaviness in the affected limb, edema, tingling, fatigue, or aching.

Lymphedema may initially be dismissed as edema, discomfort and inflammation after surgery. Axillary paresthesia and pain in the breast, chest and arm have been reported as symptoms of lymphedema (Poage et al. 2008).

Lymphedema is generally defined by the consistency of the tissues, not the volume of fluid that accumulates or the degree of limb distortion (size).

Four stages may be used to describe lymphedema (National Cancer Institute 2014 – see Table 6.4).

Clinical Consideration

Early detection and treatment of lymphedema may limit the progression and risks associated with more pronounced lymphedema. While subclinical lymphedema can be detected using methods such as perometry and bioimpedance spectroscopy, these technologies are not widely available. Alternatively, several studies indicate that patients' self-reported symptoms are accurate indicators of early lymphedema. Early intervention (e.g. manual lymph treatment, compression garments) – during the more easily manageable stage – has been shown to result in effective outcomes.

As noted in Chapter 3, lymphedema is classified as primary or secondary. Secondary lymphedema – seen in conjunction with the surgical removal of lymph nodes or the use of radiation during cancer treatment – rarely happens in isolation. Scarring (soft tissue fibrosis), deficits in muscle strength, flexibility and hypersensitivity are usually present. These symptoms are due to damage sustained to the supporting and organizational aspects of the fascial and CT structures and their response to the healing process (Fourie 2008).

There are a number of tissue composition changes in secondary lymphedema due to the

Stage	Description
Zero	Commonly referred to as latent, subclinical or pre-lymphedema, this presentation is typically seen in conjunction with those that have undergone surgical lymph node dissection with subsequent disruption of lymphatic pathways. Although the transport capacity of the lymph system is reduced resulting in impaired lymph flow – swelling is typically not evident. Generally there are no visible changes to the affected area; however, the individual may notice a difference in feeling, such as fatigue, mild regional numbness, tingling, fullness or heaviness, which may be accompanied by low-grade discomfort. The individual may notice difficulty or discomfort fitting into clothing, and jewelry may feel tight (e.g. rings, watch bands). This stage may last for months or many years, with eventual development of more obvious signs of lymph impairment.
One	Commonly referred to as the mild, pitting or reversible stage. Accumulation of protein-rich fluid is present in the tissues, the affected region or limb appears mildly swollen and pitting is evident (i.e. when you press into the skin a temporary dent/pit is seen and persists – termed pitting edema). Elevation of an affected limb tends to resolve or reduce the swelling; however, fluid accumulation will reoccur in time once the limb is lowered. Although this stage can include an increase in proliferating cells (e.g. fibroblasts, which in turn can stimulate collagen production), this stage is considered reversible because skin and tissues have not been permanently damaged. Proper management at this stage can assist the restoration of normal extremity circumference and lymphatic function, thereby preventing or reducing the risk of further progression toward irreversible changes (Zuther 2011). Once you have acquired mild lymphedema, you are at higher risk for moderate-to-severe lymphedema than someone who has never had any symptoms and this risk can persist even if your symptoms resolve with treatment.
Two	Commonly referred to as the moderate or spontaneously-irreversible stage. In this stage regional swelling is more pronounced, there is no reduction in swelling with elevation and pressing into the skin does not leave a dent/pit (termed non-pitting edema). Inflammation and subsequent fibrosis accompany this stage. Hardening, or thickening of the tissue is evident. This stage can be managed with treatment, but any tissue damage cannot be reversed. A reduction in fluid volume and fibrosis may be achieved through proper treatment (e.g. manual techniques and compression garments) (Zuther 2011). Lymphedema often stabilizes in stage II. However, if untreated, protein-rich fluid can continue to accumulate, sometimes resulting in progression to stage 3.
Three	Commonly referred to as severe or lymphostatic elephantiasis. This – most advanced – stage is relatively rare in people with breast cancer. With stage 3, the affected limb or area of the body presents as large and misshapen, the skin takes on a leathery, wrinkled appearance and there is evident skin thickening (fibrosis), hardness and large limb volume (elephantiasis). Pitting is not present in this stage. As noted in Chapter 3, the increase in protein-rich fluid and fibrosis prevents oxygen and other essential nutrients from reaching the area and creates an ideal environment for bacteria, which in turns sets the stage for subsequent recurrent infections (lymphangitis). With this stage, fluid reduction is still possible with proper treatment, but in most cases the duration of intensive complete decongestive therapy has to be extended and repeated several times. In extreme cases the surgical removal of excess skin following the conservative therapy may be indicated.

Table 6.4

Stages of lymphedema: 0–3

stagnation of the lymphatic fluid. The skin of the lymphatic arm can change from soft and pitting to hard, heavy and fibrotic with time. Use of tomography and magnetic resonance imaging (MRI) has demonstrated a pattern of circumferential edema and 'honey combing' with infiltration of the fibrosis in the subcutaneous tissue region. An increase of adipose tissue was also discovered around the lymphatic limb (Dylke et al. 2013).

Auxillary Web Syndrome or Cording

Axillary web syndrome (AWS), also known as 'cording' in the postsurgical breast cancer patient, is characterized by painful cording or strings of hardened lymph tissue in the axilla of the affected side. It affects functioning by causing pain and restriction in arm ROM, especially abduction. Alexander Moskovitz refers to the syndrome as: 'axillary pain radiating down the ipsilateral arm, shoulder ROM limitation, and an axillary web of tissue attempts abduction of the arm.' It appears that the axillary lymph node dissection of the breast procedure is the trigger to the lymphatic disruption that causes AWS (Bock 2013).

AWS may manifest with one large cord or several distinct, smaller cords running down the arm. These cords usually start near the site of any scarring in the underarm region and extend down the inner arm to the inside of the elbow. Sometimes they can continue all the way down to the palm of the hand. In some people, cording can extend down the chest wall instead of, or in addition to, the inner arm (BreastCancer.org 2015b).

The anatomy of the axilla bears review for a full understanding of AWS. The axilla compartment is home to a fascial sheath that contains neurovascular bundles, 20–30 lymph nodes, and is bounded superiorly by the head of the humerus, covered by the coracobrachialis and the short head of the biceps. The axilla is bound anteriorly by the pectoralis major; posteriorly by the subscapularis, latissimus dorsi and teres major; and inferiorly by the ribcage which is covered by the serratus anterior (Calais-Germain 2007).

The fasciae that envelopes the regional muscles is continuous with the brachial fascia, which plays a significant functional role (Stecco et al. 2008); for example, the fascia of the clavicular head of the pectoralis major displays a thickening of collagen fibers that extend into the anterior brachial fascia, surrounding the biceps and thereby creating a continuous functional link (i.e. myokinetic chain/myofascial meridian). Additionally, the fascia from the sterna and costal heads are continuous with the axillary fascia and the medial brachial fascia (Fourie 2008).

In addition to musculature and fascia, five identifiable groups of lymph nodes are found in the axilla. These groups reside in the fatty CT of the axilla or are arranged around the blood vessels such as the lateral thoracic and subscapular arteries and the axillary vein. These nodes drain the lymphatic vessels of the ipsilateral upper quadrant (both anterior and posterior), the ipsolateral mammary gland and the ipsilateral extremity (Zuther 2011). Seventy-five percent of the lymph from the breast and areolar plexus drains into the anterior pectoral group of lymph nodes before they move to the central nodes.

When any of the lymph nodes are removed, the flow and pathway of lymphatic fluid is disrupted and fibrosis may occur contributing to the development of AWS.

As scar formation is the body's mechanism for restoring tissue integrity, all wounds are subject to the repair process. For internal tissue injuries and inflammation involving fascia, scarring and adhesions contribute to the occurrence of tissue rigidity, abnormal movement patterns and pain.

Issues after breast cancer surgery that result in AWS may arise from the maturing process of CT and the prolonged inflammatory phase of wound healing. The CT maturation could result in either a dense, non-pliable scar or a pliable mobile scar. A prolonged inflammatory phase results in hypertrophic scarring and increased fibrosis in the damaged area (Fourie 2008).

Scar tissue can develop up to 6 months after treatment is complete. The skin may become hard, thick or feel bound in the areas that have been irradiated; surgical sites can also be aggravated (MacDonald 2003).

Scarring from radiation or surgery disturbs the lymphatic flow and, if not addressed, can create an environment for fibrosis. Add to this the fact that lymphatic pathways do not re-establish themselves across scars and you could draw the conclusion that un-drained lymphatic fluid contributes to the pathogenesis of the raised and swollen tissues abutting a scar (Warren & Slavin 2007).

Although no protocols exist, several excellent case studies indicate that a combination of manual lymph drainage techniques, myofascial release, snapping or popping of the cords and ROM exercises with passive stretching can bring about productive outcomes (Bock, 2013).

Breast Cancer-Related Neuropathy

Chemotherapy-associated peripheral neuropathy is the most common cause of breast cancer-related neuropathy. Chemotherapy medications travel throughout the body, where they can cause damage to the nerves (BreastCancer.org. 2015c).

Certain chemotherapy medications can cause neuropathy. Chemotherapy-associated neuropathy may begin as soon as treatment starts, and it may worsen as treatment continues. Usually it begins in the toes, but it can expand to include the legs, arms, and hands. The most common symptoms include:

- Pain, tingling, burning, weakness, tickling, or numbness in arms, hands, legs, and feet
- Sudden, sharp, stabbing, or shocking pain sensations
- Loss of touch sensation
- Clumsiness
- Trouble using hands to pick up objects or fasten clothing.

Other possible symptoms include:

- Balance problems and difficulty walking
- Hearing loss
- Jaw pain
- Constipation
- Changes in sensitivity to temperature
- Decreased reflexes
- Trouble swallowing
- Trouble passing urine
- Blood pressure changes.

Other treatments for breast cancer can cause neuropathy as well. Surgery and radiation therapy cause damage to nerve plexuses in the chest and axillary areas that include the brachial and cervical plexuses.

Nerve plexuses serve the motor and sensory needs of the limb (Marieb 2003). To fully understand the implications of damage or impingement to these plexus, we need to take a look at how they weave through the area affected by the surgery (Fig. 6.2).

The brachial plexus is shaped by the anterior branches of the last four cervical and first thoracic nerve before they begin their peripheral distribution. The brachial plexus traverses the subclavian triangle where it rests on the posterior scalene. The brachial plexus is covered by the omohyoid muscle and the middle and deep

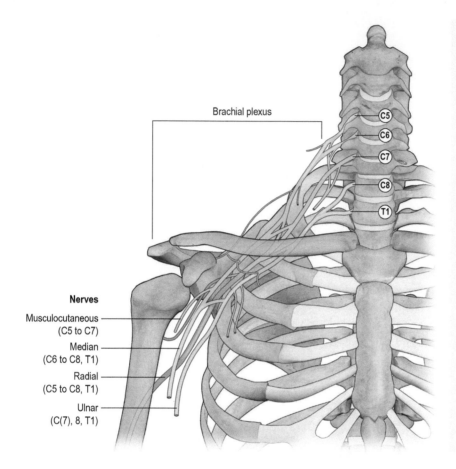

Brachial plexus

C5
C6
C7
C8
T1

Nerves

Musculocutaneous
(C5 to C7)

Median
(C6 to C8, T1)

Radial
(C5 to C8, T1)

Ulnar
(C(7), 8, T1)

Figure 6.2

Nerves plexuses in the chest and axillary areas.

cervical aponeuroses. It is separated by the subclavian muscle behind the clavicle. Its rests on the first rib and the superior digitation of the serratus anterior. It is behind the pectoral muscles, anterior to the subscapularis tendon and flanked by the two scalenes. The subclavian artery is found at the lower section of the plexus, slightly anterior to it (Croibier 1999) – see Figure 6.3.

The cervical plexus is a string of anastomoses formed by the anterior branches of the first four cervical nerves before they divide. The anterior branches are lodged in the groove that is formed by the superior surface of the transverse processes, and pass between the two

intertransverse muscles behind the vertebral artery.

The cervical plexus is situated behind the posterior edge of the sternocleidomastoid, deep to the internal jugular vein, internal carotid artery and the vagus nerve. It anastomoses with the hypoglossal, vagal and sympathetic nerves (Croibier 1999).

Trauma to these plexuses can lead to neuropathic symptoms such as pain, numbness, tingling, and/or increased sensitivity in those areas. Targeted drug therapies (Perjeta® – generic name: pertuzumab – and Kadcyla® – generic name:

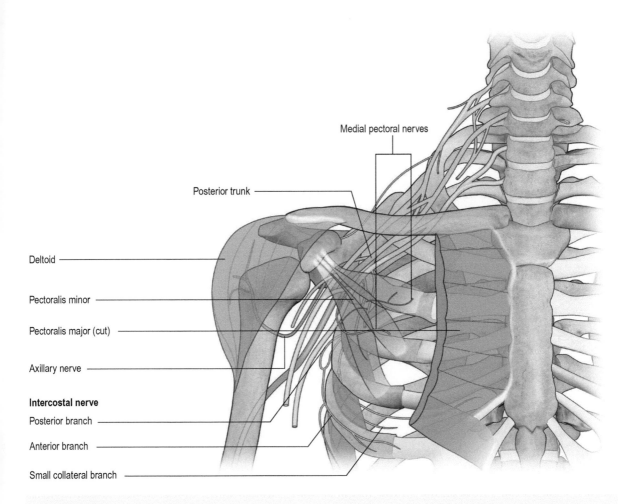

Medial pectoral nerves

Posterior trunk

Deltoid

Pectoralis minor

Pectoralis major (cut)

Axillary nerve

Intercostal nerve
Posterior branch

Anterior branch

Small collateral branch

Figure 6.3

Distribution of nerves in the thoracic region.

ado-trastuzumab emtansine) can also cause neuropathy (BreastCancer.org 2015c).

Degloving Injury

Degloving – named for the analogy of removing a glove – is a form of avulsion injury in which an extensive portion of skin and subcutaneous tissue detaches from the underlying fascia, and muscles or deeper tissues are avulsed from underlying bone or other structures. Injury classification ranges from limited avulsion with minimal tissue loss to circumferential multi-plane involvement of muscle groups and periosteum. Degloving injuries can have a devastating functional and aesthetic impact.

This type of injury typically occurs as a result of sudden shearing force trauma (e.g. explosions, falls, blunt force trauma, fractures, vehicular accidents, lacerations) and if mismanaged displays a high morbidity and mortality rate (Wójcicki et al. 2011, Latifi 2013, Yan et al. 2013). Because this type of injury is associated with violent or severe trauma, massive blood loss may occur.

While degloving injuries can occur in any region of the body, they occur more frequently in the limbs, trunk, face and genitalia, with the lower limb being the most common.

Degloving injuries are challenging to diagnose, with clinical assessment of the degloved skin being a weak predictor of the extent of injury. Ultrasound, computed tomography and MRI are indicated for proper diagnosis (Lafiti 2013).

Degloved skin that is totally avulsed from the patient's body can be reattached via a surgical procedure called *replantation*. This procedure requires great expertise and vast resources. Concurrent life-threatening injuries may not allow for a lengthy replantation and revascularization procedure (Lafiti 2013).

Because diagnosis can be delayed, degloving injuries are susceptible to infections, delayed wound healing and necrotizing fasciitis (Dearden et al 2001, Harold & Sadri 2013). Complications (e.g. multiple skin grafts, delayed wound healing and infection), existing concomitant injuries, the mechanism and the anatomy of the injury all factor into required treatment and prognosis (Latifi 2013).

Early recognition and diagnosis are key and a multidisciplinary approach is desirable. Treatment requires careful assessment of the extent of the devitalized tissue and the blood supply to the affected tissues. General treatment principles include preservation of as much of each structure as possible, measures taken to reduce risk of infection, early return of function, and

any required secondary procedures (e.g. grafting, skin flap, replantation) (Krishnamoorthy & Karthikeyan 2011, Lafiti 2013).

All MT considerations applicable to wound healing, grafting and traumatic scar tissue apply.

Liposuction

Brief consideration is given here due to the commonality of problems which may follow liposuction with incision scars, scars related to burns and subsequent fibrosis.

Liposuction is one of the most popular cosmetic surgery procedures currently performed by plastic surgeons around the world. The original concept of removing excess fat from localized areas of the body is credited to Charles Dujarrier who, in 1921, using a uterine curette, attempted to remove subcutaneous fat from the calf and knees of a ballerina. Unfortunately, an injury to the femoral vessels resulted in the amputation of the dancer's leg (Dixit & Wagh 2013).

Modern liposuction began in 1976 with the technique and instruments of Giorgio and Arpad Fischer. An otolaryngologist, Julius Newman, first used the term 'liposuction' in 1983.

Liposuction is associated with a variety of complications classified as:

- Local: such as edema, ecchymosis, seroma, hematoma, asymmetry, irregularities, skin necrosis, neural sequelae, fibrosis and adhesions

- Systemic: such as visceral perforation, DVT, infection, significant blood loss.

Local complications are more common than systemic.

Edema is considered a normal reaction to this *trauma-by-appointment*. Methods commonly employed to effectively clear edema are compression garments for 4–6 weeks post-procedure and manual lymphatic drainage in the early postoperative period (Shiffman 2006, Dixit & Wagh 2013).

Under normal, non-complicating circumstances, tissues are expected to return to normal feel and function 3 months post-procedure.

If brawny postoperative edema with heightened pain and discomfort persist beyond 6 weeks it is suggested this may be due to excessive trauma to the tissues (e.g. aggressive suctioning) and internal burn-like injury (Shiffman 2006). If this complication is present there is delayed healing and an increased risk of pathological scarring, fibrosis and surface contour irregularities (Dixit & Wagh 2013).

A higher incidence of skin necrosis, as a result of damage to the subdermal plexus of vessels, is seen in chronic smokers and with excessive superficial liposuction. Aggressive liposuction of the abdomen along with full abdominoplasty, large seromas or hematomas also increase the risk of skin necrosis.

Post-liposuction surface irregularities (waviness, dimpling) can be due to:

- Too superficial or too much liposuction

- Fibrosis and adhesions

- Redundant skin.

The scar-related problems from liposuction (aka body sculpting, lipoplasty) include:

- Poor incision placement leading to visible scars

- Depressed scars due to over-liposuctioning in the vicinity of the incision

- Hyper-pigmented scars due to skin bruising following repeated passes by the surgical instrument used

- Hypertrophic or keloid scar development associated with surgical procedures

- Skin necrosis and skin/muscle fibrosis associated with burns from over exposure to ultrasound energy (heat) emitted by the surgical instrument (liposuction cannula) (Dixit & Wagh 2013).

Neurological Sequelae

Hypoesthesia is common after liposuction. Long-standing hyperesthesia can occur due to damage to the phospholipids in the myelin sheath leading to depolarization of the cutaneous sensory nerves.

Chronic pain is rare and may be due to a neuroma or to injury to underlying fascia.

Clinical Consideration

Scar complications that are associated with liposuction show similarities to burn and mastectomy scar presentations and sequelae, therefore follow the same scar management protocols.

Traumatic Scars and MT

When working with burns, mastectomy and other traumatic scars, a clearer picture of the anatomy of the tissue involved and the nervous and lymphatic systems provides us with important information that is needed to guide treatment protocol and achieve safe and effective outcomes. Of parallel merit when considering treatment protocol is the impact on emotional well-being and quality of life – these components will be covered in greater detail in Chapter 7.

References

Akaishi S. Akimoto M, Ogawa R, Hyakusoku H (2008) The relationship between keloid growth pattern and stretching tension: visual analysis using the finite element method. Annals of Plastic Surgery 60(4): 445–451.

American Cancer Society (2010) Breast cancer. Atlanta: American Cancer Society.

Baker RH, Townley WA, McKeon S et al V (2007) Retrospective study of the association between hypertrophic burn scarring and bacterial colonization. J Burn Care Res 28(1): 152–6.

Batchelor JS, Alagappan D (2003) Pretibial wounds: a review of current practice. Trauma 5 (3): 171–177.

Berman B, Bieley HC (1995) Keloids. Journal of American Academy of Dermatology 33: 117–23.

Berman B, Perez OA, Konda S et al (2007) A review of the biologic effects, clinical efficacy, and safety of silicone elastomer sheeting for hypertrophic and keloid scar treatment and management. Dermatologic Surgery 33(11): 1291–302 [discussion 1302–3].

Bhadal N, Wall IB, Porter SR et al (2008) The effect of mechanical strain on protease production by keratinocytes. British Journal of Dermatology 158(2): 396–8.

Bock J (2013) A physical therapy directed approach for axillary web syndrome: a case study. National Lymphedema Network. Available at: http://www. lymphnet.org/resources/vol-25-no-2-a-physical-therapy-directed-approach-for-axillary-web-syndrome-a-case-study [Accessed 24 September 2014].

Bombaro KM, Engrav LH, Carrougher GJ et al (2003) What is the prevalence of hypertrophic scarring following burns? Burns 29(4): 299–302.

Bove GM, Chapelle SL (2012) Visceral mobilization can lyse and prevent peritoneal adhesions in a rat model. Journal of Bodywork and Movement Therapies 16(1): 76–82.

Box RC, Reul-Hirche HM, Bullock-Saxton JE, Furnival CM (2002) Physiotherapy after breast cancer surgery: results of a randomised controlled study to minimise lymphoedema. Breast Cancer Research and Treatment 75: 51–64.

BreastCancer.org (2015a) Available at: http://www. breastcancer.org/treatment/radiation [Accessed 24 March 2015].

BreastCancer.org (2015b) Available at : http://www. breastcancer.org/treatment/side_effects/aws [Accessed 24 March 2015].

BreastCancer.org (2015c) Side Effects-Neuropathy. Available at: http://www.breastcancer.org/treatment/ side_effects/neuropathy [Accessed 24 March 2015].

BreastCancer.org (2015d) http://www.breastcancer. org/treatment/side_effects/lymphedema [Accessed 27 May 2015].

Brissett AE, Sherris DA (2001) Scar contractures, hypertrophic scars, and keloids. Facial Plastic Surgery 17(4): 263–72.

Brown J, Bayat A (2009) Genetic susceptibility to raised dermal scarring. British Journal of Dermatology 161(1): 8–18.

Calais-Germain B (2007) The shoulder. In: Anatomy of movement, rev edn. Seattle: Eastland Press, Ch 3, p 104.

Canadian Cancer Society (CCS) (2014) Breast cancer statistics. Available at: http://www.cancer.ca/en/cancer-information/cancer-type/breast/statistics/?region=bc [Accessed 27 February 2015].

Chan KY, Lau CL, Adeeb SM et al (2005) A randomized, placebo-controlled, double blind, prospective clinical trial of silicone gel in prevention of hypertrophic scar development in median sternotomy wound. Plastic and Reconstructive Surgery 116(4):1013–20 [discussion 1021–2].

Chan MW, Hinz B, McCulloch CA (2010) Mechanical induction of gene expression in connective tissue cells. Methods in Cell Biology 98: 178–205.

Chapelle SL, Bove GM (2013) Visceral massage reduces postoperative ileus in a rat model. Journal of Bodywork and Movement Therapies, 17(1): 83–88.

Cheng B, Liu HW, Fu XB (2011) Update on pruritic mechanisms of hypertrophic scars in postburn patients: the potential role of opioids and their receptors. Journal of Burn Care Research 32(4):e118-25. Doi: 10.1097/ BCR.0b013e3182223c32.

Cheville AL, Troxel AB, Basford JR, Kornblith AB (2008) Prevalence and treatment patterns of physical impairments in patients with metastatic breast cancer. Journal of Clinical Oncology 26: 2621–2629.

Cheville AL, Beck LA, Petersen TL et al (2009) The detection and treatment of cancer-related functional problems in an outpatient setting. Support Care Cancer 17: 61–67.

Cho YS, Jeon JH, Hong A et al (2014) The effect of burn rehabilitation massage therapy on hypertrophic scar after burn: a randomized controlled trial. Burns 40(8):1513-20. Doi: 10.1016/j.burns.2014.02.005.

Crandall S, Davis M, Shibasaki D et al (2009) Sustained impairments in cutaneous vasodilation and sweating in grafted skin following long-term recovery. Journal of Burn Care and Research 30(4): 675–685.

Crandall CG, Davis SL (2010) Cutaneous vascular and sudomotor responses in human skin grafts. Journal of Applied Physiology 109(5): 1524–1530.

Croibier J-PB (1999) Cervicobrachial plexus. In: Trauma: an osteopathic approach. Seattle: Eastland Press, p 201.

Cubison TC, Pape SA, Parkhouse N (2006) Evidence for the link between healing time and the development of hypertrophic scars (HTS) in paediatric burns due to scald injury. Burns 32(8): 992–9.

Dearden C, Donnell J, Dunlop M (2001) Traumatic wounds: local wound management. Nursing Times 97: 35, 55.

Deitch EA, Wheelahan TM, Rose MP et al (1983) Hypertrophic burn scars: analysis of variables. Journal of Trauma 23(10): 895–8.

Demling RH (2005) The burn edema process: current concepts. Journal of Burn Care and Research 26(3) 207–227.

Derderian CA, Bastidas N, Lerman OZ et al (2005) Mechanical strain alters gene expression in an in vitro model of hypertrophic scarring. Annals of Plastic Surgery 55(1): 69–75.

Diamond (2012) Scars and Adhesion Panel. Lecture notes from The 3rd International Fascia Research Congress, Vancouver 28–30 March.

Diego AM, Serghiou M, Padmanabha A et al (2013). Exercise training after burn injury: a survey of practice. Journal of Burn Care and Research 34(6), e311–7.

DiEqidio P, Friedman H, Gourdie R et al (2014) Biomedical implant capsule formation: lessons learned and the road ahead. Annals of Plastic Surgery 73(4): 451–60.

Dixit VV, Wagh MS (2013) Unfavourable outcomes of liposuction and their management. Indian Journal of Plastic Surgery 46:377-92. Available at: http://www.ijps.org/text.asp?2013/46/2/377/118617 [Accessed 28 July 2014].

Dylke E et al (2013) Tissue composition changes and secondary lymphedema. Lymphatic Research and Biology 11(4): 211–218.

Engrav LH, Garner WL, Tredget EE (2007) Hypertrophic scar, wound contraction and hyper-hypopigmentation. Journal of Burn Care and Research 28(4): 593–597.

Fernandes J, Salinas H, Broelsch G (2014) Prevention of capsular contracture with photochemical tissue passivation. Plastic and Reconstructive Surgery 133(3): 571-577. Doi:10.1097/01.prs.0000438063.31043.79.

Fitch P (2005) Scars of life. Journal of Soft Tissue Manipulation 12(4): 3–6.

Fourie W (2008) Lymphatic scarring and secondary lymphoedema post breast cancer treatment. British Lymphology Society Annual Conference, Belfast, October, p. 1–6.

Fourie W (2012) In: Schleip et al. Fascia: the tensional network of the human body. Edinburgh: Churchill Livingstone Elsevier, Ch 7.17, 411–419.

Ganio MS, Gagnon D, Stapleton J et al (2013) Effect of human skin grafts on whole-body heat loss during exercise heat stress: A case report. Journal of Burn Care and Research 34(4): e263.

Gauglitz GG, Korting HC, Pavicic T et al (2011). Hypertrophic scarring and keloids: pathomechanisms and current and emerging treatment strategies. Molecular medicine 17(1–2): 113.

Gerber LH, Stout N, McGarvey C et al (2011) Factors predicting clinically significant fatigue in women following treatment for primary breast cancer. Support Care Cancer 19: 1581–1591.

Harold B, Sadri A (2013) Good practice in the management of serious degloving injuries: Beatrice Harold and Amir Sadri provide a case study involving the emergency care of a patient who had sustained a pretibial laceration after a fall. Emergency Nurse 21(4): 30–33.

Honardoust D, Varkey M, Marcoux Y et al (2012) Reduced decorin, fibromodulin, and transforming growth factor-β3 in deep dermis leads to hypertrophic scarring. Journal of Burn Care and Research 33(2): 218–227.

Huang C, Murphy GF, Akaishi S, Ogawa R (2013) Keloids and hypertrophic scars: update and future directions. Plastic and Reconstructive Surgery Global Open, 1(4).

Johns Hopkins Medicine (2014) Available at: http://www.hopkinsmedicine.org/avon_foundation_breast_center/treatments_services/breast_surgical_oncology/mastectomy.html [Accessed 10 November 2014].

Kanazawa Y, Nomura J, Yoshimoto S, Suzuki T et al (2009) Cyclical cell stretching of skin-derived fibroblasts downregulates connective tissue growth factor (CTGF) production. Connect Tissue Research 50: 323–9.

Kania A (2012) Scars. In: Dryden T, Moyer C, eds. Massage therapy: integrating research and practice. Human Kinetics Ch 15, 173–184.

Karasawa K (2014) Problems after radiation therapy. Gan To Kagaku Ryoho [Cancer & Chemotherapy] 41(1): 27–30.

Khan MS, Bann SD, Darzi A, Butler PEM (2002) Suturing: a lost art. Annals of the Royal College of Surgeons of England 84 (4): 278–279.

Kobesova A et al (2007) Twenty-year-old pathogenic 'active' postsurgical scar: a case study of a patient with persistent right lower quadrant pain. Journal of Manipulative and Physiological Therapeutics 30(3): 234–238.

Kowalske K, Holavanahalli R, Helm P (2001) Neuropathy after burn injury. Journal of Burn Care and Research 22(5): 353–357.

Krishnamoorthy R, Karthikeyan G (2011) Degloving injuries of the hand. Indian Journal of Plastic Surgery 44(2): 227–236.

Latifi R (2013) The diagnostic and therapeutic challenges of degloving soft-tissue injuries, Department of Surgery University of Arizona. Available at: http://symbiosisonlinepublishing.com/surgery/surgery01.php [Accessed 27 February 2015].

Lee TS, Kilbreath SL, Refshange KM et al (2009) Prognosis of the upper limb following surgery and radiation for breast cancer. Breast Cancer Research and Treatment 110: 19–37.

Linares HA (1996) From wound to scar. Burns 22(5): 339–352.

Lu C, Fuchs E (2014) Sweat gland progenitors in development, homeostasis, and wound repair. Cold Spring Harbor Perspectives in Medicine 4(2): a015222.

MacDonald G (2003) Cancer, radiation and massage. Available at: http://www.massagetherapy.com/articles/index.php/article_id/184/Cancer-Radiation-and-Massage [Accessed 24 March 2015].

Mancini RE, Quaife JV (1962) Histogenesis of experimentally produced keloids. Journal of Investigative Dermatology 38: 143–81.

Marieb EN (2003) Essentials of human anatomy and physiology. San Francisco: Benjamin Cummings, Ch 7, p. 234–235.

Nakagawa N, Matsumoto M, Sakai S (2010) In vivo measurement of the water content in the dermis by confocal Raman spectroscopy. Skin Research and Technology 16(2): 137–141.

National Cancer Institute (2014) Lymphedema PDQ®. General information about lymphedema. Available at: http://www.cancer.gov/cancertopics/pdq/supportivecare/lymphedema/Patient/page1.

National Institutes of Health (2015) Medline Plus. Telangiectasia. Bethesda: US National Library of Medicine. Available at: http://www.nlm.nih.gov/medlineplus/ency/article/003284.htm [Accessed 13 February 2015].

National Mastectomy Breast Reconstruction Audit (2008) A national audit of provision and outcomes of mastectomy and breast reconstruction surgery for women in England and Wales. First Annual Report of the National Mastectomy and Breast Reconstruction Audit 2008. NHS Information Center, p 23.

Neill T, Liliana Schaefer L, Renato V, Iozzo RV (2012) A guardian from the matrix. The American Journal of Pathology 181(2): 380–387.

Niessen FB, Spauwen PH, Kon M (1997) The role of suture material in hypertrophic scar formation: Monocryl vs. Vicryl-rapide. Annals of Plastic Surgery 39(3): 254–60.

Niessen FB, Spauwen PH, Schalkwijk J, Kon M (1999) On the nature of hypertrophic scars and keloids: a review. Plastic and Reconstructive Surgery 104(5): 1435–58.

Niessen FB, Schalkwijk J, Vos H, Timens W (2004) Hypertrophic scar formation is associated with an increased number of epidermal Langerhans cells. Journal of Pathology 202(1): 121–9.

Ogawa R, Akaishi S, Huang C et al (2011) Clinical applications of basic research that shows reducing skin tension could prevent and treat abnormal scarring: the importance of fascial/subcutaneous tensile reduction sutures and flap surgery for keloid and hypertrophic scar reconstruction. Journal of Nippon Medical School, 78(2): 68–76.

Oliveira GV, Chinkes D, Mitchell C et al (2005) Objective assessment of burn scar vascularity, erythema, thickness, and planimetry. Dermatologic Surgery 31(1): 48–58.

Patel T, Yosipovitch G (2010) Therapy of pruritus. Expert opinion on pharmacotherapy 11(10): 1673–1682.

Peacock EE Jr, Madden JW, Trier WC (1970) Biologic basis for the treatment of keloids and hypertrophic scars. Southern Medical Journal 63: 755–60.

Peuckmann V, Ekholm O, Rasmussen NK et al (2009) Chronic pain and other sequelae in long-term breast cancer survivors: Nationwide survey in Denmark. European Journal of Pain 13(5): 478–485.

Poage E, Singer M, Armer J et al (2008) Demystifying lymphedema: development of the lymphedema putting evidence into practice card. Clinical Journal of Oncology Nursing 12(6): 951–964.

Pohl H (2010) Changes in structure of collagen distribution in the skin caused by a manual technique Journal of Bodywork and Movement Therapies 14(1): 27–34.

Rabello FB, Souza CD, Farina Júnior JA (2014) Update on hypertrophic scar treatment. Clinics 69(8): 565–573.

Ratner D (1998) Skin grafting: from here to there. Dermatologic Clinics 16(1): 75–90.

Rockson SG (2013) The lymphatics and the inflammatory response: lessons learned from human lymphedema. Lymphatic Research and Biology 11(3): 117–120.

Roh YS, Cho H, Oh JO, Yoon CJ (2007) Effects of skin rehabilitation massage therapy on pruritus, skin status, and depression in burn survivors. Taehan Kanho Hakhoe chi [Journal of Korean Academy of Nursing] 37: 221–6.

Rosedale M, Fu MR (2010) Confronting the unexpected: temporal, situational, and attributive dimensions of distressing symptom experience for breast cancer survivors. Oncology Nursing Forum 37: E28–E33.

Salzberg S (2015) http://www.sharonsalzberg.com/ [Accessed 20 January 2015].

Schmitz KH, Ahmed RL, Troxel AB et al (2010) Weight lifting for women at risk for breast cancer-related lymphedema: a randomized trial. JAMA 304: 2699–2705.

Schmitz KH, Speck RM, Rye SA et al (2012) Prevalence of breast cancer treatment sequelae over 6 years of follow-up. Cancer 118: 2217–2225. Doi: 10.1002/cncr.27474.

Schneider JC, Harris NL, El Shami A et al (2006) A descriptive review of neuropathic-like pain after burn injury. Journal of Burn Care and Research 27(4): 524–528.

Shankar R, Melstrom Jr, KA, Gamelli RL (2007) Inflammation and sepsis: past, present, and the future. Journal of Burn Care and Research 28(4): 566–571.

Shiffman MA (2006) Prevention and treatment of liposuction complications. In Shiffman and Di Giuseppe (eds) Liposuction – Principles and Practice. 1st edn pp 333–341. New York:Springer.

Slemp AE, Kirschner RE (2006) Keloids and scars: a review of keloids and scars, their pathogenesis, risk factors, and management. Current Opinion in Pediatrics 18(4): 396–402.

Springer BA, Levy E, McGarvey C et al (2010) Pre-operative assessment enables early diagnosis and recovery of shoulder function in patients with breast cancer. Breast Cancer Research and Treatment 120: 135–147.

Spurr ED, Shakespeare PG (1990) Incidence of hypertrophic scarring in burn-injured children. Burns 16(3): 179–81.

Stanton AW, Modi S, Mellor RH et al (2009) Recent advances in breast cancer-related lymphedema of the arm: lymphatic pump failure and predisposing factors. Lymphatic Research and Biology 7(1): 29–45.

Stecco C, Porzionato A, Lancerotto L et al (2008) Histological study of the deep fasciae of the limbs. Journal of Bodywork and Movement Therapies 12(3): 225–230.

Stout Gergich NL, Pfalzer LA, McGarvey C et al (2008) Preoperative assessment enables the early diagnosis and successful treatment of lymphedema. Cancer 112: 2809–2819.

Thompson CM, Hocking AM, Honari S (2013) Genetic risk factors for hypertrophic scar development. Journal of Burn Care and Research 34(5): 477.

Torres Lacomba M, Yuste Sanchez MJ, Zapico Goni A et al (2010) Fffectiveness of early physiotherapy

to prevent lymphoedema after surgery for breast cancer: randomised, single blinded, clinical trial. BMJ 340:b5396.

Tredget EE (2008) Pathophysiology of wound healing: the basis of fibrosis and wound healing disorders. Chicago, American Burn Association.

Van der Veer WM, Bloemen MCT, Ulrich MMW et al (2009) Potential cellular and molecular causes of hypertrophic scar formation. Burns 35(1): 15–29.

Warren AG, Slavin SS (2007) Scar lymphedema: fact or fiction? Available at: http://www.ncbi.nlm.nih.gov/pubmed/17589258.

Wójcicki P, Wojtkiewicz W, Drozdowski P (2011) Severe lower extremities degloving injuries — medical problems and treatment results. Polski Przeglad Chirurgiczny 83(5): 276–282.

World Health Organization (2015) Violence and injury prevention. Available at: http://www.who.int/violence_injury_prevention/other_injury/burns/en/ [Accessed 13 February 2015].

Yan H, Gao W, Li Z, Wang C et al (2013) The management of degloving injury of lower extremities: Technical refinement and classification. Journal of Trauma and Acute Care Surgery 74(2): 604–610.

Yosipovitch G, Goon A, Wee J et al (2000) The prevalence and clinical characteristics of pruritus among patients with extensive psoriasis. British Journal of Dermatology 143: 969–73. Doi: bjd3829 [pii].

Yosipovitch G, Ansari N, Goon A et al (2002a) Clinical characteristics of pruritus in chronic idiopathic urticaria. British Journal of Dermatology 147: 32–6.

Yosipovitch G, Goon AT, Wee J et al (2002b) Itch characteristics in Chinese patients with atopic dermatitis using a new questionnaire for the assessment of pruritus. International Journal of Dermatology 41:212–6. Doi: 1460 [pii].

Zuther JE (2011) Lymphedema management: the comprehensive guide for practitioners. Stuttgart· Thieme.

Resource and further reading

The Wound Healing Society. Available at: http://woundheal.org/

Trauma

The quality of outcome must be worth the pain of survival

Fiona Wood

Trauma can be defined as an insult or injury to the physical body or psychological state (Barral & Croibier 1999). Physically, trauma can occur in the form of a wound or injury; and in psychological terms, in the form of a deeply disturbing, frightening or disquieting experience or event. Traumatic scars, as defined by the authors, embody this dual representation of trauma.

The authors submit that psychological traumatic responses can occur as a result of: a physically traumatic wound or injury; life-preserving interventions (surgery); experiences that occur during wound healing; and the impact of impairments, disabilities and disfigurements that can occur with pathophysiological scars.

As massage therapists (MTs), when we touch a person's body, we *touch* the traumatic events that their body has experienced. According to van der Kolk (1994), '*The body keeps the score*', and so we often find that our clients' bodies tell their stories to our hands (Fitch 2014).

The potential for the revealing of psychological trauma during a massage therapy (MT) scar management session, in the authors' opinion, is very high. The psychological impact of trauma may not be as immediately evident as the physical or aesthetic presentations and so therapist awareness of what to look and listen for presents particular consideration.

The aim of this chapter is to inform and offer a bridge of understanding to assist with safely and appropriately navigating the psychological impact of traumatic scar tissue, while being mindful of our scope of practice. The psychological trauma information covered in this chapter is intended to help guide the delivery of safe, effective and ethical care for people with traumatic scars. Particular relevance to this book is stress response; the impact of stress on wound healing; somatic memory; how to safely navigate emotional response/release during treatment; considerations for MT as a co-partner in health psychology and recognizing indicators for when the client may require professional psychological care.

Providing psychotherapy is not within the MT scope of practice. Over-stepping our professional boundaries constitutes professional misconduct and presents the potential risk of causing harm to the client. It is in the client's best interest that we refer out when it is clear that presentations exist that are beyond our scope of practice and the client would benefit from additional or other care.

Traumatic Events and Traumatic Response

The Diagnostic and Statistical Manual of Mental Disorders (DSM-V) defines a traumatic event as that which is outside the range of usual human experience that would markedly distress almost anyone; a serious threat or harm to life or one's physical integrity; a serious threat or harm befalling a friend or family member; sudden destruction of one's home or community or witnessing of another being seriously injured or killed. Such experiences can occur as a result of direct exposure to a traumatic event or indirectly (indirect trauma) in the form of learning about a traumatic event experienced by another.

Threat, actual or perceived, of death or serious injury to self or others results in a response of intense fear, helplessness or horror. It is not necessarily the event itself but the meaning it has for the individual that makes it traumatic. Traumatic events are emotionally shocking events that can overwhelm a person in a variety of ways (Trauma Center 2015).

Physiological Response

As discussed in previous chapters, traumatic scar tissue forms as a result of an excessive reaction from the systems responding to the trauma (Foex 2013). Physiological responses to trauma can occur as local and systemic. Individual system responses can have a synergistic effect on the other involved systems. Tissue discontinuity, infection, hypovolaemia, hypoxia or hypercarbia initiate the physiological response to trauma. The response, although necessary to maintain life, is harmful when excessive or prolonged (Black 1998).

Traumatic scarring is more likely in injuries where enough of the dermis has been compromised or destroyed to have a profound effect on numerous systems: vascular, lymph, nervous, immune, endocrine, integumentary and fascia.

Psychological Response

Psychological response to trauma exposure varies considerably from person to person.

However, certain inherent and learned *normal* responses to threatening events are part of our survival/stress response mechanism, which are covered in greater detail later in this chapter.

During times of stress, most people draw on established coping skills and support from family and friends to manage such experiences. Healing following trauma exposure often proceeds normally and there are no long-term consequences. At other times, an individual may experience temporary or long-term, mild to severe and debilitating effects from exposure to trauma, which may transition to more serious psychological conditions such as stress disorders – discussed in greater detail below (Trauma Center 2015).

Disruptive or debilitating trauma/stress response symptoms can present immediately, days, months or even years after the traumatic event. Symptoms may arise through an environmental trigger and present as emotional, cognitive or physical.

The Effects of Trauma Exposure: a General Overview

Following trauma exposure, anyone of us might experience a range of normal reactions such as anxiety, fear, shock, upset, an adrenalin rush, irritability, impatience, hyper-vigilance, exaggerated startle response, distressing thoughts, feeling overwhelmed, emotional numbness, loss of appetite, sleep disturbance, personal or social disconnection and various comorbidities associated with dissociation (Trauma Center 2015).

Some of the common characteristic feelings that arise with trauma exposure are (Colorado 2012):

- Loss of control

- Intense fear or horror

- Helplessness

- The realization that one is about to die.

Each person's trauma journey varies, depending on genetic predispositions, tissue properties, cumulative effects, previous injuries and how their CNS and psychological make-up reacts to trauma/stress stimuli (Barral & Croibier 1999).

Exposure to traumatic events can lead to varied psychological and physiological difficulties, including an increased risk for chronic physical health problems and chronic pain disorders, which are thought to be mediated through the three major biological systems involved in the human stress response: neural, endocrine and immune (Tursich 2013) – discussed in greater detail later in this chapter.

Stress

*Day in and day out, our hands feel it –
STRESS. Tissue so tightly wound and densely
compressed, we pause for a moment and con-
template … is this bone or is this flesh???*

Cathy Ryan RMT

Lazarus and Folkman (1984) define stress as: *'a
relationship between the person and the environment that is appraised by the person as taxing or
exceeding his/her resources and endangering his/
her wellbeing'.* Appraisal and coping are key to this
definition and lead to the subjective experience of
stress. And generally speaking, the degree of perceived threat (appraisal) influences the magnitude of the stress response.

Stress response is psychobiologically complex,
involving the individual's appraisal of the situation, coping skills/behaviors and the resources
the individual has available to draw on. Resources
include both extrinsic (e.g. social support) and
intrinsic in the form of the functioning of the
involved systems. When an individual can no
longer cope with stressful situations, affective,
behavioral, and physiological changes result
(Cohen et al. 1997, Lucas 2011).

Whether you are human, cat, dog or mouse,
experiencing stress is simply a part of life. But
neither stress nor stress response are inherently
harmful and certainly stress response does have
its time and place, such as when we need to run
fast or leap far to avoid some calamity. Therefore,
it is important to differentiate between acute
stress, a beneficial adaptation response and
chronic stress, which can prove detrimental.

Stress Response and Stress Hormones

Stress response encompasses the hormonal and
metabolic changes that are activated by real or
perceived danger, injury or trauma (Desborough

2000). Human stress response is innately
intended to enhance coping, adaptation and-
chances of survival. Stress response is rooted in
the capacity for rapid recognition of potentially
harmful stimuli and the ability to mobilize a
defense/stress response. Mobilization of stress
response is adaptive and resilient and normally
terminates as soon as the danger has passed
(Friedman 2015).

Stress Adaptation Response

A vast array of potential stress responses exist. In
any given circumstance one may run like crazy,
fight when cornered, stand perfectly still so as not
to be seen or gather with others; commonly referred
to as fight, flight or freeze and tend/befriend.

The phrase *fight or flight* was coined by Cannon
in the 1920s to describe the typical behaviors
that occur in the context of perceived threat. A
freeze response, or tonic immobility, may occur
in some threatening situations (Gallup 1977,
Barlow 2002). *Tend and befriend* refers to coping with stress through social or group support
(i.e. befriending) and providing or receiving
protection, nurturing or emotional support (i.e.
tending to others or being tended to). Social isolation significantly enhances risk of mortality,
whereas securing social support results in beneficial health outcomes, including reduced risk of
illness and death (Cohen & Willis 1985).

Fight, flight or freeze are recognized as the initial
stage of stress response adaptation. Fight may
manifest not only as a physical exchange but also
as vocally aggressive or argumentative behavior.
Flight can occur as escaping in either a sensory
way (e.g. social withdrawal, substance abuse or
television viewing – Friedman & Silver 2007) or a
physical way (e.g. running away from something
perceived as threatening or toward something
that is needed or feels safe).

Freeze response may occur when fleeing or
aggressive responses are perceived to likely be

ineffective (Barlow 2002). For example, tonic immobility may be useful when attack is further provoked by movement or when immobility may increase the chance of escaping, such as when a predator believes its prey to be dead and releases it. Tonic immobility is hypothesized to be an inherent biological response to extreme stress and shows some correlation with the experience of extreme fear. High basal cortisol levels, which are related to heightened stress responses, are predictive of freeze responses in the presence of threat (Kalin et al. 1998; Schmidt et al. 2008).

Schmidt and colleagues suggest that freeze response is more highly associated with certain cognitive symptoms of anxiety (e.g., confusion, unreality, dissociation and inner shakiness) (Schmidt et al. 2008). Levine (2010) suggests that freeze response is an oxymoron, where as simultaneously one *foot* is on the brake and one on the accelerator. Externally we are still, but internally our nervous system (NS) is racing, resulting in a tornado of energy in the body:

When imminent danger has passed animals can be observed 'shaking off' the energy following the freezing period and then go happily about their business with apparently no ill effects. However for a number of reasons humans have lost the instinctual ability to discharge this residual energy leading to a wide variety of symptoms following trauma; i.e., anxiety, depression, psychosomatic and behavioral problems. In extreme cases this can manifest as posttraumatic stress disorder or PTSD which is incredibly debilitating.

Post-traumatic stress disorder (PTSD) is discussed in greater detail later in this chapter.

Stress Response Physiology

Stress places demands on the body that are initially met by the activation of two systems: the hypothalamic–pituitary–adrenal (HPA) axis and the sympathetic nervous system (SNS). Stressful events trigger simultaneous activation of both

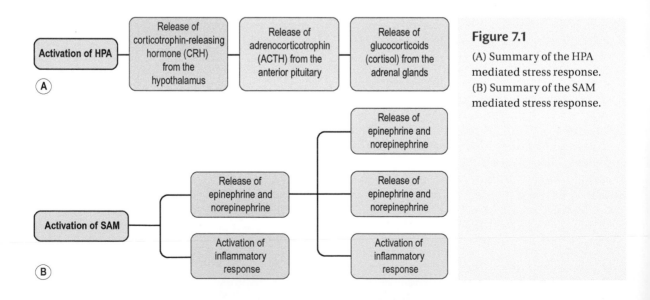

Figure 7.1

(A) Summary of the HPA mediated stress response. (B) Summary of the SAM mediated stress response.

the HPA axis in the CNS and the sympatho-adre-nomedullary (SAM) axis in the SNS, which in turn mediate a series of neural and endocrine adaptations associated with stress response or the stress cascade (see Fig 7.1).

The stress cascade assists the body with making the necessary physiological and metabolic changes required to cope with the demands of a homeostatic challenge/stressor. If the stress cascade progresses normally there is a return to homeostasis (Miller & O'Callaghan 2002).

HPA and Stress Response

Stress activation stimulates the HPA to orchestrate the release of various stress hormones, with the eventual return to homeostasis (see Fig. 7.2).

The body strives to maintain glucocorticoid levels within certain boundaries. Interference at any level will influence the other components via feedback loops. Dysregulation of the HPA axis can have adverse health consequences including the deposition of visceral fat, a feature of cardiovascular diseases such as atherosclerosis (Miller & O'Callaghan 2002).

SNS and Stress Response

When an actual or perceived threat occurs, our normal stress response kicks in, often involving some aspect of flight, flight and freeze, which is largely mediated by the SNS.

The SNS orchestrates a cascade of events, including the release of stress hormones (see Fig. 7.1b).

In times of acute stress, SNS mediated release of hormones readies us to respond to threat, real or perceived, by driving a host of physiological and psychological changes. Heart rate, blood pressure and respiration rate changes enable quick actions to be taken (e.g. fight or flight). Skeletal muscle acquires additional energy from adipose and hepatic cells. Suppression of normal thought

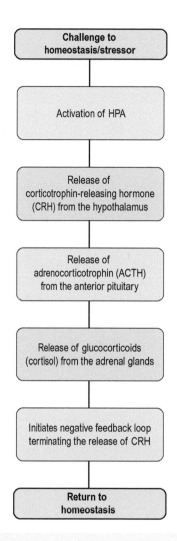

Figure 7.2

Summary of the normal stress cascade with return to homeostasis.

functions enables our brain to switch into survival mode, further supporting the ability to react quickly without the *usual* time taken for evaluation and planning. Such changes are considered beneficial adaptations.

In the absence of stress or under normal circumstances, the parasympathetic nervous system (PSNS) governs self-preservative functions, such as homeostasis and wound healing (van der Kolk 1994). During stress response, SNS predominance will suppress or alter functions that are normally governed by the PSNS.

As previously noted, stress response is generally short-lived, lasting only long enough to get us out of harm's way. All *inessential* activity in-the-moment (e.g. digestion, reproduction, feeding and *growth*) will be supressed, largely through actions exerted by glucocorticoids (Vitlic et al. 2014). Typically there is an eventual return to homeostasis as the PSNS returns to the *driver's* seat. Although stress response is normally short-lived, certain circumstances can set the stage for prolonged or chronic (pathophysiological) stress response and in turn this can adversely impact wound healing – more on this later in this chapter.

Chronic Stress Response

Chronic stress response occurs when stress stimulus exceeds our natural regulatory capacity and ability to return to homeostasis (Koolhaas et al. 2011). Overwhelming psychological stressors commonly result in chronic stress response. Without proper intervention a chronic stress state can persist indefinitely.

Chronic stress response is characterized by the prolonged and/or elevated presence of stress hormones. The physical and psychological ramifications of chronic stress presents a host of clinical problems and the chronic propagation of stress response mechanisms have deleterious long-range effects (Miller & O'Callaghan 2002, Friedman 2015).

If the stress response system fails to return to homeostasis or *reset* (i.e. remains hyperaroused or in a state of excess SNS activation and deficient PSNS activation) the individual is at risk for allostatic overload, exhausting various systems and leading to the development of stress-related physiological and psychological disorders

(Padgett & Glaser 2003, Lusk & Lash 2005, Starkweather 2007, Von Ah & Kang 2007, Rosenberger et al. 2009, Lucas 2011, van der Kolk 2014, Payne et al. 2015).

Many of the impairments that MTs address in clinic are clearly and inextricably linked with the effects of chronic stress and trauma on the body.

Pathophysiological Consideration

A systematic review (Linton 2000) showed that stress, distress and anxiety are significant factors in the development of neck and back pain and another study demonstrated a strong correlation between a diagnosis of anxiety and chronic widespread pain. Recent brain imaging studies show that emotions have a powerful effect on modulating pain – when experimental subjects were shown pictures that provoked different emotional states, this caused corresponding changes in relevant structures involved in pain processing in the brain (Roy 2009).

Pathophysiological Consideration

Chronic stress response can comprise the hormonal and metabolic changes which follow trauma or injury, a systemic reaction which encompasses a wide range of endocrinological, immunological and haematological effects – impacting normal wound healing.

Pathophysiological Consideration

Various innate re-setting or recalibration mechanisms assist us with return to homeostasis following stress response; for example, crying has been recognized as a spontaneous biological activity which can lead to the restoration of balanced autonomic tone (Graèanin 2014). Similarly, seeking comfort (tend and befriend) or shaking off/discharging the internal tornado of

Pathophysiological Consideration (Cont.)

energy following a threat are also innate mechanisms for restoring autonomic balance. If behavioral conditioning or circumstances prevents or interferes with our innate restoration mechanisms, our ability to return to a normal state of autonomic nervous system (ANS) functionality is impacted (Payne et al. 2015).

Clinical Consideration

Prolonged stress response has been shown to suppress the immune system, disturb diurnal rhythm, stimulate or sustain obesity, adversely impact the body's pH balance and increase the incidence of chronic myofascial tension.

Clinical Consideration

Stress and the myofascial system; psychological distress and anxiety have clearly been identified as a source of *unnecessary* muscular tension. Unnecessary muscle tension being; the confusing intermediate between a non-voluntary muscle contraction (spasm) and viscoelastic tension showing no EMG activity (Simon & Mense 2007). According to Chaitow (2013):

...the shortened fibers of the soft tissues may be the result of a combination of structural anomalies, trauma, and/or physical or emotional stress, and are always influenced by underlying nutritional and behavioral elements. Some of these shortened fibers and tender spots (i.e. trigger points) may be the source of reflex symptoms and pain. All such soft tissue dysfunctions respond to manual pressure in the form of modalities like massage therapy.

Clearly MT fulfils a number of the strategies for stress support (e.g. tend and befriend, providing a safe and calming environment) and is a means by which to safely and effectively address the adverse impact of prolonged stress response on the softtissues.

Psychological Stress and Wound Healing

Studies over the last 30 years have shown that the effects of psychological stress on healing are moderate to large, resulting in poor surgical outcomes and poor wound healing associated with other forms of trauma (Padgett & Glaser 2003, Lusk & Lash 2005, Starkweather 2007, Von Ah & Kang 2007, Rosenberger et al. 2009, Lucas 2011, Broadbent & Koschwanez 2012).

Substantial data suggest that psychological stress and the subsequent immune system disruption can negatively impact wound healing, both directly and indirectly, with the most prominent impact occurring due to the effects of stress on cellular immunity.

Cellular immunity plays an important role in wound healing through the production and regulation of pro- and anti-inflammatory cytokines, which mediate many of the complex intricacies of wound healing. Dysregulation of various cytokines disrupts normal wound healing leading to delayed or improper healing, increased healing time, increased risk of infection, prolonged edema and wound complications, such as pathophysiological scars (Glaser et al. 1999, Broadbent et al. 2003, Ebrecht et al. 2003, Lucas 2011).

Psychological considerations, such as distress, depression and anxiety, have also been shown to slow wound healing. Patients reporting greater than average symptoms of depression or anxiety were four times more likely to be categorized as slow healers compared with patients reporting less distress. Heightened distress, associated with unhealthy behaviors, such as smoking, substance abuse, poor nutrition and alteration of normal sleep patterns, can impact wound healing in a variety of ways. The impact of smoking on wound healing was discussed in Chapter 5, most notably reduced proliferation of macrophages and a decrease in the levels of oxygen capable of reaching the periphery. Increased alcohol use can reduce angiogenesis, delay deposition of collagen at the wound site and slow wound healing by adversely impacting cardiac and immune function. Poor nutrition, such as protein deficiency, can impact capillary formation, collagen synthesis and wound remodelling. Alteration in sleep patterns impacts growth hormone (GH) release, which may down-regulate wound healing processes such as immune response. Even relatively mild sleep disruption can alter proinflammatory cytokines and GH secretion (Benveniste & Thut 1981, Silverstein 1992, Leproult et al. 1997, Vgontzas et al. 1999, Cole-King & Harding 2001, Rose et al. 2001, Irwin 2002, Christian et al. 2006, Posthauer 2006, Bosch et al. 2007, Lucas 2011, House 2015).

According to Christian and co-workers (Christian et al. 2006):

> *Greater exploration of the role of glucocorticoids, GH, oxytocin, and other hormones/ growth factors will provide a clearer understanding of the multiple biological pathways by which stress affects healing. Similarly, we know that the nervous system substantially influences healing. However, little attention has been paid to delineating the influences of stress on the nerves in injured tissue, but it would be no surprise to discover that their neuropeptides and neurotransmitters play an important role in the stress-healing link.*

During trauma, mechanoreceptors are subjected to harsh treatment and may react to strong mechanical force by relaying incoherent or misinformation to local, regional, or central nerve centers. The various nerve centers may under- or overestimate the mechanical stimuli information during truamtic events, and nerve receptors can become confused by the milieu of the traumatic insults occurring simultaneously (Barral & Croibier 1999).

Pathophysiological Consideration

Normal levels of glucocorticoids are believed to be immunomodulatory. However, when stress increases levels of glucocorticoids, suppression of inflammatory and immune responses occur. Cortisol has been shown to decrease circulating leukocytes and inhibit the migration of leukocytes to the site of injury or infection by decreasing capillary permeability and inhibiting chemotaxis. Elevated cortisol levels have also been found to inhibit certain cytokines such as interleukin 1– prolonging the wound healing process (Lusk & Lash 2005, Guyre et al. 2008, Lucas 2011).

Pathophysiological Consideration

Elevated levels of cortisol and other glucocorticoids, produced by the adrenal glands during prolonged stress are associated with SNS hyperarousal which can lead to suppressed immunity, sleep disturbance, inappropriate inflammatory response, and increases in the level of substance P (Fritz 2013).

Pathophysiological Consideration

Stress response to surgery comprises a number of hormonal changes initiated by neuronal activation of the HPA. The magnitude and duration of the response is proportional to the degree of surgical injury and development of complications such as sepsis (Desborough 2000).

Pathophysiological Consideration

Those patients who experience greater postsurgical pain take longer to heal, suggesting that pain perception may impact wound healing. In addition to the physical disruption of tissue, pain perception can be influenced by psychological stress, and the heightened distress, in response to pain perception, can contribute to slower healing (Kiecolt-Glaser et al. 1998, Christian et al. 2006, McGuire et al. 2006).

Clinical Consideration

According to Christian et al. 2006:

A variety of stress paradigms, wounding techniques, and methods of healing assessment have clearly established that psychological stress slows healing. Dysregulation of both glucocorticoid and cytokine function are key biological links between stress and healing. The potential clinical impact of stress on wound healing is notable, with important implications in the context of surgery and other wounds. Therefore, evidence suggests that interventions designed to reduce stress and its concomitants can prevent stress-induced impairments in healing.

Research supporting MTs impact on stress and anxiety as well as emerging research suggesting MT may improve immune function, affirm MT as a worthwhile consideration in wound healing protocols.

Clinical Consideration

Multiple studies show that therapeutic massage helps with various trauma and/or chronic stress-related

Clinical Consideration (Cont.)

considerations, such as pain, depression, fatigue, sleep quality and anxiety, and it is well accepted that massage therapy promotes feelings of relaxation, peacefulness and comfort (Grealish et al. 2000, Cassileth & Vickers 2004, Hernandez-Reif et al. 2005, Jane et al. 2009, Smith et al. 2009, Wentworth et al. 2009, Parlak et al. 2010, Castro-Sanchez et al. 2011, Karlson et al. 2014, Celebioğlu et al. 2014). Highly educated and skilled MTs can assist the medical management team in achieving better patient outcomes.

Clinical Consideration

Evidence suggests that sleep disturbance has a negative impact on immune function. Cancer treatment and stress can impact cytokine secretion. Circulating cytokine levels play a role in regulating sleep by interacting with the HPA axis. Cytokines can cause cortisol fluctuations and abnormal levels of cortisol can cause sleep disturbance, therefore improving sleep quality can have a positive impact on immunity. In a study conducted on breast cancer patients (Kashani & Kashani 2014), medical MT was found to promote health and significantly improve sleep quality. It appears that sleep quality improvement results from the sedation effect of massage on the NS. Additionally, massage has been found to improve blood circulation, stimulate the lymphatic system, reduce serum cortisol, chromogranin A in saliva (a carcinoid indicator) and heart rate. When massage is performed by properly trained providers, treatment is a safe, non-pharmacological (lower cost and no side-effects) method to improve care quality and outcomes (Cox & Hayes 1998, Davidson et al. 2002, Smith et al. 2002, Soden et al. 2004, Ouchi et al. 2006, Pruthi et al. 2009, Reza et al. 2010, Sprod et al. 2010, Kashani et al. 2012, Kashani & Kashani 2014).

Clinical Consideration

Listing and colleagues suggest that MT may lead to a short-term reduction of stress perception and cortisol levels and impact mood disturbances (Listing et al. 2010). It is suggested that one explanation for stress reduction after MT could be the activation of brain areas involved in relaxation processes, for example Diego and co-workers suggest that MT stimulates PSNS activity (Diego et al. 2005). Another explanation for stress reduction after MT could be the inhibitory effect of intracerebraloxytocin on the stress-induced activity of the HPA axls, including attenuated secretion of adrenocorticotropin, catecholamines, and corticosterone (Heinrichs et al. 2003).

Clinical Consideration

According to Tejero-Fernández and colleagues:

> *High-quality but preliminary evidence supports the possibility that massage exerts immunological effects by virtue of influence on the PSNS – inducing a more relaxed/less distressed state*

(Crane et al. 2012, Tejero-Fernández et al. 2014)

Although the physiologic effects of touch are not fully understood, it appears to sustain social bonds and to increase cooperative behaviors. Oxytocin is known to facilitate social bonding and has been shown to play an important role in the modulation of stress response (Wikstrom et al. 2003, Uvnas-Moberg & Petersson 2005, Listing et al. 2010). As touch is linked to increased levels of oxytocin, in part, certain beneficial responses to massage are attributed to the release of oxytocin. Oxytocin secretion has been reported to significantly increase after a 15-minute

Clinical Consideration (Cont.)

moderate-pressure back massage in association with a significant decrease in the stress hormone adrenocorticotropic hormone. Oxytocin has also been shown to significantly enhance the analgesic placebo response to pain. Oxytocin is also thought to modulate inflammation by decreasing certain cytokines and attenuating stress-induced cortisol levels. Therefore, it is suggested that increased release of oxytocin has the potential to speed healing (Sen et al. 2002, Detillion et al. 2004, Christian et al. 2006, Morhenn et al. 2012, Kessner et al. 2013, Turkeltaub et al. 2014).]

Clinical Consideration

Rapid developments in brain imaging techniques and expanded understanding of stress biology support that altering the threat value of an injury procedure or pain-state beneficially influences brain plastic changes and biological coping leading to improved healing (Melzack & Katz 2004, 1999, Butler 2000, Moseley 2005, Janig et al. 2006, Wand et al. 2011).

Clinical Consideration

The effects of stress on health outcomes in general and immune outcomes tend to differ throughout the life span. For example, in terms of wound healing, older adults, experiencing distress, tend to heal more slowly and are at greater risk of wound infection (Ghadially et al. 1995, Graham et al. 2006a,b,c, Christian et al. 2006). Therefore interventions aimed at stress reduction ought to be considered an important component in the care of elder populations.

Stress Disorders

Following a traumatic event, stress reactions are common and the majority subside within a short timeframe, posing no substantial interference with our ability to carry on with our daily lives. However, under certain circumstances, an individual can experience severe or pathological stress reactions that may lead to stress disorders, wherein the various stress response mechanisms are sustained and remain active long after imminent danger is no longer present (DSM-V 2013).

Diagnosing stress disorders is beyond the massage therapist's scope of practice. The following information is provided to assist the massage therapist with recognizing indicators associated with severe stress reactions for the purpose of determining who may benefit from a referral out for proper diagnosis and the implementation of early interventions with proven efficacy, as early and appropriate treatment can attenuate significant suffering and distress. People who experience trauma cope with the memories and painful effects in a variety of ways. For many, their trauma responses gradually diminish over time. Some find it helpful to talk about what happened and their feelings, to get support from people who can be trusted, or to be involved in other activities that help them to reconnect with people and find meaning in their lives.

For some people, the symptoms and disturbing reactions persist or even worsen over time. This can lead people toward coping behaviors that are not so helpful, such as substance abuse and withdrawing from friends and family. Seeking appropriate, professional help can be helpful when important areas of life, such as relationships, work or school are impacted, or when quality of life and activities of daily living are being affected by traumatic stress.

Interprofessional collaboration and referring out are covered in greater detail in Chapter 8. That said, there is emerging data and support for MT as a viable co-partner in health psychology – discussed in greater detail later in this chapter.

Traumatic situations can challenge a person's sense of personal safety and control, leaving them feeling less secure and more vulnerable. Physical health may suffer as well, they may experience increased fatigue, headaches, and other physical impairments that fall within the scope of MT. Some may experience aches and pains without detectable physical cause (somatization) (van der Kolk 2014, Trauma Center 2015).

Trauma produces physiological changes including a recalibration of the brain's alarm system, an increase in stress hormone activity and alterations in the system that filters relevant information from irrelevant. With normal threat-response, as soon as the threat is over, stress hormones dissipate and the body returns to normal functioning (PSNS dominance). Stress hormone levels in traumatized individuals, in contrast, take much longer to return to baseline and spike quickly and disproportionately in response to even mild stressful stimuli. Additionally, long after a traumatic experience is over, stress response may be reactivated at the slightest hint of danger and mobilize disturbed brain circuits that trigger the secretion of massive amounts of stress hormones (van der Kolk 2013).

Trauma can compromise the brain area that communicates the physical embodied feeling of being alive, associated with interoception, explaining why traumatized individuals can become hypervigilant to threat at the expense of fully engaging in their present day lives. Not being fully alive in the present keeps the individual more firmly imprisoned in the past.

New methods that utilize the brain's own natural neuroplasticity can help survivors feel fully alive in the present and move on with their lives (van der Kolk 2014).

Clinical Consideration

According to van der Kolk (2014):

The biology of safety and danger, one based on subtle interplay between the visceral experiences of our own bodies and the voices and faces of the people around us – explains why a kind face or a soothing voice can make us feel calm and safe. Focused attunement with another person can shift us out of disorganized and fearful states (Tomkins 1962, Porges

Clinical Consideration (Cont.)

2011, van der Kolk 2014). Porges' polyvagal theory looks beyond the effects of fight/flight and puts social relationships front and center in understanding trauma. When the message is 'you are safe here' tension eases and relaxation occurs. Being able to feel safe with other people is probably the single most important aspect of mental health. Social support (e.g. being truly heard and seen by those around us, feeling that we are held in someone else's mind and heart) is the most powerful protection against becoming overwhelmed by stress and trauma. For our physiology to calm down and in order to heal we need a visceral feeling of safety. There is no prescription for this.

Clinical Consideration

Certainly it is no new revelation to the MT profession that the body and mind are intimately linked, communicating and coexisting, sometimes harmoniously-supportive and sometimes not. According to Sagar et al. (2007):

Available evidence is sufficient to indicate that therapeutic massage is a useful discipline for the relief of a variety of symptoms that affect both the body and the mind.

Clinical Consideration

Mainstream trauma treatment has paid scant attention to helping terrified people to safely experience their sensations and emotions. Medications such as serotonin reuptake blockers, Respiridol and Seroquel increasingly have taken the place of helping people to deal with their

Clinical Consideration (Cont.)

sensory world. However, the most natural way that we humans calm our distress is by being touched. Touch, the most elementary tool that we have to calm down, is proscribed from most therapeutic practices. Yet you can't fully recover if you don't feel safe in your skin. Therefore, I encourage all my trauma patients to engage in some sort of bodywork, such as therapeutic massage

(van der Kolk 2014).

Van der Kolk's clinical treatment approach, considered unconventional, also includes therapeutic yoga (calming and getting in touch with dissociated bodies), theatre, pranayama, chanting, martial arts, drumming, dancing and singing.

Acute Stress Disorder (ASD) and PTSD

The major distinguishing factor between ASD and PTSD is the duration of symptoms (Koren et al. 2002; Isserlin et al. 2008; DSM-V 2013).

ASD is recognized as a potentially transient disorder, whereas PTSD is presumed to be a disorder that persists beyond a timeframe when the majority of people will experience remission of severe reactions following trauma (Bonanno et al. 2002, Lichtenthal et al. 2004, DSM-V 2013).

ASD

ASD is characterized by the development of severe anxiety, dissociative, and other symptoms that occur within 1 month after exposure to an extreme traumatic stressor such as an injury, unplanned or planned (surgery).

ASD symptoms include (DSM-V 2013):

- Intense or prolonged psychological distress or physiological reactivity at exposure to internal or external cues that symbolize or resemble an aspect of the traumatic event

- A subjective sense of numbing, detachment, altered emotional responses

- Altered sense of one's surroundings or oneself

- Inability to remember at least one important aspect of the traumatic event –not associated with head trauma or substance abuse

- Recurrent and intrusive distressing memories and/or dreams of the event

- Dissociative reactions

- Persistent and effortful avoidance of thoughts, conversations, feelings, activities, places or physical reminders that arouse recollections of the trauma

- Sleep disturbance

- Hypervigilence

- Irritable, angry or aggressive behavior

- Exaggerated startle response

- Agitation or restlessness.

To be classified as ASD, these physiological, emotional, cognitive and behavioral changes must impose significant impact on important areas of functioning (e.g. social, occupational or the ability to obtain and use support) and occur within a month of the incident, and last for at least 2 days, but not more than 4 weeks.

ASD may be conceptualized as severe distress in the acute phase but without the presumption that it will develop into PTSD. ASD diagnosis is a means to describe acute stress responses that are severe enough to warrant clinical attention. In many health systems, receiving a diagnosis can facilitate access to mental health services, and so the ASD diagnosis may allow people in need of mental health services to receive adequate care (DSM-V 2013).

Additional ASD Considerations for Various Phases of Recovery

ASD can occur as a result of medical trauma, including surgeries or other invasive procedures or events that are perceived as invasive or frightening. There is substantial data on medical trauma, in particular pediatric medical trauma. Pediatric medical traumatic stress refers to a set of psychological and physiological responses of children and their families to pain, injury, serious illness, medical procedures, and invasive or frightening treatment experiences. These responses may include symptoms of SNS hyperarousal, re-experiencing and/or avoidance. They may vary in intensity, are related to the subjective experience of the event, and can become disruptive to functioning.

Box 7.1

Why do medical events potentially lead to traumatic stress? (Adapted from NCTSN 2014):

- These events challenge beliefs about the world as a safe place; they are harsh reminders of one's own or family members' vulnerability

- There can be a realistic (or subjective) sense of life threat

- High-tech, intense medical treatment may be frightening, and the patient or family members may feel helpless

- There may be uncertainty about course and outcome

- Pain or observed pain is often involved

- Exposure to injury or death of others can occur

- The patient and/or family are often required to make important decisions in times of great distress.

Phases of recovery from a traumatic injury are well documented (Blakeney et al. 2008). It is important to identify where your client is at in their process.

The critical care phase

A patient may experience one or all of the following upon being admitted to the hospital after a traumatic injury: anxiety, terror, pain, sadness and grief. Whether admitted to general in-hospital care or the intensive/critical care unit, clients may also experience ASD.

In-hospital recuperation

Clinical experience has shown traumatic scar clients usually spend a large amount of time recuperating in the hospital. Their hospital stay usually involves increased pain with exercise, and signs of anger and rage toward their circumstances. It is typical to go through grief, depressive episodes and rapid emotional shifting.

Rehabilitation and reintegration

This phase occurs after a hospital stay and, in some cases, may take years. During this phase there are adjustment difficulties, PTSD manifestations, additional anxiety and depression.

Unless the MT works in a hospital setting, most therapists will see the traumatic scar patient in the rehab and reintegration phase.

PTSD

PTSD is associated with a wide range of psychiatric comorbidity, poor quality of life, and social dysfunction.

PTSD is characterized by three predominant categories of symptoms.

- Re-experiencing symptoms including: flashbacks, frightening thoughts and disturbing dreams

- Avoidance symptoms including: staying away from places, events, or objects that are reminders of the experience, feeling emotionally numb, experiencing strong guilt, depression, or worry, losing interest in activities that were enjoyable in the past, difficulty remembering the dangerous event

- Hyperarousal symptoms including: being easily startled, feeling tense or 'on edge', sleep disturbance, and/or having angry outbursts.

A diagnosis of PTSD is considered when chronic alterations in the physiological stress response and classic PTSD symptoms persist beyond a month after the traumatic event. PTSD symptoms can persist indefinitely.

According to van der Kolk (2014), what distinguishes people who develop PTSD from people who are temporarily overwhelmed by trauma is that people who develop PTSD keep reliving it in thoughts, feelings or images. It is the constant, intrusive reliving – not the actual trauma – that causes PTSD.

In those with PTSD, sustained SNS hyperarousal can affect the ongoing evaluation of sensory stimuli. Although memory is ordinarily an active and constructive process, in PTSD failure of declarative memory may lead to organization of the trauma on a somatosensory level (as visual images or physical sensations). The inability of people with PTSD to integrate traumatic experiences and their tendency, instead, to continuously relive the past are mirrored physiologically and hormonally in the misinterpretation of innocuous stimuli as potential threats (van der Kolk 1994).

Pathophysiological Consideration

According to van der Kolk:

Trauma victims are alienated from their bodies by the cascade of events that begins in the amygdala, which triggers a fight-or-flight response and consequent flood of stress

Pathophysiological Consideration (Cont.)

hormones. Stress response usually persists until the threat is vanquished. But if the perception of threat isn't vanquished, the amygdala keeps sounding the alarm and we keep producing stress hormones. It's similar to what happens in chronic stress response, except that in traumatic stress, the memories of the traumatic event invade patients' subconscious thoughts, sending them back into fight-or-flight mode at the slightest provocation. Traumatized individuals will attempt to avoid the emotional pain by 'dissociating'– taking leave of their bodies, so much so that they often cannot describe their own physical sensations.

(Interlandi 2014).

Clinical Consideration

van der Kolk (2014) suggests that massage therapy may serve to assist the trauma patient with establishing positive sensory experiences that assist with improving bodyawareness and feeling more in-the-present.

Clinical Consideration

According to Falkensteiner et al. (2011):

Qualitative data shows that the effectiveness of interventions such as MT are increased if the patient is treated with empathy and if a therapeutic relationship is established prior to treatment. This observation may support the hypothesis that desired or undesired effects of a massage are not only dependent on the

Clinical Consideration (Cont.)

interventions themselves but also by the therapist/client relationship. Patients whose social network is poor especially consider MT a precious offer. Those patients who experience little physical contact, affection and security may be more responsive to MT. Therefore, it should especially be made available for socially isolated patients. MT is to be considered a cost-efficient, non-invasive intervention positively influencing and contributing to the reduction of pain, anxiety, and depression (Wilke et al. 2000, Cassileth & Vickers 2004, Nagele & Feichtner 2005, Kutner et al. 2008, Russell et al. 2008, Downey et al. 2009, Kutner et al. 2010).

Clinical Consideration

MT is commonly used for relaxation and pain relief, and it can also be an effective therapy for aspects of mental health. Research suggests that symptoms of stress, anxiety and depression may be positively affected with MT. According to AMTA (2014), MT may:

- Reduce trait anxiety and depression with a course of care providing benefits similar in magnitude to those of psychotherapy

- Increase neurotransmitters associated with lowering anxiety and decrease hormones associated with increasing anxiety

- Significantly decrease heart rate, systolic blood pressure, and diastolic blood pressure

- Reduce depression in individuals with HIV, lessen anxiety in cancer patients, and reduce anxiety and depression in military veterans and lower work-related stress for nurses.

Dissociation

Dissociation is described as an abnormal sense of psychological, emotional or physical detachment, experienced as a sense of unusual separation from the body (depersonalization) and/or unusual separation from the surrounding physical environment (derealization). Generally speaking, people experience dissociation as part of a psychological defense mechanism against overwhelming traumatic events. Some affected individuals develop any one of several diagnosable conditions known collectively as dissociative disorders. However, others develop dissociation-related symptoms in the context of ASD or PTSD (ptsdtraumatreatment.org 2014).

Depersonalization is experienced as sensations which include being 'outside' of the body, looking down at the body from a distance, and a partial disconnection of the body–mind link that forms the basis for emotional responses.

Derealization experiences are commonly associated with the feeling of being stuck within a dream, a perception of objects in the environment as 'unreal' and a more generalized feeling of distance or separation from people or things (ptsdtraumatreatment.org 2014).

According to van der Kolk (2014):

Dissociation is the essence of trauma. The overwhelming experience is being split off and fragmented and the sensory fragments of memory can intrude into the present. As long as the trauma is not resolved, the stress hormones that the body secretes to protect itself keep circulating and the defensive movements and emotional responses keep getting replayed. If the elements of the trauma are replayed again and again the accompanying stress hormones engrave those memories ever more deeply in the mind.

When stimulated in the present day, the amygdala makes no distinction between past and present and reactivation triggers powerful stress hormones and NS responses (e.g. sweating, trembling, racing heart rate and elevated BP). With an amygdala that is primed to go into overdrive – the resulting SNS driven hypersensitivity responses disrupt present day life and pose long-term (stress hormone driven) health considerations (van der Kolk 2014).

Clinical Consideration

According to Korn (2013): MT can provide many benefits (e.g. improved: body awareness, sense of self, sense of connectedness/socialization, selfcare and selfregulation behaviors) for the issues seen in conjunction with diseases of dissociation.

Scope of Practice Considerations

We began Chapter 1 with a quote from esteemed massage therapist and educator Pamela Fitch – *we are not just treating scars; we are treating people with scars* – because this encapsulates the very essence of our work –the totality of the person must be considered during treatment.

People who survive injuries that lead to traumatic scarring can face a series of multiple sources of distress which include emotional and monetary challenges, disfiguring and debilitating scars and functional limitations and the challenge of vocational and community reentry along with a feeling of isolation and feeling alone after discharge from hospital or treatment center (Wiechman et al. 2015).

It is beyond the MT's scope of practice to diagnose or treat psychological symptoms. However, we routinely find ourselves at the treatment table assisting those with traumatic scars and addressing how their distress manifests as impairments that impact them on many levels.

It is well established that the mind and body are not separate, but intimately intertwined, and thus MTs must be present and attentive to the person and their scar on every level. It is beyond our scope of practice to provide psychological counseling but it is not beyond our scope of practice to provide empathy, compassion and care. And it is certainly not at all uncommon for the therapist to be required to navigate somatic memory and emotional responses that occur during treatment.

Somatic/Tissue Memory

In addition to trauma memory being stored in the various memory centers of the brain, various parts of the CNS and nerve plexus, trauma can also be stored as a form of somatic/tissue memory and expressed as changes in the biological stress response (Barral & Croibier 1999, van der Kolk et al. 1997, Pert 1999).

Tissues can retain trauma memory and symptoms which may arise long after the traumatic event, with or without apparent cause or direct stimulation (Minasny 2009, Bordoni & Zanier 2014).

According to Pert (1999), the science behind mind–body medicine suggests that not only does the brain carry memories but that cells and neuropeptides hold and transport memories throughout the entire body. According to Levine (1997), memories are not literal recordings of events but rather a complex of images that are influenced by arousal, emotional context, and prior experience. Levine asserts that psychological wounds are reversible and that healing comes when physical and mental release occurs.

Intense emotions at the time of trauma initiate the long-term conditional response to reminders (triggers) of the event, which are associated with both chronic alterations in physiological stress response and dissociative disturbances. Animal research suggests that intense emotional memories are processed outside of the hippocampus mediated memory system and are difficult to extinguish (van der Kolk et al. 1997, van der Kolk 2014).

The individual's perception of the danger, the force of collision, reactive lesions, pain and other alarm sensations, all combine to create the preserved, intense, information. The stored information may get triggered, resulting in reactions such as fear, panic, syncope (partial or complete loss of consciousness), and somatization – a tendency to experience and communicate psychological distress in the form of physical symptoms.

MT may spark a somatic response or implicit tissue memory. Unexplained or atypical responses relate to the client's trauma history memories (e.g. recall of the traumatic event, the moment of injury, consequent surgeries or other lifesaving interventions) rather than to the MT intervention or technique (Andrade 2013, Fitch 2014).

For example: during a session with a burn survivor who had traumatic scarring decades old, upon a release of a thick scar band, the patient experienced a memory of being 7 years old in the Huber Tank at the burn unit, some 40 years in the past. The sights, smells and feelings of that experience were replicated, as if she were in the tank in the present day.

Autonomic discharge may also occur in tandem with somatic memory, and be expressed in the form of autonomic phenomena, such as fasciculation, tremor, shaking, nystagmus, tears, skin color changes, sweating, clamminess, laughing, crying and emotions like anger, aggression or irritation.

Such responses may cause a client to feel surprised, vulnerable and confused. The conversation we have with the client during such an experience can be of value to their therapeutic process. Conversely, if not well navigated the client may feel unsettled or distressed and not trust the therapeutic process. And heightened distress can further drive SNS hyperarousal, essentially opposite to a common therapeutic goal or intention.

Many studies show that the therapeutic value of MT increases when a connection or rapport is established between client and therapist prior to commencing with treatment. When working with traumatic scar tissue clients the solidness of the established therapeutic relationship (e.g. rapport, safety and trust) lays a foundation for the therapist to better navigate emotional or somatic memory responses that may occur during treatment. The therapeutic relationship is covered in greater detail in Chapter 8.

Clinical Consideration

According to Payne et al. (2015):

When the SNS is stuck in hyperarousal, any situation which in any way looks or feels like the original trauma can lead to a re-experiencing of symptoms. This is vital to understand as there is a high possibility that bodywork can trigger such re-experiencing.

This underpins why it is important that we understand the fundamentals of how to create a safe space for each client, develop strategies for safe navigation of all aspects of therapeutic interaction and determine when referral out is appropriate.

Clinical Consideration

Following an overwhelming, stressful situation, the SNS may drive unremitting stress response until the body-mind perceives that it is safe and recognizes that it can let down its guard. According to van der Kolk (2014):

an important aspect of trauma treatment is to be in the present without feeling or behaving according to demands belonging to the past, meaning that traumatic experiences need to be located in time and place and distinguished from current reality.

A powerful therapeutic approach used by trauma-specialist psychotherapists is helping trauma patients develop body awareness, which enhances a person's ability to be in the present. Assisting patients with body awareness development is one of the most common reasons the authors have received referrals from psychotherapists. MT is known to improve body awareness and body literacy, which in turn assists with the development of a person's ability to identify and articulate sensory experiences in the present (Kabat-Zinn, 1990, Smith et al. 1999, Kosakoski 2003, Moyer et al. 2004, Price 2005, Kahn 2007, Price et al. 2007).

Somatoemotional Response

During treatment, traumatic scar clients may display responses that are containing (e.g. holding of breath, swallowing, tensing) or releasing (tearing up, sighing, fasciculation, shaking) and the realm of response can span subtle to intense and overt. In MT this is termed somatoemotional response.

When working with trauma survivors, there is a greater likelihood that emotional responses occur as intense or overt. It is important for the therapist to be prepared for such responses and important to develop a comfort level that supports their ability to navigate client emotional response well. Additional training, beyond the scope of this book, might be necessary to assist the therapist with being better able to navigate such situations in a manner that can facilitate the clients healing process and enhance their health and well-being.

Some basic strategies for navigating emotional responses are provided in Box 7.2.

Box 7.2

Basic strategies for navigating somatic memory and emotional responses. Establish in-the-moment connection – let the client know you are present, focused on them and their needs

- Be calm and grounded

- Be attentive to subtle verbal and non-verbal cues and respond empathetically

- Respect the client's need to contain or release, do not direct or guide their experience (e.g. do not insist that they 'relax' if displaying signs of containment, do not 'correct' their breathing pattern) – simply provide a safe space for them to have their experience

- Be empathetic, use a calm quiet voice

- In an unobtrusive way, ask the client what they need (e.g. Kleenex, pause the treatment or continue, relocate treatment to another region of their body)

- Proceed slowly

- Do not specifically initiate conversation or ask questions that would intensify the client's emotional state

- If the therapist begins to feel overwhelmed, do not abandon the client by suddenly disengaging as this may be distressing, but do find a way to reground (e.g. stop applying techniques, instead simply maintain touch contact, take a few slow breaths, talk calmly to the client)

- Stay connected to the client but distanced from the client's experience, support them in an empathetic and quiet way

(Continued)

Box 7.2 (Continued)

- Once the client's emotional response has dissipated, in most cases treatment can continue – exercising good judgement comes into play here

- If the client asks what happened or if you see that the client is confused or apologetic – provide a simple explanation of triggered somatic memory and emotional response to a degree that will satisfy the client

- If the client still seems unsettled and is having difficulty coping with their experience, a conversation around referral out for counseling may be required

- Do not exceed your therapeutic comfort level as this puts both the client and you at risk – if you find yourself in a situation where the client's emotional response to treatment is beyond what you can handle, do your best in-the-moment to navigate. When treatment has concluded have an honest conversation with the client about this and discuss the possibility of referral out to another therapist in a way that supports the client's needs and does not imply that they have done something inappropriate or wrong

Adapted from Fritz 2013, Andrade 2013 and Fitch 2014.

MTs are not trained in psychotherapy. However, therapeutic listening skills and compassionate response are important components in MT. It is important to note that we stay within our professional scope of practice and training when attending to the client and recognize when a referral for psychological care/counseling is appropriate.

Clinical Consideration

For some who have experienced a traumatic event, positioning on the table may warrant special consideration. Some clients may prefer to be positioned supine rather than prone, or if side-lying they may feel safer if they are facing the therapist. Other treatment considerations will be covered in greater detail in Chapter 9.

Clinical Consideration

Working with both body and mind is becoming widely recognized as the way forward for stress disorders such as PTSD and other mental health symptoms

Clinical Consideration (Cont.)

that do not respond to the sole use of bodywork or talk therapy alone. According to van der Kolk (2014), 'trauma therapy requires you to work with the whole person, their body and their NS'. Van der Kolk's Trauma Clinic and Levine's Somatic Experiencing (SE) utilize a combination of somatic and talk therapy directed at re-setting or recalibrating the stress response system, and both approaches require specialized training.

Interoception

Damasio (2003) and Craig (2010) suggest a link between sense of self and interoceptive awareness. Interoception, subconscious signaling from free nerve endings in the body's viscera and other tissues, informs the brain about the physiological state of the body. Interoception is central to regulation of homeostasis and thus to motivated behavior, emotion and sociality (Schleip & Jäger 2012, Warner et al. 2014).

According to Schleip and Jäger (2012):

> *While sensations from proprioceptive receptors are usually projected via their somatomotor cortex, signalling from interoceptive endings is processed via the insula region in the brain, and is usually associated with an emotional or motivational component. Attentiveness to one's physical and emotional inner bodily experience is a result of good interoceptive awareness. Refining interoceptive awareness can help improve emotional understanding and self-regulation: a big step toward overall health.*

A potentially integral but under-researched approach to building self-awareness and self-regulatory capacity is the development of interoceptive awareness of attunement to and skills for shifting SNS-driven hyperarousal. Emotional regulation strategies, particularly those focused on somatic experience, facilitate the reduction of stress disorder presentations, such as those associated with PTSD (Cloitre et al. 2012, Warner et al. 2014).

Unfortunately, somatic approaches to trauma therapy are not commonly included as first or second line treatment protocols; the gap likely a by-product of a dearth of somatic intervention research outcomes and failure of intervention developers to consider and utilize somatic-based approaches (Warner et al. 2014). Although current understanding of complex trauma presentations highlights somatic dysregulation as a major area of difficulty in trauma recovery, utility of somatically-based approaches has been under-addressed in the emerging models of treatment (D'Andrea et al. 2013, Ford et al. 2013, Kisiel et al. 2014, Warner et al. 2014).

Given the impact of trauma on the brain and NS, somatic-based approaches to treatment seem to warrant heightened consideration. Somatic interventions can assist with improving interoceptive awareness and be assistive tools or components for improving self-regulation (van der Kolk 2014, Warner et al. 2014).

According to van der Kolk (2014):

> *Trauma victims can't fully recover until they become familiar with and befriend the sensations in their bodies. In order to change, one needs to be aware of their sensations and the way their bodies interact with the world around them. Physical self-awareness is the first step in releasing the tyranny of past trauma and this begins with people being able to describe what they feel in their body, not emotions (e.g. fear, anger, anxiety) but physical sensations like pressure, heat, muscular tension, tingling etc.*
>
> *If the body keeps the score, if memory of trauma is encoded in the viscera, in heartbreaking and gut-wrenching emotions, in autoimmune disorders, and skeletal/muscular problems and if mind/brain/visceral communication is the royal road to emotion-regulation, this demands a radical shift in therapeutic assumptions and approaches.*

Clinical Consideration

A number of somatic, non-linguistically dependent interventions demonstrate some degree of effectiveness; for example, trauma-sensitive yoga (Emerson et al. 2009, Emerson & Hopper 2011, Spinazzola et al. 2011, Van der Kolk et al. 2014). Additionally, MT can be an effective tool in teaching interoceptive awareness with respect to trauma and non-trauma patients.

Clinical Consideration

According to Payne et al. (2015), clear links have been found between compromised interoceptive function and psychiatric disorders including depression

MT: A Co-Partner in Health Psychology

There is increasing recognition that health psychology and MT encompass overlapping areas of focus regarding diverse client/patient populations and the health conditions treated (Hymel & Rich 2013). Health psychology, according to Hockenbury and Hockenbury (2011):

> ... focuses on the role of psychological factors in the development, prevention, and treatment of illness and includes such areas as stress and coping, the relationship between psychological factors and physical health, and ways of promoting health-enhancing behaviors.

A meta-analysis of MT research suggests that some of the positive responses to MT may be attributable to the warmth and positive regard of the therapist toward the client and the development of an alliance between the therapist and the client – factors considered to be associated with psychotherapeutic interactions (Andrade 2013). Moyer et al. (2004) state that 'MT may have more in common with psychotherapy than was previously considered. Such evidence puts considerable responsibility on the therapist to respond to clients in a supportive and compassionate way' – and this demands maturity and deep understanding of the nature of the therapeutic relationship.

As noted, practitioners who use massage techniques are generally not trained in psychotherapy and psychotherapy is not part of the entry-to-practice education and training for even the most extensively trained registered or licensed MTs. However, good hands-on therapy involves the therapist's ability to listen, observe, assist clients with body awareness, appropriately respond to discomfort, modify interventions according to the client's needs and requests, and reinforce client selfcare behaviors (Andrade 2013).

Despite whatever bodily changes the therapist hopes to achieve on behalf of the client, MT clients are often seeking significant, professional, interpersonal experiences such as caring, connectedness and compassion along with therapist competence and productive treatment outcomes (Fitch 2004, Moyer et al. 2004, Andrade 2013). According to van der Kolk: 'The single most important issue for traumatized people is to find a sense of safety in their own bodies'.

MT can be an effective partner in the traumatic scar client's during and aftercare health program. It is also important for the therapist to take measures not to become overwhelmed by others suffering or take responsibility for the feelings, thoughts or behaviors of others. Considerations for compassion fatigue and therapist selfcare strategies will be covered in greater detail in Chapter 10.

The Massage Therapist and Trauma

The trauma information, specifically stress disorders, is provided for your consumption and understanding. It is in no way meant for you to venture outside your scope of practice and 'help' the client psychologically.

It is not necessary for a massage therapist to know explicit details of the client's trauma history in order to provide productive treatment. It is of utmost importance to recognize your limits of care – stay within your scope of practice. If you observe your client consistently displaying stress disorder behaviors, ask if they would like a referral for support or counseling (Fitch 2014).

As MTs, we have a vital role to play in assisting with healing of traumatic scarring. The goals we set as therapists with these particular clients are no different than with our other clients: to diminish the impact of stress, provide pain management care and selfcare strategies, assist the healing process, improve sleep and physical function. What does set traumatic scar clients apart are the psychological and patho-physiological changes associated with traumatic scarring.

When working with these clients the massage therapist may need to be more vigilant with regard to responding empathically, making informed choices that ensure client safety and continually provide opportunities for the traumatic scar client to select how the treatment proceeds during each session. These points are essential to providing client-centered care and can ensure that clients feel validated and safe in your treatment room (Fitch 2014).

Your client's recovery from trauma is associated with a good deal of pain along with many challenges. Traumatic scar clients may incur life-changing events, such as altered physical appearance, amputations, compromised functional abilities, changes in daily activities that may impact quality of life, and such may increase their need for social support and assistance. The potential for psychological distress is heightened when scars result in appearance alteration (Fauerbach et al. 2007, Badger & Royse 2013).

Those who experience disability and disfigurement, no matter at what age, must recreate themselves. They require new ways of moving their changed bodies in order to complete tasks that once were accomplished with ease. They must find new identities to fit their new body image. This process can be complex and difficult (Blakeney & Creson 2002).

Along with the physical tissue changes, the psychological memory of the trauma can become interwoven into the fabric of the client's life and can become a significant part of who they are or perceive themselves to be and how they interact out in the world. Compassion is vital when working with those with traumatic scars.

It is imperative that MTs are able to communicate effectively during intake, treatment and encourage/guide client health-enhancing behaviors. When working with clients where emotional or psychological trauma is present, excellent communication skills can further enhance client outcomes. Communication and therapeutic relationship considerations and strategies are covered in Chapter 8.

References

Altemus M, Rao B, Dhabhar FS et al (2001) Stress-induced changes in skin barrier function in healthy women. Journal of Investigative Dermatology 117:309–317.

AMTA (2014) American Massage Therapy Association. http://www.amtamassage.org/research/Massage-Therapy-Research-Roundup.html [Accessed 15 December 2015].

Andrade CK (2013) Outcome-based massage: putting evidence into practice, 3rd edn. Philadelphia: Lippincott Williams & Wilkins.

Avery JA, Drevets WC, Moseman SE et al (2013) Major depressive disorder is associated with abnormal interoceptive activity and functional connectivity in the insula. Biological Psychiatry 76: 258–266. Doi:10.1016/j.biopsych.2013.11.027.

Badger K, Royse D (2013) Describing compassionate care: the burn. Journal of Burn Care Research.

Barlow DH (2002) Anxiety and its disorders. 2. New York: Guilford Press.

Barral JP, Croibier A (1999) Trauma: An osteopathic approach. Seattle: Eastland Press.

Benveniste K, Thut P (1981) The effect of chronic alcoholism on wound healing. Proceedings of The Society for Experimental Biology and Medicine 166:568–575.

Black J (1998) Physiological responses to trauma. Plastic Surgical Nursing 18(3): 143–145.

Blakeney P, Creson D (2002) Psychological and physical trauma: treating the whole person. The Journal of ERW and Mine Action 6: 88–9.

Blakeney PE, Rosenberg L, Rosenberg M, Faber AW (2008) Psychosocial care of persons with severe burns. Burns 34(4): 433–440.

Bonanno GA, Wortman CB, Lehman DR et al (2002) Resilience to loss and chronic grief: a prospective study from preloss to 18-months postloss. Journal of Personality and Social Psychology 83:1150–1164.

Bordoni B, Zanier E (2014) Skin, fascias, and scars: symptoms and systemic connections. Journal of Multidisciplinary Healthcare 7:11.

Bosch JA, Engeland CG, Cacioppo JT, Marucha PT (2007) Depressive symptoms predict mucosal wound healing. Psychosomatic Medicine 69(7): 597–605.

Broadbent E, Petrie KJ, Alley PG, Booth RJ (2003) Psychological stress impairs early wound repair following surgery. Psychosomatic Medicine 65:865–869.

Broadbent E, Koschwanez H (2012) The psychology of wound healing. Current Opinion in Psychiatry 25(2): 135–140.

Broadbent E, Kahokehr A, Booth R et al (2012) A brief relaxation intervention reduces stress and improves surgical wound healing response: a randomised trial. Brain Behavior and Immunity 26(2): 212–217.

Butler DS (2000) The sensitive nervous system. Adelaide: NOI Group Publishing.

Butler DG, Moseley GL (2003) Explain pain. Adelaide: NOI Group Publishing.

Cassileth BR, Vickers AJ (2004) Massage therapy for symptom control: outcome study at a major cancer center. Journalof Pain and Symptom Management 28(3): 244–249.

Castro-Sanchez AM, Mataran-Penarrocha GA, Granero-Molina J et al (2011) Benefits of massage-myofascial release therapy on pain, anxiety, quality of sleep, depression, and quality of life in patients with fibromyalgia. Evidence-based Complementary and Alternative Medicine (2011) Article 561753.

Celebioğlu A1, Gürol A, Yildirim ZK, Büyükavci M (2014) Effects of massage therapy on pain and anxiety arising from intrathecal therapy or bone marrow aspiration in children with cancer. International Journal of Nursing Practice [Epub ahead of print].

Chaitow L (2013) Soft tissue manipulation: diagnostic and therapeutic potential. http://leonchaitow.com/2013/04/27/soft-tissue-manipulation-diagnostic-and-therapeutic-potential/ [Accessed July 2015].

Christian LM, Graham JE, Padgett DA et al (2006) Stress and wound healing. Neuroimmunomodulation 13(5–6): 337–346.

Cloitre M, Courtois C, Ford J et al (2012) ISTSS expert consensus guidelines for treatment of complex PTSD in adults. Journal of Traumatic Stress 24(6): 615–627.

Cohen S, Wills TA (1985) Stress, social support, and the buffering hypothesis. Psychological Bulletin 98(2): 310.

Cohen S, Kessler RC, Gordon LU (1997) Strategies for measuring stress in studies of psychiatric and physical disorders. In: Cohen S, Kessler RC, Gordon LU, eds. Measuring stress: a guide for health and social scientists. New York: Oxford University Press, pp 3–26.

Cole-King A, Harding KG (2001) Psychological factors and delayed healing in chronic wound. Psychosomatic Medicine 63(2): 216–220.

Colorado MHA (2012) Colorado Mental Health Advocates' Forum - Trauma. Available at: http://www.colorado.gov/cs/Satellite?blobcol=urldata&blobheadername1=Content-Disposition&blobheadername2=Content-Type&blobheadervalue1=inline%3B+filename%3D%-22Consensus+Statement+on+Trauma+Informed+Care.pdf%22&blobheadervalue2=application%2Fpdf&blobkey=id&blobtable=MungoBlobs&blob-where=1251834088204&ssbinary=true [Accessed Jan 12, 2015].

Cox C, Hayes J (1998) Experiences of administering and receiving therapeutic touch in intensive care. Complementary Therapies in Nursing and Midwifery 4:128–32.

Craig AD (2010) The sentient self. Brain Structure and Function 214: 563–577. Doi: 10.1007/s00429-010-0248-y.

Crane JD, Ogborn DI, Cupido C et al (2012) Massage therapy attenuates inflammatory signaling after exercise-induced muscle damage. Science Translational Medicine 4(119): 119ra13–119ra13.

Damasio A (2003) Feelings of emotion and the self. Annalsof the New York Academy of Sciences 1001: 253–261. Doi:10.1196/annals.1279.014.

D'Andrea W, Bergholz L, Fortunato A, Spinazzola J (2013) Play to the whistle: a pilot investigation of a trauma informed sports-based intervention for girls in residential treatment. Journal of Family Violence 28(8): 739–749.

Davidson JR, MacLean AW, Brundage MD, Schulze K (2002) Sleep disturbance in cancer patients. Social Science and Medicine 54:1309–21.

Desborough JP (2000) The stress response to trauma and surgery. British Journal of Anaesthesia 85(1): 109-117. Doi:10.1093/bja/85.1.109.

Detillion CE, Craft TKS, Glasper ER et al (2004) Social facilitation of wound healing. Psychoneuroendocrinology 29:1004–1011.

DeVries AC, Craft TKS, Glasper ER et al (2006) Curt P. Richter award winner: Social influences on stress responses and health. Psychoneuroendocrinology 32:587–603.

Diego MA, Field T, Hernandez-Reif M (2005) Vagal activity, gastric motility, and weight gain in massaged preterm neonates. Journal of Pediatrics 147:50–55.

Downey L, Diehr P, Standish LJ et al (2009) Might massage or guided meditation provide 'means to a better end'? Primary outcomes from an efficacy trial with patients at the end of life. Journal of Palliative Care 25(2): 100–108.

DSM-V (2013) American Psychiatric Association. Diagnostic and statistical manual of mental disorders, (DSM-5®). Arlington, VA: American Psychiatric Publishing.

Ebrecht M, Hextall J, Kirtley L et al (2003) Perceived stress and cortisol levels predict speed of wound healing in healthy male adults. Psychoneuroendocrinology 29(6): 798–809.

Emerson D, Hopper E (2011) Overcoming trauma through yoga. San Francisco: North Atlantic Press.

Emerson D, Sharma R, Chaudhry S, Turner J (2009) Yoga therapy in practice. Trauma sensitive yoga: principles, practice, and research. International Journal of Yoga Therapy 19: 123–128.

Emery CF, Kiecolt-Glaser JK, Glaser R et al (2005) Exercise accelerates wound healing among healthy older adults: a preliminary investigation. Journal of Gerontology: Biological Sciences 60:1432–1436.

Falkensteiner M, Mantovan F, Müller I, Them C (2011)The use of massage therapy for reducing pain, anxiety, and depression in oncological palliative care patients: a narrative review of the literature. ISRN Nursing vol. 2011, Article ID 929868, 8 pages. Doi:10.5402/2011/929868.

Farb NAS, Segal ZV and Anderson AK (2013) Mindfulness meditation training alters cortical representations of interoceptive attention. Social Cognitive and Affective Neuroscience 8:15–26. Doi:10.1093/scan/nss066.

Fauerbach JA, Pruzinsky T, Saxe GN (2007) Psychological health and function after burn injury: setting research priorities. Journal of Burn Care and Research 28(4): 587–592.

Fitch P (2004) Nurturance, intimacy and attachment. Journal of Soft Tissue Manipulation 12(1): 6–9.

Fitch P (2014) Talking Body, Listening Hands: a guide to professionalism, communication and the therapeutic relationship. Saddle River, New Jersey: Prentice Hall.

Foex (2013) Surgical Tutor UK Available at: http://www.health.harvard.edu/mind-and-mood/relaxation-techniques-breath-control-helps-quell-errant-stress-response [Accessed 31 May 2015].

Ford JD, Grasso DJ, Hawke J, Chapman JF (2013) Polyvictimization among juvenile justice-involved youths. Child Abuse and Neglect 10(37): 788–800.

Friedman HS, Silver RC (2007) Foundations of health psychology. New York: Oxford University Press.

Friedman M (2015) The human stress response. A practical guide to PTSD treatment: Pharmacological and psychotherapeutic approaches [e-book]. Washington, DC:

American Psychological Association; 2015:9-19. Ipswich, MA: sycINFO.

Fritz S (2013) Mosby's Fundamentals of therapeutic massage, 5th edn. Maryland Heights, MO: Elsevier Mosby.

Gallup GG (1977) Tonic immobility: the role of fear and predation. Psychological Record 27:41–61.

Ghadially R, Brown B, Sequeira-Martin S, Feingold K, Elias PM (1995) The aged epidermal permeability barrier: structural, functional, and lipid biochemical abnormalities in humans and a senescent murine model. Journal of Clinical Investigation 95:2281–2290.

Glaser R, Kiecolt-Glaser J, Marchucha P et al (1999) Stress-related changes in proinflammatory cytokine production in wounds. Archives of General Psychiatry 56(5): 450–456.

Graèanin A (2014)Is crying a self-soothing behavior? Frontiers in Psychology 5:502. Doi: 10.3389/fpsyg.2014.00502.

Graham JE, Christian LM, Kiecolt-Glaser JK (2006a) Close relationships and immunity. In: Ader R, ed. Psychoneuroimmunology. Amsterdam: Academic Press Elsevier, pp 781–798.

Graham JE, Christian LM, Kiecolt-Glaser JK (2006b) Stress, age, and immune function: toward a lifespan approach. Journal Behav Med 2006; 29:389–400.

Graham JE, Robles TF, Kiecolt-Glaser JK et al (2006c) Hostility and pain are related to inflammation in older adults. Brain Behavior and Immunity 20:389–400.

Grealish L, Lomasney A, Whiteman B (2000) Foot massage: a nursing intervention to modify the distressing symptoms of pain and nausea in patients hospitalized with cancer. Cancer Nursing 23: 237–243.

Guyre P, Yeager M, Munk A (2008) Glucocorticoid effects on immune responses. In: del Rey A, Chousos G, Besedovsky H, eds. NeuroImmune Biology: The Hypothalamus-Pituitary-Adrenal Axis. vol. 7, pp 147–167. Amsterdam:Elsevier.

Heinrichs M, Baumgartner T, Kirschbaum C, Ehlert U (2003) Social support and oxytocin interact to suppress cortisol and subjective responses to psychosocial stress. 54:1389–1 Biological Psychiatry 398.

Hernandez-Reif M, Field T, Ironson G et al (2005) Natural killer cells and lymphocytes increase in women with breast cancer following massage therapy. International Journal of Neuroscience 115: 495–510.

Hockenbury DH, Hockenbury SE (2011) Discovering psychology. New York: Worth Publishers.

Holzel BK, Carmody J, Vangel M et al (2011) Mindfulness practice leads to increases in regional brain gray matter density. Psychiatry Research 191: 36–43. Doi:10.1016/j.pscychresns.2010.08.006.

House S (2015) Psychological distress and its impact on wound healing: an integrative review. Journal of Wound,

Ostomy, And Continence Nursing: Official Publication of the Wound, Ostomy and Continence Nurses Society / WOCN [serial online]. January, 42(1):38-41. Available from: MEDLINE with Full Text, Ipswich, MA. [Accessed 15 January 2015].

Hymel G et al (2013) Health psychology as a context for massage therapy: a conceptual model with CAM as mediator. Journal of Bodywork and Movement Therapies 18(2): 174–182.

Interlandi J (2014) A revolutionary approach to treating PTSD. The New York Times, 22 May 2014. Available at: www.NYTimes.com [Accessed 30 May 2014].

Irwin M (2002) Effects of sleep and sleep loss on immunity and cytokines. Brain Behavior and Immunity 16:503–512.

Isserlin L, Zerach G, Solomon Z (2008) Acute stress responses: a review and synthesis of ASD, ASR, and CSR. AmericanJournal Orthopsychiatry 78:423–429.

Jane SW, Wilkie DJ, Gallucci BB et al (2009) Effects of a full-body massage on pain intensity, anxiety, and physiological relaxation in Taiwanese patients with metastatic bone pain: A pilot study. Journal of Pain and SymptomManagement 37: 754–763.

Jänig W (2006) Integrative action of the autonomic nervous system: Neurobiology of Homeostasis. Cambridge:-Cambridge University Press.

Kabat-Zinn J (1990) Full catastrophe living: using the wisdom of your body and mind to face stress, pain, and illness. New York: Dell Publishing.

Kahn J (2007) Massage Clients' Perceptions of the Effects of Massage. MTI Foundation and Massage Therapy Research Consortium.

Kalin NH, Shelton SE, Rickman M, Davidson RJ (1998) Individual differences in freezing and cortisol in infant and mother rhesus monkeys. Behavioral Neuroscience 112:251–254.

Karlson CW, Hamilton NA, Rapoff MA (2014). Massage on experimental pain in healthy females: a randomized controlled trial. Journal of Health Psychology 19(3), 427–440.

Kashani F, Babaee S, Bahrami M, Valiani M (2012) The effects of relaxation on reducing depression, anxiety and stress in women who underwent mastectomy for breast cancer. Iranian Journal of Nursing and Midwifery Research 17 (1): 30.

Kashani F, Kashani P (2014) The effect of massage therapy on the quality of sleep in breast cancer patients. Iranian Journal of Nursing and Midwifery Research 19(2): 113–118.

Kessner S, Sprenger C, Wrobel N et al (2013) Effect of oxytocin on placebo analgesia: a randomized study. Analgesic Lett. JAMA 310:1733–1735.

Kiecolt-Glaser JK, Page GG, Marucha PT et al (1998) Psychological influences on surgical recovery: perspectives from psychoneuroimmunology. American Psychology 53:1209–1218. [PubMed:9830373]

Kisiel CL, Fehrenbach T, Torgersen E et al (2014) Constellations of interpersonal trauma and symptoms in child welfare: implications for a developmental trauma framework. Journal of Family Violence 29(1): 1–14. Doi:10.1007/s10896-013-9559-0.

Koolhaas J et al (2011) Stress revisited: a critical evaluation of the stress concept. Neuro science and Biobehavioral Reviews 35: 1291–1301.

Koren D, Arnon I, Lavie P, Klein E (2002) Sleep complaints as early predictors of posttraumatic stress disorder: a 1-year prospective study of injured survivors of motor vehicle accidents. American Journal Psychiatry 159: 855–857.

Korn L (2013) Keynote: Somatic empathy - restoring community health with massage. Lecture notes from the International Massage Therapy Research Conference. Boston, MA, April 25–27.

Kosakoski J (2003) Massage: hands down, a treatment for addiction. Counselor: The Magazine for Addiction Professionals 4: 36–38.

Kutner JS, Smith M, Mellis K et al (2010) Methodological challenges in conducting a multi-site randomized clinical trial of massage therapy in hospice. The Journal of Palliative Medicine 13(6): 739–744.

Kutner JS, Smith MC, Corbin L et al (2008) Massage therapy versus simple touch to improve pain and mood in patients with advanced cancer: a randomized trial. Annals of Internal Medicine 149(6): 369–379.

Lazarus R, Folkman S (1984) Stress, appraisal and coping. New York: Springer.

Leproult R, Copinschi G, Buxton O, Van Cauter E (1997) Sleep loss results in an elevation of cortisol levels the next evening. Sleep 20:865–870.

Levine PA (1997) Waking the tiger: healing trauma – the innate capacity to transform overwhelming experiences. Berkeley, CA: North Atlantic Books.

Levine PA (2010) In an unspoken voice: how the body releases trauma and restores goodness. Berkeley, CA: North Atlantic Books.

Lichtenthal WG, Cruess DG, Prigerson HG (2004) A case for establishing complicated grief as a distinct mental disorder in DSM-V. Clinical Psychology Review 24:637–662.

Linton SJ (2000) A review of psychological risk factors in back and neck pain. Spine 25(9): 1148–1156.

Listing M, Krohn M, Liezmann C, Kim I et al (2010) The efficacy of classical massage on stress perception and cortisol following primary treatment of breast cancer. Archives of Women's Mental Health 13:165–173 [DOI 10.1007/s00737-009-0143-9].

Lucas VS (2011) Psychological stress and wound healing in humans: what we know. Wounds 23: 76–83.

Lusk B, Lash AA (2005) The stress response, psychoneuro-immunology and stress among ICU patients. Dimensions of Critical Care Nursing 24(1): 25–31.

May A, Stewart J, Tapert S, Paulus M (2014) Current and former methamphetamine-dependent adults show attenuated brain response to pleasant interoceptive stimuli. Drug and Alcohol Dependence 140, e138. Doi: 10.1016/j.drugalcdep.2014.02.391.

McGuire L, Heffner KL, Glaser R et al (2006) Pain and wound healing in surgical patients. Annals of Behavioral Medicine 31: 165–172.

Melzack R (1999) From the gate to the neuromatrix. Pain 82: S121–S126.

Melzack R, Katz J (2004) The gate control theory: reaching for the brain. In: Hadjistavropoulos T, Craig KD, eds. Pain: psychological perspectives. pp 13–34. Hillsdale: Lawrence Erlbaum.

Miller DB, O'Callaghan JP (2002) Neuroendocrine aspects of the response to stress. Metabolism 51(6): 5–10.

Minasny B (2009) Understanding the process of fascial unwinding. International Journal of Therepeutic Massage Bodywork 2(3): 10–17.

Morhenn V, Beavin LE, Zak PJ (2012) Massage increases oxytocin and reduces adrenocorticotropin hormone in humans. Alternative Therapies in Health and Medicine 18: 11–18.

Moseley GL (2005) Widespread brain activity during an abdominal task markedly reduced after pain physiology education: fMRI evaluation of a single patient with chronic low back pain. Australian Journal of Physiotherapy 51(1): 49–52.

Moyer CA, Rounds J, Hannum JW (2004) A meta-analysis of massage therapy research. Psychological Bulletin 130(1): 3–18.

Nagele S, Feichtner A (2005) Lehrbuch der Palliativpflege, Facultas, Wien, Austria.

NCTSN (2014) National Child Traumatic Stress Network. Available at: http://www.nctsn.org/ [Accessed 17 December 2014].

Ouchi Y, Kanno T, Okada H et al (2006) Changes in cerebral blood flow under the prone condition with and without massage. Neuroscience Letters 407: 131–135.

Padgett D, Glaser R (2003) How stress influences the immune response. Trends in Immunology 24(8): 444–448.

Parlak A, Polat S, Akçay MN (2010) Itching, pain, and anxiety levels are reduced with massage therapy in adolescents with burns. Journal of Burn Care and Research 31: 429–432.

Paulus MP, Stein MB (2010) Interoception in anxiety and depression. Brain Structure and Function 214 451–463. Doi:10.1007/s00429-010-0258-9.

Payne P, Levine PA, Crane-Godreau MA (2015) Somatic experiencing: using interoception and proprioception as core elements of trauma therapy. Frontiers in Psychology 6: 93.

Pert C (1999) Molecules of emotion: the science behind mind-body medicine. New York: Simon and Schuster.

Porges SW (2011) The polyvagal theory: neurophysiological foundations of emotions, attachment, communication, and self-regulation (Norton Series on Interpersonal Neurobiology). 1e. New York: WW Norton & Company.

Posthauer ME (2006) The role of nutrition in wound care. Adv Skin Wound Care 19: 43–52.

Pressman SD, Cohen S (2005) Does positive affect influence health? Psychological Bulletin 131: 925–971.

Price CJ (2005) Body-oriented therapy in recovery from child sexual abuse: an efficacy study. Alternative Therapies in Health and Medicine 11(5): 46–57.

Price CJ, McBride B, Hyerle L, Kivlahan DR (2007) Mindful awareness in body-oriented therapy for female veterans with post-traumatic stress disorder taking prescription analgesics for chronic pain: a feasibility study. Alternative Therapies in Health and Medicine 13(6): 32–40.

Pruthi S, Degnim AC, Bauer BA et al (2009) Value of massage therapy for patients in a breast clinic. Clinical Journal of Oncology Nursing 13: 422–5.

Ptsdtraumatreatment.org (2014) PTSD Trauma Treatment. Available at: http://www.ptsdtraumatreatment.org/?s=-dissociation [Accessed 14 December 2014].

Reza H, Kian N, Pouresmail Z (2010) The effect of acupressure on quality of sleep in Iranian elderly nursing home residents. Complementary Therapies in Clinical Practice 16: 81–5.

Rose M, Sanford A, Thomas C, Opp MR (2001) Factors altering the sleep of burned children. Sleep 24(1): 45–5.

Rosenberger, PH, Ickovics JR, Epel E etal (2009) Surgical stress-induced immune cell redistribution profiles predict short-term and long-term postsurgical recovery. A prospective study. Journal of Bone and Joint Surgery 91(12): 2783–2794.

Roy M, Piché M, Chen JI et al (2009) Cerebral and spinal modulation of pain by emotions. Proceedings of the National Academy of Sciences 106(49): 20900–20905.

Russell NC, Sumler SS, Beinhorn CM, Frenkel MA (2008) Role of massage therapy in cancer care. The Journal of Alternative and Complementary Medicine 14(2): 209–214.

Sagar S, Dryden T, Wong RK (2007) Massage therapy for cancer patients: a reciprocal relationship between body and mind. Current Oncology 14: 45–56.

Schleip R, Jager H (2012) Interoception: a new correlate for intricate connections between fascial receptors, emotion and self recognition. In: Schleip R, Findley TW,

Chaitow L, Huijing P, eds. Fascia: the tensional network of the human body. Edinburgh: Churchill Livingstone Elsevier, pp 89–94.

Schmidt NB, Richey JA, Zvolensky MJ, Maner JK (2008) Exploring human freeze responses to a threat stressor. Journal of Behavior Therapy and Experimental Psychiatry 39(3): 292–304Doi: 10.1016/j.jbtep.2007.08.002.

Sen CK, Khanna S, Gordillo G et al (2002) Oxygen, oxidants, and antioxidants in wound healing. Annals of the New York. Academy of Sciences 957: 239–249.

Silverstein PS (1992) Smoking and wound healing. American Journal Med 93: 22S–24S.

Simon DG, Mense S (2007) Understanding and measurement of muscle tonus as related to clinical muscle pain. In Fascia Research: basic science and implications for conventional and complementary health care. (eds Findley T and Schleip R). Ch. 6.1.1, pp 144–161. Elsevier Urban & Fischer: Munich.

Smith MC et al (1999) Benefits of massage therapy for hospitalized patients: a descriptive and qualitative evaluation. Alternative Therapies, Health and Medicine 5(4): 64–71.

Smith MC, Kemp J, Hemphill L, Vojir CP (2002) Outcomes of therapeutic massage for hospitalized cancer patients. Journal of Nursing Scholarship 34: 257–62.

Smith JM, Sullivan SJ, Baxter GD (2009) The culture of massage therapy: Valued elements and the role of comfort, contact, connection and caring. Complementary Therapies in Medicine 17(4): 181–189.

Smith PG, Liu M (2002) Impaired cutaneous wound healing after sensory denervation in developing rats: effects on cell proliferation and apoptosis. Cell Tissue Research 307: 281–291.

Soden K, Vincent K, Craske S et al (2004) A randomized controlled trial of aromatherapy massage in a hospice setting. Palliative Medicine 18: 87–92.

Spinazzola J, Rhodes A, Emerson D et al (2011) Application of yoga in residential treatment of traumatized youth. Journal of American Psychiatric Nurses Association 17(6): 431–444.

Sprod LK, Palesh OG, Janelsins MC et al (2010) Exercise, sleep quality, and mediators of sleep in breast and prostate cancer patients receiving radiation therapy. Community Oncology 7:463–71 [PMCID: PMC3026283].

Starkweather AR (2007) The effects of exercise on perceived stress and IL-6 levels among older adults. Biological Research for Nursing 8(3): 186–194.

Tejero-Fernández V, Membrilla-Mesa M, Galiano-Castillo N, Arroyo-Morales M (2014) Immunological effects of massage after exercise: a systematic review. Physical Therapy in Sport [Epub ahead of print].

Tomkins SS (1962) Affect, imagery, consciousness: Vol. I. The positive affects. London: Tavistock.

Trauma Center (2015) First Responders and traumatic events: normal distress and stress disorders. Available at: www.traumacenter.org [Accessed 5 January 2015].

Turkeltaub PC, Yearwood EL, Friedmann E (2014) Effect of a brief seated massage on nursing student attitudes toward touch for comfort care. Journalof Alternative and Complementary Medicine 20(10): 792–9. Epub 2014 Aug 20.

Tursich M (2013) Relationships between psychological distress and immune function in women with a history of childhood maltreatment[e-book]. US: ProQuest Information & Learning Available from: PsycINFO, Ipswich, MA [Accessed January 14, 2015].

Uvnas-Moberg K, Petersson M (2005) Oxytocin, a mediator of antistress, well-being, social interaction, growth and healing. Zeitschrift für Psychosomatische Medizin und Psychotherapie 51: 57–80.

Van der Kolk B (1994) The body keeps the score: memory and the evolving psychobiology of posttraumatic stress. Harvard Review of Psychiatry 1(5):253–65. [online] http://informahealthcare.com/doi/abs/10.3109/10673229409017088.

Van Der Kolk B (2014) The Body Keeps the Score: brain, mind, and body in the healing of trauma. New York:Viking Penguin.

Van der Kolk B, Burbridge JA, Suzuki J (1997). The psychobiology of traumatic memory: clinical implications of neuroimaging studies. Annals of the New York Academy of Sciences 821: 99–113.

Vgontzas AN, Papanicolaou DA, Bixler EO et al (1999) Circadian interleukin-6 secretion and quantity and depth of sleep. Journal Clinical Endocrinology and Metabolism 84: 2603–2607.

Vitlic A, Lor, JM, Phillips AC (2014) Stress, ageing and their influence on functional, cellular and molecular aspects of the immune system. AGE: 1–17.

Von Ah D, Kang DH, Carpenter JS (2007) Stress, optimism and social support: Impact on immune response in breast cancer. Research in Nursing and Health 30(1): 72–83.

Wand BM, Parkitny L, O'Connell NE et al (2011) Cortical changes in chronic low back pain: current state of the art and implications for clinical practice. Manual Therapy 16(1): 15–20.

Warner E, Spinazzola J, Westcott A et al (2014) The body can change the score: empirical support for somatic regulation in the treatment of traumatized adolescents. Journal of Child and Adolescent Trauma DOI: 10.1007/s40653-014-0030-z.

Weine S, Danieli Y, Silove D et al (2002) Guidelines for International Training in Mental Health and Psychosocial Interventions for Trauma Exposed Populations in Clinical and Community Settings. For the task force on international trauma training of the international society for traumatic stress studies. Psychiatry 65(2): Summer: 156–164.

Wentworth LJ, Briese LJ, Timimi FK, et al (2009) Massage therapy reduces tension, anxiety, and pain in patients awaiting invasive cardiovascular procedures. Progress in Cardiovascular Nursing 24(4): 155–161.

Wiechman SA, Carrougher GJ, Esselman PC et al (2015) An expanded delivery model for outpatient burn rehabilitation. Journal of Burn Care and Research 36(1): 14–22.

Wikstrom S, Gunnarsson T, Nordin C (2003) Tactile stimulus and neurohormonal response: a pilot study. Int Journal Neurosci 113: 787–793.

Wilkie DJ, Kampbell J, Cutshall S et al (2000) Effects of massage on pain intensity, analgesics and quality of life in patients with cancer pain: a pilot study of a randomized clinical trial conducted within hospice care delivery. The Hospice Journal 15(3): 31–53.

Wood F (2015) Available at: http://www.fionawoodfoundation.com/our-challenge/burns-journey/ [Accessed 26 March 2015].

Resources and Further Reading

Korn LE (2012) Rhythms of recovery: trauma, nature, and the body. New York: Routledge

Ptsdtraumatreatment.org: http://www.ptsdtraumatreatment.org/

Trauma Center: http://www.traumacenter.org/

Communication and the therapeutic relationship

Anything that's human is mentionable, and anything that is mentionable can be more manageable

Fred Rogers

Before starting any treatment, gathering thorough information from the client is important, and how the therapist begins the conversation is a crucial first step in the therapeutic process.

Every scar has a story, and not always one that is easy to talk about. Along with aesthetic and physical impairments, traumatic scars may represent many emotions and a mixture of feelings.

When a therapist is aware of the client's sensitivities, concerns and potential reactions to receiving touch and knows how to ensure client safety, the treatment will yield a more productive outcome (Fitch 2014).

Internationally, massage therapy (MT) education/training and regulation/licensing requirements vary widely in this area. This book provides basic tools, guidelines and concepts to be mindful of when working with people with traumatic scars. As professional ethics, communication and the therapeutic relationship are complex topics, supplemental education may be helpful. Many professional associations, licensure agencies and regulatory colleges provide continuing education in this area. Additionally the authors highly recommend Pamela Fitch's book, *Talking Body, Listening Hands – A Guide to Professionalism, Communication and the Therapeutic Relationship*, as a comprehensive resource, written specifically for MTs.

This chapter aims to provide strategies to guide, creating a safe, therapeutic environment and developing professional/ethical therapeutic

Drop an unkind word, or careless: in a minute it is gone; But there's half-a-hundred ripples- circling on and on and on.

They keep spreading, spreading, spreading from the center as they go, And there is no way to stop them, once you've started them to flow.

James W. Foley

relationships. Additionally, some guidelines on how to engage in interprofessional communication, for the benefit of the client, are also provided.

Aspects of initial intake, assessment and evaluation of the person, their scar and its history are also covered in Chapter 9.

The Therapeutic Relationship

The therapeutic relationship is an amalgam encompassing the client's spoken and unspoken wishes and what the therapist perceives to be feasible, appropriate and helpful (Andrade 2013).

The nature of the client–therapist therapeutic relationship is a fiduciary one – the client trusts that the therapist will act in his/her best interests and the professional must, at all times, put the client's best interests at the forefront of every interaction and intervention.

Establishing trust, safety and rapport between therapist and client are central to a professional practice and the therapeutic relationship. The therapeutic relationship comprises a number of components: decision-making (a therapist/client collaborative process); providing a safe therapeutic environment; and interpersonal and ethical considerations.

Informed Consent and Intake

Informed consent constitutes an important component in professional practice and in the development of the therapeutic relationship.

Specifics pertaining to obtaining and documenting informed consent (e.g. legal requirements and standards) vary depending upon the massage therapist's licensing/registration requirements. However, the very essence of informed consent is universal; ensuring the client has the information they need to participate in the collaborative process of determining course of therapeutic action and understanding that they can halt or refuse all or any aspect of care at any time (right of refusal).

The Free Medical Dictionary defines informed consent as: 'consent of a patient or other recipient of services based on the principles of autonomy and privacy'. This has become the requirement at the center of morally valid decision making in health care and research. Seven criteria define informed consent:

1. Competence to understand and to decide

2. Voluntary decision-making

3. Disclosure of material information

4. Recommendation of a plan

5. Comprehension of terms (3 & 4)

6. Decision in favor of a plan

7. Authorization of the plan.

A comprehensive intake procedure is an important part of the therapeutic process. A needs assessment, based on the client's history and physical assessment, is used to devise a treatment plan and identify therapeutic goals, and outline the proposed measures taken to meet those goals. Effective therapists systematically collect, document and analyze

information from their clients throughout the therapeutic process and so it is important to utilize an objective method for measuring progress and identifying when goals have been reached (Andrade & Clifford 2012, Fritz 2013).

Needs assessment, treatment planning and measuring progress are covered in greater detail in Chapter 9.

Providing a Safe Therapeutic Environment

As professional healthcare providers, massage therapists (MTs) carry the responsibility to neither harm nor exploit and to provide a safe therapeutic environment. A safe therapeutic environment is essentially two-fold; the physical treatment space and therapist demeanor.

Numerous elements factor into a safe treatment space (e.g. free of potential hazards and a quiet/low stimulation environment with calm lighting and décor). In terms of therapist demeanor, creating a safe environment begins with establishing rapport with the client through respectful, collaborative, client-centered discussion – a partnership grounded in the point of view and experiences of the client. Good rapport helps build trust and the client's sense of safety.

Clinical Consideration

It is important that every client understands that they are in charge in the treatment room; that nothing occurs without their consent and that any aspect of interaction or intervention can be halted at any time. Because those who have experienced traumatic events may feel particularly vulnerable, this understanding warrants heightened consideration.

It is important that the client understands that if anything does not feel right to them, in any way, they need to inform the therapist so that treatment can be paused, changes/modifications discussed and carried out in a manner that is satisfactory to the client. This affirms that the client's voice matters – they are in control.

In addition to verbal direction from the client, it is the professional's responsibility to be attentive and appropriately responsive to client non-verbal cues that indicate discomfort and/or unease.

Establishing the treatment room and therapist/client interaction as a safe environment enhances the therapeutic process and treatment outcomes.

Client-Centered Care

A safe therapeutic environment ensures that the client has opportunities to express their needs and priority concerns.

Client-centered care looks beyond the mere delivery of services to the client to include advocacy, empowerment, respect for the client's autonomy and participation in decision-making (Andrade 2013).

The authors embrace a clinical philosophy that encompasses a collaborative position of working *with* a client rather than *on* a client. Respecting that, while the therapist is the professional in the therapeutic relationship with expertise to help guide the treatment process, clients are experts on their own lives and bodies and what they feel and experience.

There is no hierarchy in a client-centered therapeutic relationship, it is a collaborative partnership that supports the perspectives and experiences of the client along with the therapist's knowledge and expertise – with absolute commitment to *what is in the best interest of the client.*

Therapeutic Closeness and Vulnerability

MT is a therapeutically intimate experience that occurs in a unique environment. Typically, MT sessions occur as a one-to-one experience within a closed room. The nature of such a setting can contribute to the therapeutic potential of a MT treatment and at the same time heighten client vulnerability. Although the concept of client vulnerability is often viewed as a precarious part of MT care, when managed respectfully, the intention and outcome of vulnerability is trust and connection (Brown 2010).

In a professional context, trust and connection can be powzerful contributors to the therapeutic process. Although vulnerability can enhance therapeutic productivity, MT professionals need to ensure utmost care is taken to ensure client dignity and respect, and not to exploit a client's vulnerability. Safeguarding client vulnerability is a fundamental element of the therapeutic relationship.

In the MT environment, therapist/client closeness occurs in a number of ways: physical closeness; extended periods of therapeutic touching; disclosure; client in various degrees of undress; and client emotional responses that may occur during treatment. Although client emotional responses can present uncomfortableness for the client and therapist, such experiences are an important part of the therapeutic process. And the therapist's ability to effectively navigate a client's emotional response is an important part of care. What to or not to share requires the therapist to engage in good discernment.

Disclosure, essentially sharing, often occurs progressively in the therapeutic environment and the act of sharing can be a source of profound therapeutic value and can contribute to the precariousness of vulnerability. Disclosure can include personal information, an emotional state, a point of view, circumstances or context for the client's state of health. Although it is generally considered inappropriate for the therapist to share personal information with a client, if disclosure of certain information provides therapeutic value for the client, then such sharing is considered acceptable. An experience of closeness achieved through sharing can contribute to the therapeutic process. What to or not to share requires the therapist to engage in good discernment as inappropriate sharing can be detrimental to the therapeutic process and well-being of the client. Therapist oversharing is unprofessional and can lead to client distrust, culminating in deterioration of the therapeutic relationship.

Safeguarding client vulnerability and the delivery of safe and ethical care are dependent upon the therapist establishing and maintaining professional boundaries.

Boundaries

Over the course of our lives we can learn from our parents, guardians, teachers and friends what is deemed appropriate boundaries in various interpersonal relationships and social environments. If there are issues, problems, or trauma during the time that our boundaries are being formed, our ability to establish and maintain healthy boundaries is compromised (Kluft et al. 2000).

The health of the therapeutic relationship is reliant on both the therapist and client understanding the nature and importance of professional boundaries.

The therapeutic relationship differs from a personal relationship in essentially two ways:

- The interests of the client always come first

- There is an imbalance of power between the therapist/client and this difference in power means that it is not usually possible to maintain a therapeutic and personal relationship with a patient at the same time (CPTO 2013).

It is the professional's responsibility to establish and maintain appropriate therapist–client boundaries at all times, and demonstrate through their behavior and communication what is appropriate in a therapeutic relationship.

Establishing professional boundaries through clear communication during the initial informed consent procedure or clearly outlining important points in document form that can be presented to the client as part of initial intake will help circumvent potential pitfalls, conflict or ethical dilemmas.

If a professional, for any reason, cannot respect a client's boundary needs, the professional should refer the client to another practitioner (Fritz 2013).

Even when the professional is conscientious about establishing boundaries with the client during the initial intake procedure, those boundaries can become blurred as the professional interaction progresses. Should a client attempt to cross boundaries, it is the professional's responsibility to effectively manage this immediately as waiting only allows the problem to escalate, leading to the development of conflict (Fritz 2013).

Common boundary considerations include issues of transference and countertransference, which can diminish the effectiveness of the therapeutic relationship. Transference is the personalization of the professional relationship by the client. Countertransference is the inability of the professional to separate the therapeutic relationship from personal feelings and expectations for the client, resulting in the professional's personalization of the therapeutic relationship (Fritz 2013).

Additional resources on professional boundaries can be found in the Appendix.

Box 8.1

Aside from obvious sexually inappropriate boundary crossing, the following are some examples of less conspicuous boundary crossings:

- Extending treatment time beyond what is needed to meet the client's therapeutic needs

- Maintaining a client on a treatment program longer than is required to meet their needs

- Disclosing personal problems to a client

- Discussing personal information that provides no therapeutic value to the client

- Therapist-guided casual conversation that provides no therapeutic value to the client.

Professional Ethics

The purpose of practicing our profession ethically is to promote and maintain the welfare of the client. Through their behavior, professionals can comply both with the law and with professional codes. If compliance with the law is the only motivation in ethical behavior, the person is said to be practicing mandatory ethics. If, however, the professional strives for the highest possible benefit and welfare for the client, he or she behaves with aspirational ethics (Corey et al. 2006, Fritz 2013), see Box 8.2.

Box 8.2

Eight principles that guide professional ethical behavior (adapted from Fritz 2013):

- Respect (esteem and regard for clients, other professionals, and oneself)

- Client autonomy and self-determination (the right to decide and the right to sufficient information to make the decision)

- Veracity (the right to the objective truth)

- Proportionality (benefit must outweigh the burden of treatment)

- Non-maleficence (the profession shall do no harm and prevent harm from happening)

- Beneficence (treatment should contribute to the client's well-being)

- Confidentiality (respect for privacy of information)

- Justice and non-judgement (ensures equality among clients).

Ethical therapist behavior and clear communication are essential for a productive therapeutic relationship. The technical and interpersonal aspects of care are symbiotic. Touch demands intimate human contact, interaction and response. The therapist's interactions and responses to the client are of parallel importance to skillful assessment and treatment (Fitch 2005).

A few rules in the professional setting are absolutes: a professional does not breach sexual boundaries with a client; clients are to be referred when the skills required are out of the scope of practice or training of the professional; all care must focus on giving help and avoiding harm; and clients are to be given complete information about the treatment (Fritz 2013).

Communication

Ethical and professional dilemmas tend to occur as a result of ineffective or mis-communication. Without a direct communication approach, ethical dilemmas tend to escalate and both parties suffer in the process. To make ethical decisions and resolve ethical dilemmas, we must communicate effectively. Good communication skills are required to retrieve information, maintain charting and client records, and provide information effectively so that the client can give informed consent (Fritz 2013).

A traumatic scar injury can have multiple physical, neurological and cognitive consequences (Grigorovich et al. 2013). Many traumatic scar clients bring experiences of multiple surgeries, doctors' appointments and physiotherapy visits before they walk through your clinic door. Or other consultations may be concurrent; the client may have just arrived at your door after such a visit.

With this understanding, it is imperative to gather a more complete picture of the client's needs prior to each session. Pay attention to their mood and physical condition as they step through your clinic door. These are clues to open up dialogue about the pain they are experiencing and how to proceed in the session; for example, if the client presents tense and displays a more deliberate gait or holding pattern, ask about their day. Knowledge about their day-to-day life and prior experiences leading up to their session may indicate a need for changes in pressure and depth.

It is important to actively listen and emphatically respond to the client as a whole person, not just the area of injury or symptom and create an appropriate set of protocols for each treatment session (Fitch 2014).

Effective Listening and Empathetic Response

Effective listening involves the development of focusing skills. You cannot listen effectively if you are distracted in anyway (e.g. planning or preparing your response). Reflective listening involves restating the information to indicate that you have received and understood the message. Active listening may clarify a feeling attached to the message but does not add to or change the message (Fritz 2013).

Active listening is an important part of the therapeutic process. Listening carefully to the clients responses and making the client feel they are heard enables them to describe their situation more fully (Fitch 2014). Using your active listening and observation skills to validate client discomfort helps to build the therapeutic relationship.

Supportive, active listening when taking a case history (e.g. being non-judgmental and maintaining good eye contact) and asking open-ended questions, enables your client to provide responses in their own words.

There are some key concepts to the therapeutic listening relationship. When engaging a client during the intake, truly listen to the answer and the body language in which the statement is presented. Asking questions concerning the client's history can sometimes feel uncomfortable and intrusive to the therapist and the client; however, asking direct questions is necessary for client

safety. Active listening skills along with attention to the responses will give the therapist the information needed to formulate the proper protocol for the treatment session (Fitch 2014).

As massage therapists, we are visual and palpatory observers of the body. We may see scars that no-one in the client's family or friends have seen and we may touch scars that no-one else, including the individual themselves, have touched. Traumatic scars carry their story within the tissue and mechanics of the body. Flexibility, comfort, edema and movement can play a significant role in the quality of life of the client (Fitch 2014).

Clinical experience has shown that gaining knowledge about the traumatic scar provides the therapist with important data, which helps shape protocol and enhance follow-up questions during each intake prior to the beginning of the session.

Clinical Consideration

Never underestimate the far-reaching, therapeutic value of attentive and compassionate listening. A critical turning point in a client's healing journey can occur when he/she feels as if their story has been heard. The authors have experienced numerous times, over decades of practice, the client (and sometimes therapist) reduced to tears when the client discloses; *'you are the first care provider to take the time to, really, listen to my story'*. In that moment something within the client shifts, hope is sparked and where there is hope, change begins to unfold. Herein lies one of the unique aspects of a MT practice, the *luxury* of time. Our clinical structure differs from many forms of healthcare in that appointments are typically an hour long, providing the opportunity for clients to more thoroughly share the complexities of their experience. This, in combination with therapeutic touch, can impact the client in significant ways beyond the physical/functional value of the work.

Active listening intentionally focuses on the client. The therapist should be able to repeat back, in his/her own words, what the client has communicated, to the client's approval. This affirms that the therapist fully comprehends what the client has communicated and conveys to the client that his/her voice matters and that their perspective is of value (Study Guide and Strategies 2014).

Understanding the journey of the traumatic scar patient, empathizing and acknowledging the steps they have taken to recovery will build trust in the therapeutic relationship. As much as therapists may empathize with their clients and appreciate their pain conditions, therapists do not experience a client's pain in the same way the client does (Fitch 2014). The client description is meant to offer ways for the therapist to educate the clients on how the changes in their muscles, structures, posture, and quality of daily life can benefit from the therapeutic massage they are about to receive.

If a client is silent during the treatment, engage the client with questions on pressure, comfort and breath. Listen carefully with your ears and your hands to gather information for the session.

If you observe the client reacting to pressure by holding their breath or tension in their body (a protection mechanism), suspend the treatment immediately. Inquire about pressure, depth of touch and pain. Seek their guidance about how much pressure and depth they can tolerate without displaying this type of protective response. This process not only empowers the client and reaffirms the therapist's trustworthiness, it also presents an opportunity for the client to know what to expect from the therapeutic experience. By engaging the client in this way, the therapist teaches the client what to expect and knowing what to expect can greatly diminish any anxiety related to the *unexpected*, which is common in those who have experienced trauma (Fitch 2014). Additionally, as noted in Chapter 7, trauma survivors commonly experience PTSD-type presentations and stimulating the protection mechanism not only detracts

from the productiveness of the treatment, this also may trigger complex consequences for the client.

Clinical Consideration

As manual therapists, it is important that we adapt and respond to client needs immediately, during every treatment session. Client response varies from one client to the next and may vary from one session to the next. For example, you may work with two different burn survivors on similar parts of the body. Each one will bring their own interpretation of pain and experience of the traumatic event to the table and client interpretation can vary over the life-span of treatment. Each individual's expressed (verbal or non-verbal) response to treatment must be considered when formulating treatment protocol and ongoing treatment.

Interview Skills and Communication of Goals

One of the first questions a traumatic scar client should be asked is the reason for their visit. Some will answer that their doctor sent them; others may describe a pain, sensation, restriction or condition as the reason for the visit. Exploring those reasons will help to set up a conversation on goals.

Paying attention to the client's goals and wishes is an important key when working with someone with a traumatic scar. Recognizing and understanding how the client's quality of life has been altered is a springboard into discussing realistic therapeutic goals.

Learning to listen is often a difficult challenge for massage therapists. It is also about asking the right questions of clients to get them to open up about their real issues. This isn't psychotherapy but getting people to become more aware of their bodies –

Julie Onofrio, 31 March 2013

Each circumstance requires thoughtful questioning and active listening, not only during the first but at the beginning of every session. Quality of life may have changed since the last session; medication changes and new diagnosis should be fleshed out at the beginning of each session so alterations in the protocol can be made immediately.

Constructive questions that lead to the client's awareness of what they are presently feeling in the physical, physiological and internal areas of their body will help to focus the conversation on how the injury or traumatic scar tissue related impairments are manifesting on that given day (Fitch 2014). Simply asking, 'How is _____ manifesting in your body?', helps set a focus for the MT session and helps to springboard an end to the conversation and the beginning of the hands-on part of treatment.

Box 8.3

Interview example

Mary is a client with mastectomy scars on her right chest wall. She states she has pain in her neck, upper back and shoulder. Restriction of movement in her right shoulder limits her ability to move her steering wheel properly, reach for items above the first shelf in her kitchen and causes her issues with sleep.

After going through initial range of motion (ROM) and muscle testing assessments, I asked Mary about her medications. She was on two types of anti-depressants and narcotic pain medication.

Our conversation:

- Therapist (T): 'Mary, thank you for being patient during the assessment. Before we begin the session, I need to know more about your medications. Can you tell me what these medications are used for?'

- Mary: 'My oncologist put me on this anti-depressant after my breast cancer surgery. The other anti-depressant I've been taking since my daughter passed away a few years ago.'

- T: 'I'm sorry for your loss. How did this loss affect you physically?'

- Mary: 'I didn't move for months. It hurt too much.'

- T: 'It must have been difficult for you to do daily tasks.'

- Mary: 'Yes, it was.'

- T: 'What daily tasks are difficult for you now?'

- Mary: 'I would love to reach the second shelf in the kitchen. I would love to make a full rotation on my steering wheel in the truck. I would love to play softball again at the 4th of July picnic.'

- T: 'Those are great goals. Let's take them one by one. With the assessment, the scarring from the surgery is showing some restriction across your chest wall and is inhibiting the movement you use to reach. I would like to work on the chest wall scar tissue today and take some measurements to document the progress. If, at any time, you are uncomfortable or feel discomfort at any time, please let me know immediately. I never want to go beyond your pain threshold.'

- Mary: 'Ok. I'll let you know.'

Summary

Several pieces of information were gathered in this 4-minute conversation. Mary had a cancer diagnosis, the loss of a breast, huge quality of life change and the loss of a child within a short amount of time. Her medication side-effects cause muscle soreness and some tissue dehydration issues. Mary had also continued her pain medication 4 years after her surgery.

Listening to Mary and negotiating her treatment for the session empowered the therapeutic relationship we had started. Agreement was made on goals, treatment protocol and pain tolerance.

Box 8.4

According to Broas (2008), MT treatment for traumatic scarring requires five things in order to assure client sense of safety, comfort and acceptance of the session.

Our conversation:

- **Creating a container of safety**. Is your clinic environment pleasing, calming, free of distractions and potential hazards? Are window blinds drawn or secured in a manner that respects privacy? Has good rapport been established prior to commencing hands-on? The next step in creating a container of safety is to make meaningful contact with the client. Approach the area you are going to work on with the intention of kindness and respect. A light touch at first sends the signal of non-threatening, appropriate therapeutic touch.

- **Access and being attentive to the traumatic scarred area**. What is happening to the tissue? What is the response to the pressure and touch being used? Is there a hypersensitive response, no response? Ask questions during this time. How's the pressure? What are you noticing in your body when I'm working in this area? How does the area feel after some work has been provided? Ask the client what they are feeling in their body, in the area being treated and in general. Feedback not only helps the therapist guide delivery of care but also helps the client develop better body awareness.

- **Processing the therapy**. How is the client's posture during the treatment? Are they holding their breath? Are they stiffening under your touch? Do you notice any holding patterns? This is another great opportunity to ask questions on how their body is receiving and processing the work.

- **Transformation**. After negotiating the appropriate amount of pressure and technique, do you notice a change in the client's breathing? Has something changed in the tissue/area you are working?

- **Integration/completion**. Knowing when to say 'when' is key in working with traumatic scar tissue clients. Too little work and nothing changes in the tissue. Too much work and there could be damage to the tissues or the client could unnecessarily experience post-treatment soreness. The client may request you go deeper with the technique, or stay in the area longer. Professional discernment is key to avoiding the risk of over-treatment. Knowing when to leave an area and move on to another is crucial for the overall assimilation of the sessions work and helps to create a base to build on for the next session.

Interprofessional Collaboration

Interprofessional collaboration is a mutual and coordinated approach to shared decision-making around health and social issues (CIHC 2010).

The World Health Organization (WHO) defines collaborative practice in healthcare as occurring 'when multiple health workers from different professional backgrounds provide comprehensive services by working with patients, their families, caregivers and communities to deliver the highest quality of care across settings.'

Traumatic scar clients presenting with complex health needs and complex medical issues can be best served by interprofessional teams (Bridges et al. 2011). An interprofessional approach allows for the sharing of expertise and perspectives to form a common goal of restoring or maintaining an individual's health and improving outcomes (Barker & Oandasan 2005, Lumague et al. 2008, Bridges et al. 2011).

Patients receive safer, high quality care when health professionals work effectively in a team, communicate productively and understand each other's roles (Rao 2003, Morrison 2007, Bridges et al. 2011). Conversely, poor interprofessional collaboration can have a negative impact on the quality of patient care (Zwarenstein et al. 2005).

Successful collaborative interactions exhibit a blending of professional cultures and are achieved though cooperation, effective communication, knowledge and information sharing, collaborative decision-making and mutual trust and respect.

Understanding the professions of others and your own role in the healthcare team is critical. It is this partnership that creates an interprofessional team designed to work on common goals to improve patient outcomes (Bridges et al. 2011).

Skills in working as an interprofessional team, gained through interprofessional education, are important for high quality care. Training future healthcare providers to work in such teams will help facilitate this model resulting in improved healthcare outcomes for patients (Bridges et al. 2011).

In 1998, The College of Family Physicians in Canada published an article, the 'Physicians' perspective of massage therapy'(Verhoef & Page 1998) - citing:

> *Physicians demonstrated a discrepancy between their knowledge of MT and their opinions of, and referrals to, the profession. Physicians who referred patients to massage therapists generally held more positive opinions and had more knowledge of the discipline.*

Although a more heightened awareness of MT has come to fruition in the present day, it still often falls to the MT professional to educate clients and other medical professionals on the benefits of MT and what you as a professional can bring to the team. It is our professional responsibility to advocate on behalf of our clients and in order to further MT inclusion in interprofessional collaboration, we must all be keenly proactive.

Interprofessional Communication: Speak the Language

Across healthcare providers there exists variations in terminology and language when documenting and discussing patient outcomes. When working interprofessionally, it is important to become familiar with common or universal medical terms, whether writing progress notes, detailed reports or an introductory letter.

It is important to use proper medical terminology when communicating, written or verbal, with other healthcare professionals. When other healthcare providers become familiar with your expertise and understanding of the patients' needs, good interprofessional rapport will be established.

Various online medical terminology resources (e.g. http://www.medilexicon.com) and medical terminology/abbreviation apps are useful tools to assist with communication.

Referrals

For MTs, knowing when to refer to another MT, physiotherapist or mental health professional is an important part of client-centered care.

Join professional business organizations in your community to get to know others in your area. Gather information from your clients about their healthcare team and, with the clients consent, make contact through letters, emails or phone calls.

Open dialogue with your traumatic scar tissue client about the reason for the referral is very important. Explain in detail why you feel they should see a particular professional and how it will help them achieve their goals.

Referring a client to a mental health professional can take some navigation and finesse. If a client expresses symptoms of depression, a simple question of 'Do you feel you would benefit in speaking with a professional counselor or clergy?' may be appropriate. If you feel posing this type of question is inappropriate, leave cards of professionals you have a relationship with in your clinic room. Display them conspicuously before clients' appointments. If they are inclined to seek help, this gesture will be appreciated (see Box 8.5).

Box 8.5

Referral example

Tonya, a 21-year-old healthy woman, receives twice-monthly relaxation sessions with a focus on her shoulders.

Tonya always feels great after the sessions, but each session I observe extreme rounded shoulders and palpate adhesions in her platysma, subclavius, sternocleidomastoid (SCM) and anterior scalenes. For several visits inquiry is made as to her activities to try and pinpoint contributing factors. Tonya's response is always 'too much computer work.'

Then, during one session, without questioning or remarking on the adhesions, Tonya began to weep. I asked if she wanted me to stop. She said, 'No, but I have to tell you something – I think the reason for the adhesions is because I purge after every meal. I spend 20 minutes sometimes over the toilet. I can't seem to straighten up after that.'

She continued to cry as I held her head and again asked if she wanted to continue. She responds 'yes.' After the session, after making sure Tonya felt calm, I asked if she wanted to seek help from a professional. She said she would think about it. At our next session, I did not mention it nor did she. But she did take one of the psychotherapy business cards I left on the intake table.

Networking with massage therapists in your area and discovering their area of expertise or particular practice focus will enhance and assist your clients' care (see Box 8.6).

Box 8.6

Referral example

A common example of scar-related, intraprofessional referral occurs when working with someone living with cancer (Fitch 2014). Referring to another massage therapist that has vast experience or more advanced training in working with someone with cancer facilitates trust and appreciation in the therapeutic relationship.

Reaching out to your clients' healthcare team with progress notes and treatment plans will assist with future client referrals.

Additionally, advocating on behalf of your client can help reduce the individual's anxiety about seeing another care provider, help establish good interprofessional respect and affirm the therapist's commitment to client-centered care (see Box 8.7).

Box 8.7

Referral example

Jane experienced medical trauma following a severe motor vehicle accident in which she was involved as a child. Multiple injuries, addressed by numerous surgeries, resulted in extensive scarring that contributed to musculoskeletal impairments she experienced as an adult. Abrupt, forceful type treatment techniques (PT administered grade 4/5 mobilizations) triggered distress and subsequent protection mechanism fallout. She disclosed this during a MT treatment a couple of days after experiencing this and indicated that she was reluctant to receive further physiotherapy. I asked if she had spoken with the physical therapist about her experience. She said she had not. I discussed with Jane why it is important to share this kind

Box 8.7 (Cont.)

of information with a care provider, that such information is appreciated by the therapist as it an important consideration for the provision of safe and effective treatment. She agreed. I asked if she was comfortable speaking directly with the PT and if not, with her consent, I would be willing to advocate on her behalf.

A collaborative, client-centered approach is key to the delivery of ethical, high quality healthcare.

A number of components factor into the individual providers delivery of ethical high quality care: establishing and maintaining professional therapeutic relationships; sound clinical decision-making; and the provision of evidence-informed/based practices. Throughout this book, clinical and pathophysiological considerations have been provided as a basis for evidence. In the next chapter assessment procedures and treatment protocols will be provided to help guide sound clinical decision-making and treatment planning in order to achieve consistently safe and predictable clinical outcomes.

References

Andrade CK, Clifford P (2012) In: Dryden T, Moyer C (eds) Massage therapy: integrating research and practice. Human Kinetics, p. 31.

Andrade CK (2013) Outcome-based massage: putting evidence into practice. Baltimore: Lippincott Williams & Wilkins.

Barker K, Oandasan I (2005) Interprofessional care review with medical residents: lessons learned, tensions aired – a pilot study. Journal of Interprofessional Care 19: 207–14.

Bridges D, Davidson R, Soule-Odegard P et al (2011) Interprofessional collaboration: three best practice models of interprofessional education. Medical Education Online 16: 6035. Doi: 10.3402/meo.v16i0.6035.

Broas M (2008) The theory and practice of sensorimotor psychotherapy. Lecture notes from Trauma and the Body Conference, Gainesville, Florida.

Brown B (2010) TEDx talk: The power of vulnerability - Brené Brown, June 2010. Available at: http://www.ted.com/talks/brene_brown_on_vulnerability.

CIHC (Canadian Interprofessional Health Collaborative) (2010) A national interprofessional competency framework; February 2010. Available at: http://www.cihc.ca/files/CIHC_IPCompetencies_Feb1210.pdf [Accessed 31 May 2015].

Corey G, Corey MS, Callanan P (2006) Issues and ethics in the helping professions, 7e. Pacific Grove, CA: Wadsworth Publishing.

CPTO (College of Physiotherapists of Ontario) (2013) Guide to therapeutic relationships and professional boundaries. Available at: http://www.collegept.org/Assets/registrants'guideenglish/standards_framework/standards_practice_guides/Therapeutic_Relationships_Prof_Boundaries_Guide130527.pdf [Accessed 31 May 2015].

Fitch P (2005) Scars of life. The Journal of Soft Tissue Manipulation, Summer, p 3.

Fitch P (2014) Talking body, listening hands: a guide to professionalism, communication and the therapeutic relationship. Upper Saddle River, NJ: Prentice Hall.

Foley JW (n.d.) Drop a pebble in the water. Available at: http://www.ripplemaker.com/pebbles.htm [Accessed 26 March 2015].

Free Medical Dictionary (2015) Available at: http://medical-dictionary.thefreedictionary.com/informed+consent[Accessed 31 May 2015].

Fritz S (2013) Mosby's Fundamentals of therapeutic massage, 5th edn. Mosby, pp 45–46.

Grigorovich A, Gomez M, Leach L, Fish J (2013) Impact of posttraumatic stress disorder and depression on neuropsychological functioning in electrical injury survivors. Journal of Burn Care and Research 34 (6): 659–665.

Kluft RP, Bloom SL, Kinzie JD (2000) Treating traumatized patients and victims of violence. New Directions for Mental Health Services (86): 79–102.

Lumague M, Morgan A, Mak D et al (2008) Interprofessional education: the student perspective. Journal of Interprofessional Care 20: 246–53.

Morrison S (2007) Working together: why bother with collaboration? Work Bas Learn Prim Care 5: 65–70.

Rao R (2003) Dignity and impudence: how should medical students acquire and practice clinical skills for use with older people? Medical Education 37: 190–1.

Study Guide and Strategies (2014) Study Guides and strategies-active listening. http://www.studygs.net/listening.htm [Accessed 11 December 2014].

Verhoef MJ, Page SA (1998) Physicians' perspectives on massage therapy. Canadian Family Physician 44: 1018.

Zwarenstein M, Reeves S, Perrier L (2005) Effectiveness of pre-licensure interprofessional education and post-licensure collaborative interventions. Journal of Interprofessional Care 2005 19: 148–65.

Assessment and treatment

Healing is a matter of time, but it is sometimes also a matter of opportunity

Hippocrates

When considering therapeutic strategies to improve or restore damaged tissues, it is crucial to realize that most wound-healing pathologies are due to a combination of underlying systemic disease (e.g. diabetes) and/or regional and anatomical factors that cause undue mechanical tension (Eming et al. 2014). Although treating pathologies is outside our scope of practice, influencing mechanical tension is most certainly and clearly massage therapy (MT) territory. Control of tissue tension or tone is predominantly mediated by the nervous system and the integrin/mechanotransduction pathway, and so techniques that interface with these regulators are our ticket 'in'.

In addition to existing pathologies, outcomes following wounding (planned or unplanned) vary depending on the injured tissue type, the type and extent of trauma or injury, and genetic factors. The impact on the client can range from a mild functional deficit to biopsychosocially debilitating. Poor cosmetic or disfigurement, emotional and functional outcomes can extol a heavy economic burden as a result of direct cost of care or due to future readmissions and surgeries. In the US alone, adhesion-related health costs exceed $1 billion annually (ASRM Committee 2013, Fourie 2014).

Facilitating the healing of planned and unplanned wounds and injuries and minimizing the aesthetic and/or cosmetic, emotional and functional impact on the patient constitutes a central focus of clinical care (Eming et al. 2014). Facilitating the healing process and restoring function are elements that fall squarely into the realm of MT efficacy – the ability to make a difference or direct change. Minimization of the aesthetic impact presents multiple considerations, some of which may be improved by MT. The most notable of these is early intervention to improve scar quality and, subsequently, how this may impact the client's emotional state. And in all cases, measures taken to minimize or prevent the occurrence of pathophysiological scars is in every patient's best interest.

Sadly, however, it is most likely that several days, weeks, months or even years will pass before we treat the client for the first time. Access to the client may be hindered while they are in hospital or other treatment centers, post-trauma referrals for MT still lag and, simply, it may not occur to the individual that MT could be a valuable part of their post-trauma care.

On a grand scale, it is the authors' intention that outlining an evidence-informed approach will serve to improve delivery of care and outcomes, support the acknowledgment and inclusion of MT as a viable component in scar management and, most importantly, ensure that those in need have access to and receive the safe and effective MT treatment that could make a tremendous difference in their trauma recovery.

Previous chapters have provided a solid base for understanding traumatic scar tissue, its formation, physiological tissue changes, structural changes and the psychosocial issues that may or may not present with the traumatic scar tissue client. Additionally, throughout the book, clinical considerations have been interjected as a means to create a nexus, linking science (evidence base) to our work in the treatment room.

The aim of this chapter is to provide a solid, evidence-informed approach to scar assessment procedures and scar management protocols that take into consideration the unique, MT clinical environment.

The assessment approach and treatment protocols presented in this book are supported by basic science, current research, the authors' (collective) 45+ years of clinical practice and other clinician's important work. Much effort has been taken to ensure the safety and advisability of the information provided; however, it is possible to injure people by performing almost any type of intervention. This is more likely when a procedure is performed without judicious precautions, or when the recipient of the intervention has unique biological or other factors that make them more vulnerable to negative reactions/responses to MT. Additionally, sometimes people have a negative reaction to MT that is wholly unpredictable, or their health becomes compromised at the same time an intervention is performed or shortly thereafter as a result of unrelated factors.

An evidence-based approach to practice is not solely about using the best research evidence to choose and apply our therapeutic actions – it also means using our clinical expertise and it fully embraces the importance of and incorporates what our clients' value from us (Sackett et al. 2000). See Box 9.1.

The authors encourage further learning to support how best to practice in an evidence-based informed way – incorporating the best available scientific evidence and blending that with your client's unique biological factors, needs and desires, and your own clinical judgment. Some suggested resources for further learning can be found in the Appendix, p. 255.

Box 9.1

Evidence-based and evidence-informed practice

In practice it is desirable to be as evidence-based as possible, and evidence-informed when definitive evidence does not exist. Evidence-informed practice includes:

- Practice knowledge and experience
- Opinions of colleagues and other professionals
- Wishes and experience of clients and
- Evidence from research in massage or other similar disciplines.

Evidence can be used to:

- Explain and justify reasons for a decision relating to a treatment approach
- Help choose between different approaches
- Explain the potential benefits that MT may provide to a particular client and
- Raise your awareness about a condition or illness.

(Adapted from Fritz 2013)

Traumatic Scars and Associated Impairments

Before we discuss assessment and treatment, we need to identify what we are assessing and treating. In clarifying the focus of this book, it is important to make a distinction between postsurgical abdominal and visceral adhesions and the authors' defined traumatic scars. Postsurgical abdominal/visceral adhesions and manual visceral work are not discussed as the authors' acknowledge that this area is comprehensively covered elsewhere.

This is not to imply that we do not address the abdominal region; as a region it is addressed, but the work is directed to the skin, fascia, muscles, vessels and nerves rather than, specifically, the adherences between viscera and articulating tissues and structures.

Clinical Consideration

One important note on postsurgical abdominal and visceral adhesions is made by Chapelle. In personal email correspondence, in her research with Bove, she indicated that:

> … no specific time course for intervention has been clearly identified; however, it appears that adhesion formation occurs 6–12 hours after surgery. Early manual mobilization is a hypothesis of prevention – keep things moving to avoid adherence and subsequent complications. Mostly, once established, adhesions are difficult to affect.

Seems the old adage applies – an ounce (manual mobilization) of prevention outweighs a pound (subsequent surgical lysing) of cure. One can reasonably surmise that 'keeping things moving' as a means to prevent adherences can also apply to other tissues and the sliding layers between tissues and structures.

As massage therapists we are not called upon, nor is it within our scope of practice, to treat medical conditions and illnesses (e.g. diabetes, cancer) or acute critical trauma. Our primary role is to provide treatment that is designed to facilitate the wound-healing process or elicit a desired change in consequent complications in the form of impairments, such as any loss in body function or abnormal body structures that occur as a result of a medical condition or trauma (Andrade & Clifford 2008, Andrade 2013, Dryden & Moyer 2012).

Specific to this book are impairments associated with pathophysiological scars, such as adherences, contractures, fibrosis, postural and movement adaptations, edema, pain, anxiety, sympathetic nervous system (SNS)-hyperarousal, disturbed sleep and altered or impaired body awareness, which are representative of the realm of considerations that accompany the aftermath of trauma and poor wound healing outcomes.

Clinical Consideration

Reduction of anxiety and musculoskeletal pain are among the most established outcomes for massage (Moyer et al. 2009).

Clinical Consideration

In a cancer patient study it was determined that while both healing touch and massage lowered anxiety and pain, massage also reduced the need for pain medicine (Post-White et al. 2003).

Clinical Consideration

MT has been found to be effective for reducing burn-related depression, pain, pruritus and state anxiety, and positively impacting scar characteristics such as thickness, melanin deposition, erythema, transdermal water loss, and elasticity/tissue mobility (Eti et al. 2006, Roh et al. 2007, Goutos et al. 2009, Gürol et al. 2010, Cho et al. 2014).

Clinical Consideration

It is hypothesized that massage can impact cellular structural and signaling milieu, thereby inducing beneficial effects through the ability to affect fibroblast apoptosis and remodeling (Derderian et al. 2005, Bhadal et al. 2008, Chan et al. 2010, Cho et al. 2014).

Clinical Consideration

Massage can help soften and desensitize scars. When combined with stretching, massage can make the scar looser, softer and more comfortable (MSKTC 2011).

Clinical Reasoning

Over the life-span of our MT practice, we will work with clients with all types of scars at various stages of formation and in a variety of settings. Different scar types and stage of formation requires specific treatment considerations. Additionally, the extensive range of settings makes MT available to wide-ranging population that includes those in frail health, those in overall great health, and those somewhere in between. And as such this requires massage therapists to weigh multifactorial considerations and adjust treatment protocol accordingly (Walton 2011).

In order to generate, implement and evaluate care, a sound reasoning process must be carried out. When working with scar tissue clients all clinical reasoning components apply: client health history and interview; physical assessment and scar evaluation; treatment planning; choosing methods to implement the treatment plan; and record keeping/documentation (Fritz 2013).

Health History and Interview

A standard health history form that covers musculoskeletal, neurological, cardiopulmonary, psychological and psychoneuroimmunologic information provides a good starting point for more detailed conversation with your client.

Specific to traumatic scar clients, it will be important to gather further detailed information about the extent of the injuries and any procedures, surgeries and postsurgical complications (e.g. infection, prolonged inflammation, delayed healing) they experienced and subsequent care provided, including medications.

Medications

If you are seeing a client for the first time, ask them to bring their list of medications. Ask the client what the medications are for and if they are experiencing any known side-effects. Then, make sure you look up each medication yourself. Some medications may have side-effects that will have a direct effect on manipulation of the tissue and some that perhaps the client is unaware of – ones that may be the cause of the symptoms the client is experiencing. A classic example is the spectrum of statin medications prescribed for high cholesterol (e.g. Lipitor and Crestor) as potential sources of muscle pain, tenderness and weakness.

If your client is on pain medication, ask them how often they take it and if the prescribed dose was taken prior to the session as this would alter the client's perception of what they are experiencing during the session. As an example, you may ask about pressure being used and they may say 'fine' or 'you can go deeper.' Because the client's pain perception is altered, be sure to take the necessary precautions. When in doubt, please remember less is more.

Clinical Consideration

Anything that suppresses inflammatory response potentially impacts the healing process. The use of anti-inflammatory medication can be helpful and

Clinical Consideration (Cont.)

necessary at times; however, with regard to the healing process, there are potential 'negative' considerations (Cohen et al. 2006, Magra & Maffulli 2006, Tortland 2007, Van den Berg 2012), most notably the impact on tissues that are less vascular (e.g. tendons, ligaments and fascial attachments). This negative effect on healing also results from analgesic medication because the individual is likely to be confused by masked pain levels and so exceeds load on healing tissues – further impacting the natural healing process.

Record Keeping and Documentation

Keeping a record of client care is a requirement for professional healthcare providers.

Documenting client expressed concerns, therapist findings and treatment outcomes supports sound clinical decision-making (Fitch 2014). The more thorough and complete the client record is, the easier it is for the therapists to make sound protocol decisions.

Record the date, time and length of each session and include all correspondence from a referral or other health care professionals and any diagnostic information, such as X-ray, computed tomography scan, MRI and ultrasound reports.

Traumatic events may result in unique and unusual considerations; for example, metal pins and plates, staples and/or sutures may be present in the tissue. During the initial intake, be sure to gather as much information as possible about the presenting condition(s) (Tappan & Benjamin 1998). Ask the client to bring a copy of their surgical report(s) so you can understand which muscle or muscle groups were affected so you may proceed safely. Prior knowledge of any surrounding muscle structures that were altered during surgery, hardware used and medications

given is important in order to provide safe and effective treatment.

Documentation should be made for each session and should be transparent and clear; so much so that another care provider could read your notes and have an understanding of your procedures and protocol for the client. Use standard, accepted professional clinical intake forms (e.g. patient health history, disability index, range of movement (ROM) charts, postural scan), abbreviations and terminology in your notes. If you do create your own form of shorthand, make a chart of those abbreviations for the file (Fitch 2014).

Remember, too, that regular communication with the client's healthcare team is critical for optimal and ethical client-centered care.

Assessment and Evaluation

It is important that healthcare professionals use up-to-date information and tools to guide clinical decision-making. Simple, valid and reliable assessment and evaluation methods will help the therapist to proceed with confidence in providing safe and effective care, tracking progress and then communicating results to stakeholders (e.g. the client, other care providers, benefit providers) (Gowan-Moody 2011).

Outcome measurement, the systematic collection and analysis of information, is used to evaluate the efficacy of a treatment intervention (Clark & Gironda 2002, Gowan-Moody 2011). An important idea in health sciences' research on efficacy is that the outcomes measured are client- or patient-centered; namely, pain, function, quality of life and satisfaction with care (Philadelphia Panel 2001, Gowan-Moody 2011).

Professional MTs must continually ask if their care is safely and effectively aiding in the resolution or management of the client's presenting concerns and issues. As clinicians we need to have valid, reliable and responsive tools to establish a baseline and monitor change as a result of our treatment. Using these simple tools also aids in identifying appropriate dose-related variables, such as the frequency, duration and number of treatments required to achieve clinically significant outcomes (Ezzo 2007, Gowan-Moody 2011).

Outcome measures are also invaluable for the therapist wishing to write and publish case reports and case series, and also for those wishing to engage in clinical audit.

Assessment and evaluation procedures for traumatic scar tissue clients will encompass the usual spectrum: palpation, local and global functional assessment (including postural and movement evaluation); neurological and special tests; and any measures to evaluate impact on activities of daily living. All assessment and evaluation information is to be properly documented in the client's file.

Standard assessment and evaluation procedures will not be included in this book; however, certain key points with particular relevance to traumatic scars will be provided.

Assessment and evaluation will vary depending upon the stage of healing and if we are gathering information about the scar itself, the tissue around the scar or the scar-associated impairments.

In general, consideration of the client's emotional state, traumatic scar tissue and surrounding and underlying tissues, and any compensatory presentations, need to be evaluated and documented before and after each treatment session.

Observation

There are many layers to traumatic scar tissue – somatic and psychological and therefore observing client behavior is an essential part of assessment (Fitch 2014). For proper assessment and evaluation, the MT needs to pick up cues from verbal and non-verbal communication.

Tone of voice, body language, posture and physiological responses give us valuable clues about how the traumatic scar tissue client is feeling. Add to this, the quality of the client's tissue, their posture, how they respond to your questions and touch let you know what their comfort level is that particular day.

> *The most important thing in communication is hearing what isn't being said. The art of reading between the lines is a lifelong quest of the wise.*
>
> Shannon L. Alder

Words transmit one dimension of information through language. Non-verbal communication can give multiple messages that can be both deliberate and outside the conscious awareness of the client (Fitch 2014).

The ability to read non-verbal messages from traumatic scar tissue clients is a complex skill and takes time. A pioneer in the study of non-verbal communication, psychologist Albert Mehrabian conducted fascinating research on communication and how it is received. According to Mehrabian, the receiver interprets the communication based on the following (adapted from Fitch 2014):

- 7% verbal (the actual words spoken)

- 38% par verbal – this encompasses tone and pitch of the voice with other vocal sounds

- 55% non-verbal – body language, facial expressions, stance and posture, and hand gestures.

Observation plays an important role in the assessment process because posture, behaviors, attitudes, emotional state and associated affect contribute to the health or lack of health of the client (Fitch 2014).

Keep in mind that the therapist's interpretation of the client's non-verbal and verbal communication can help to clarify a clinical impression, but interpretation is subjective. It is important to confirm impressions with the client and alter the clinical observation as needed.

Be mindful that therapist-to-client communication also occurs in a direct/physical manner via our hands and in an indirect/energetic manner through our touch and that this conveys our presence, state or mood.

Posture and Movement

Observe the client as they enter your treatment room. Watch their walk, how they hold their purse, briefcase; what is the body trying to tell you? It is possible to observe imbalances and asymmetries that the client carries daily if you pay attention to their postural cues.

Traumatic scar tissue may have adhesion tentacles that reach in any direction and depth. And

Box 9.2

The MT's ability to use their senses analytically to collect information involves three key concepts:

- **The ability to visualize what is happening in your client's body**. *For example*: you observe scar tissue from a burn injury that has enveloped the client's upper thoracic region. Can you envision how scarring in this area might affect the client's movement and activities of daily living? In addition to the more obvious shoulder range of movement (ROM) issues, how might the scarring relate to the client's other expressed complaint of low back pain? Could the limitation of arm swing be altering her gait? In addition to observing straight-up shoulder ROM assessment, consider if she is limited in her ability to wash her hair, reach for items above her head or put on her car seat-belt? The ability to visualize can often lead the therapist to ask important questions as the client may not readily provide some information.

- **The ability to listen critically**. Critical listening, a form of critical analysis, is fundamental to learning. Listening critically involves analyzing or evaluating the information received, and ultimately formulating an opinion that will reinforce good critical thinking, informed decision-making and problem-solving. When listening critically it is important to keep an open mind and not be biased by preconceived ideas and personal judgments. *For example:* a client is describing the impact on her body from sitting at a computer for 8 hours a day. Your questions seem to illicit the same responses you have heard from other clients in a similar situation. You find yourself not listening because you've heard it before (a preconception), thereby blocking the ability to listen fully and comprehend the information in a critical manner and perhaps in ways that you learn something new even though the client's response *sounds* the same (Lewis 2015).

- **Touch/palpate with a critical eye and hands**. Palpation provides important information on tissue: structure, form, density and mobility. Continuous evaluation during the session is important. What is different several minutes into a treatment in comparison with when the treatment started? What is happening in the surrounding structures, when the tissue under your hands is palpated? Like critical listening, critical palpation requires us to not preconceive. Approach each session with an open mind and hands; what was true for the client in the last session may not manifest in the next session.

(Fitch 2014)

even seemingly minimally invasive key-hole incisions can result in adhesion formation that may result in chronic pain, obstruction and functional deficits (Lee et al. 2008). *For example*: a teenage ballet dancer with a small appendectomy scar complains of difficulty in raising the leg on the side of the scar. Ask the client to demonstrate the movement. Is there compensation for the pain? How is her posture? Consider which muscles are involved in that movement (e.g. iliopsoas, quadratus abdominis, gluteal muscles, abdominals). Are adherences impacting the intestines? Ask the client if they are having bowel or voiding problems. This will give you the necessary answers about depth and length of the scar, and adhesions, without benefit of an ultrasound or other imaging technique, although access to diagnostic reports is helpful.

Take these observations with you when the traumatic scar tissue client is on the table. Check the height of the hips, length of the legs, shoulder elevation, head tilt and skin color around the scarred area. Note your observations for reference post-session.

Palpation

Palpation assessment ought to include the scar itself and surrounding and associated tissue. Often certain local observations are made along with palpation. A method of tracking progress is to measure and document palpable and observable pre-treatment presentations and post-treatment changes. Palpation assessment includes soft tissue barrier evaluation (covered in more detail later in this chapter).

Scar Assessment and Evaluation

When assessing the scar itself, note what the scar feels like – is it smooth, rough, lumpy, hard, pliable, stiff? Is the tissue mobile, pliable, dense or thickened? Upon challenge does the nearby tissue dimple or pucker; can strain be seen in nearby or distant tissues? Is the scar region tender, sensitive?

Scar evaluation and documentation considerations include:

- Age of the scar (mature, immature)

- Location of the scar (near/across joint margins, visible/hidden by clothing)

- Incision line features (thick or thin, linear or tortuous)

- Feel of the scar (lumpy, elevated, hard, thickened)

- Scar color/discoloration (e.g. redness or blanching/banding with stretch and movement)

- Scar temperature (hot, warm, cold)

- Scar and surrounding tissue pliability, mobility

- Strain exerted on surrounding tissue

- Any pain associated with the scar (local and referred)

- Pruritus.

Standardized, valid and reliable assessment tools (measurement instruments) can be utilized to assist the MT with monitoring changes in scar quality and evaluating the effectiveness of treatment (see Box 9.3).

Pre-treatment assessment/evaluation and documentation

Before starting the treatment session, measure the width, length and, if possible, the depth of the scar above the skin. This can be done with a simple measuring tape. The same tape measure can be used to measure volume of edema. Pre- and post-volume measurements are a great indicator of how effective the protocol is for reducing edema.

Box 9.3

Scar assessment tools

As with other assessment procedures, scar assessments can be objective or subjective. Objective assessments provide a quantitative measurement of the scar, whereas subjective assessments are observer dependent.

Quantitative assessment of scars requires devices to measure their physical attributes. Subjective methods to assess scar provide a qualitative measurement of scar by a patient or clinician.

Semiquantitative methods to assess scars have been developed by using scales to make subjective methods more objective.

Scar scales

Scar scales can be used to quantify initial scar appearance and track changes over time. There are currently five commonly used scar scales designed to assess subjective parameters in an objective way: the Vancouver Scar Scale (VSS), Manchester Scar Scale (MSS), Patient and Observer Scar Assessment Scale (POSAS), Visual Analog Scale (VAS) and Stony Brook Scar Evaluation Scale (SBSES). These observer-dependent scales are best used to determine change within an individual rather than between individuals.

None of these scar scales measure:

- Amount of total body surface area that is scarred
- Functional disability caused by the effects of pain and pruritus
- Subsequent impact on quality of life and activities of daily living.

Therefore it is recommended that no one assessment tool be used exclusively as several tools will be necessary in order to capture all the necessary information needed to monitor changes and evaluate treatment effectiveness.

Three of the most accessible and appropriate scales for use in MT practice include the POSAS, the VSS and the VAS. PDF copies of these scales and instructions on how to use them can be readily found on the internet.

POSAS

POSAS is aimed at measuring the quality of scar tissue and includes a comprehensive list of items, based on clinically relevant scar characteristics. The observer scores: vascularization, pigmentation, thickness, surface roughness, pliability and surface area. The patient scores: pain, pruritus, color, thickness, relief, and pliability.

All included items are scored on a 10-point scale:

- 1 is given when the scar characteristic is comparable to 'normal skin'
- 10 reflects the 'worst imaginable scar'.

All items are summed to give a total scar score and, therefore, a higher score represents a poorer scar quality (van der Wal et al. 2012, POSAS Group 2015).

(Continued)

Box 9.3 (Continued)

POSAS can be used to assess burn, keloid and linear scars (e.g. surgical and hypertrophic).

VSS

Specific to burn scars, VSS assesses four variables: vascularity, height/thickness, pliability and pigmentation. Unlike POSAS, patient perception is not factored in to the overall score. VSS is typically used to evaluate therapy and measure outcomes in burn studies.

VAS

VAS, a photograph-based scale derived from evaluating standardized digital photographs, correlates intraobserver, photographic and histologic findings.

VAS is used to assess pigmentation, vascularity, contour and texture. It sums the individual scores to get a single overall score ranging from excellent to poor. VAS can be used to assess burn and linear scars.

Devices to objectively quantify scars (Fearmonti et al. 2010)

Various devices are available to assess parameters such as pliability, firmness, color, perfusion, thickness, and 3-dimensional topography. Although most of these devices are not likely to be on hand in a MT clinic nor within our scope of practice, this information is provided simply to *inform*. Such devices may be available to massage therapists in a research environment.

Pliability

Two of the most popular tools used to assess pliability are the pneumatonometer and cutometer:

- Pneumatonometer: uses pressure to objectively measure skin pliability.
- Cutometer: is a non-invasive suction device that measures the viscoelasticity of the skin by analyzing its vertical deformation in response to negative pressure. It has been used to measure the effects of treatments on burn scars and to assess scar maturation.

Firmness

The durometer applies a vertically-directed indentation load on the scar to measure tissue firmness. Originally described for use in scleroderma, it has since been applied to the analysis of induration in burn scar assessment,

Color

Tools that objectively measure scar color include the Chromameter®, DermaSpectrometer®, Mexameter®, and the Tristimulus colorimeter. These devices use spectrophotometric color analysis to calculate erythema and melanin index.

Thickness

Ultrasound scanners, such as the tissue ultrasound palpation system (TUPS), have been used to quantify scar thickness. The primary drawback with ultrasonography is that it requires technical training and experience in image interpretation and is relatively expensive compared to other modalities.

Box 9.3 (Continued)

Perfusion

Laser Doppler perfusion imaging is an established technique for the measurement of burn scar perfusion that aids in early determination of burn depth and subsequent treatment course. Laser Doppler perfusion imaging offers a non-invasive alternative to burn wound biopsy.

3-dimensional topography

3-dimensional systems capture scar surface characteristics with high definition and reproducibility.

One benefit of the digital age is that most of us own some form of instant photo-taking device, making it relatively easy to document your client's progress with photographs of their scar. If possible, document different angles pre- and post-session. Depending on your professional judgment, photographs at every session may be necessary; or pictures every third session may give you a better understanding of the body's adaptation to the scar release. This of course is done with your client's permission. If a cell phone is used to take photos it is recommended that any client photos are downloaded off the phone on to a more secure device, for the sake of preserving client confidentiality.

Another useful pre-treatment measurement tool is to ask the client to provide body awareness information once they are on the treatment table. Ask them to check-in with their body and notice any areas of discomfort or any other sensation they may feel (compressed, tight, body region not making contact with the table) and identify any movement that elicits pain, restriction, nerve sensations or paresthesia.

During and post-treatment assessment/ evaluation and documentation

Periodically, during treatment and at the conclusion of the session, ask your client to repeat any movement that is restricted or that elicits sensations (pain or paresthesia). Note any change in movement quality and movement range. What changes does the client feel? Post-treatment, repeat the measurements and photos. Compare the results. Did your protocol for the session result in measureable/visible changes? If not, consider what might need to be done differently in the next session? If there have been changes, consider what client home or selfcare measures will be productive in supporting treatment outcome sustainability and progress.

Note the pressure used during the session and apply standardized outcome measures to track the progress of the client goals and therapist-intended outcomes.

Progress can be measured in a number of ways:

- Pain changes (less, none, intermittent versus constant, location)

- Functional changes (more functional with less discomfort during activity and/or less discomfort following activity – client's will often describe this as 'less having to pay for it')

- Agitation (recurrence) occurs less frequently

- Agitation (recurrence) is less intense

- Recuperates or recovers more quickly after agitations

- Client self-management strategies are more productive.

Connective Tissue (Ct) and Fascia/Myofascia Assessment and Evaluation

Widespread use of medical diagnostic testing specific to identifying/assessing CT and fascia (encompassing skin, superficial fascia (SF), deep fascia (DF) and the myofascial envelopes) dysfunction is essentially non-existent (Prendergast & Rummer 2012).

However, some CT and fascia researchers and clinicians (e.g. Fourie, Langevin, Pohl, Rodríguez & del Río and the Steccos, to name a few) are now using ultrasonography to measure the structure and organization of the CT network – in normal and pathological states and to visualize pre- and post-treatment changes in tissue density and glide. The ability to visualize moving (or not) live tissue and to substantiate positive pre/post tissue changes is of profound importance to the manual therapy fields.

Soft tissue mobility and barriers

In terms of CT and fascia assessment/evaluation and treatment, one fundamental component is determining and evaluating tissue *barrier* and *bind*.

Similar to joints, soft tissues also have a specified range of available mobility (Andrade 2013). But unlike joint ROM testing, no instrument exists (goniometer, inclinometer) for soft tissue barrier assessment/evaluation.

Barrier is defined as the point where the therapist perceives the first slight resistance to their manually applied tissue challenge (Lewit & Olsanska 2004). Engaging barrier is commonly used as both an assessment/evaluation and treatment method. Barrier as a treatment method is covered in more detail later in this chapter.

In the context of an assessment/evaluation method, soft tissue barriers can be classified as either normal or pathological (Table 9.1).

Normal soft tissue has three barriers: physiologic (normal, available tissue range); elastic (barrier reached when all available tissue slack is taken-up); and anatomic (final resistance to normal ROM beyond this barrier will result in tissue damage). Pathological barriers occurring in skin, CT, fascia, muscles and other soft tissues are associated with tissue dysfunction, such as adhesions and scars. Pathological barriers change the quality and availability of movement and can lead to dysfunctional movement patterns (Andrade 2013) – see Table 9.1.

Bind

Once barrier is reached or surpassed, tissues shift from a state of relative ease when challenged by therapist-applied motion/glide to a state of bind. Skin and fascia display increased bulk, firmness and tension when bind is reached (Pilat 2003, Fritz 2013).

Local and global assessment and evaluation considerations

One of the most difficult or complex aspects of assessment is putting all the pieces together to create a complete picture of what is happening in order to deliver comprehensive treatment that will result in sustainable outcomes.

In terms of scar-associated impairments, the authors have found it useful to begin by addressing local concerns and eventually map out and address the bigger, global picture.

Once a scar is fully matured, manual manipulation may not be effective in changing the physicality or aesthetics of the scar. However, over-use type impairments that occur as a result of restrictions at the scar site are amenable to MT. As noted in the opening of this chapter, one aspect of care that massage therapists provide is treatment of impairments that occur as a result of traumatic scars. Generally speaking this is the type of care provided for chronic or long-standing scars (see Box 9.4).

With each client create an individual 'body story' by documenting all your findings: visual observation, palpation, objective findings and

Normal barrier	Pathological barrier
Three normal barriers: • Physiologic (normal, available tissue range) • Elastic (barrier reached when all available tissue slack is taken-up) • Anatomic (final resistance to normal range, motion beyond this barrier will result in tissue damage)	Pathological barriers occurring in skin, CT, fascia, muscles and other soft tissues are associated with tissue dysfunction, such as adhesions and scars. Pathological barriers change the quality and availability of movement and can lead to dysfunctional movement patterns
Is gradual	Is abrupt – like hitting a wall of resistance
When engaged, the therapist will feel: • Some tissue give/springyness • Tissue is mobile/pliable	When engaged the therapist will notice: • The feel of little or no give/springyness • Tissue feels stiff, dense • Observable dimpling or other irregularities, like lines or planes of adherence
When engaged the client tends to feel: • No pain • Slight to moderate pressure • Possible slight to moderate prickling sensation	When engaged the client may feel moderate to strong: • Pain or varying degrees of discomfort • Prickling • Burning • Tingling • Itching

Table 9.1

Comparative of normal and pathological barrier

Box 9.4

Over-use/impairment example (Ryan 2013)

When we are not able to change the scar itself, we still may be able to significantly impact the client's pain and assist with improving function.

At the Level I Fascial Manipulation (FM) training in Vancouver 2013, Dr Antonio Stecco was asked about the effectiveness of FM in treating scoliosis. Stecco's approach to treating scoliosis is to address the over-use type impairments that occur as a result of the spinal deviation, and is not specifically aimed at correcting the deviation.

Stecco shared one of his clinical cases and used an X-ray image to illustrate this. The X-ray showed a patient with a dramatic, 87° spinal deviation. Prior to treatment by Stecco, the patient had experienced significant neck, headache and low back pain, resulting in missed work time and preventing her from engaging in recreational activities. Following FM treatment the patient was able to function (return to work and resume activities of daily living and sport/recreation) with significantly less pain.

(Continued)

Box 9.4 (Continued)

When asked about how much the actual curvature of her spine changed post FM treatment, Stecco replied:

There was no significant change in the degree of her scoliosis following treatment. Scoliosis [spinal deviation] is not necessarily correlated with pain. With this patient, there are 3 important components to look at; the scoliosis, hyperkyphosis and hyperlordosis. The impact of the spinal deviations essentially present as 'overuse' type syndromes in the paraspinal and other associated musculature's sliding mechanism, which appears to be the predominant source of the presenting musculoskeletal pain and dysfunction. This patient still experiences some low back pain but not at the debilitating degree she experienced prior to FM treatment (e.g. missing time at work, stopping all activity). Occasional use of paracetamol (mild analgesic) (2–3 times a month) manages her back pain well, while FM treatment 2–3 times a year effectively addresses her [compensatory] neck pain. Following treatment she experiences no neck pain between treatments and her episodes of neck pain are occurring less frequently and are quicker to resolve.

client subjective account. Locally assess which components may factor into the client's presenting impairments and consequent pain and dysfunction.

Clinical Consideration

Chronic and/or fully matured scars, much like significant spinal deviations, may not be significantly changed by manual manipulation. However, much like Stecco's approach to working with scoliosis (see Box 9.5), treating the scar-mediated impairment can result in changes that positively impact the client's pain and functional deficits.

Thinking about and putting a global approach into action will ultimately assist the client in achieving more sustainable outcomes. As noted in Chapter 2, myokinetic or myofascial chains/meridians are a grouping or sequence of tissues and structures – structurally and neurologically linked together to support functional and perceptive continuity. Restriction or fixation at any point along the chain/meridian can impact function at distant segments resulting in tensional compensations along the chain/meridian. Additionally, antagonistic chains/meridian components can be impacted, and often are.

Myers' *Anatomy Trains* (2013) and the Steccos' *Fascial Manipulation for Musculoskeletal Pain and Fascial Manipulation – the Practical Part*

Box 9.5

Myofascial meridian example

Superficial Front Arm Line: pectoralis major, latissimus dorsi, medial intermuscular septum, forearm flexor group, carpal tunnel/flexor retinaculum.

Using Myers' meridian example, one can surmise the global consequences following breast cancer procedures. Even *less invasive* lumpectomy or partial mastectomy incisions can result in shoulder, elbow and wrist impairments.

Adapted from *Anatomy Trains* (Myers 2013).

(Stecco & Stecco 2009) both provide excellent illustrations of the myofascial global picture and excellent assessment protocols. The authors highly recommend studying some form of global assessment and treatment approach.

Boxes 9.5 and 9.6 provide two examples: one from Myers and the other from Stecco. In both examples muscular terms are used as a common reference, but it is to be noted that the corresponding myofascial envelopes are

---

Box 9.6

Myofascial sequence example

Anatomical continuity of the myofascial sequence on the sagittal plane of the lower limb – producing antemotion talus (dorsiflexion of the foot) – include the following: tibialis anterior, extensor digitorum longus, extensor halluces longus.

The antemotion sequence continues proximally, connecting the quadriceps tendon, intermuscular septa of the vastus medialis and lateralis, sartorius (knee antemotion), fascia lata, iliopsoas/iliopsoas fascia (hip antemotion), iliacus, psoas minor, inferior rectus abdominis (pelvis antemotion).

The inferior rectus abdominis is surrounded by the lateral raphe which connects the abdominal muscles to the middle and posterior layers of the thoracolumbar fascia. The anterior continuity and connection between the abdominal muscles and thoracolumbar fascia presents a hypothesis for the connection between ankle and knee dysfunction and low back pain/dysfunction. (adapted from Stecco & Stecco 2009)

Clinical Consideration

Knee and back relationship example

A client who had knee surgery presented with edema, gait issues and back pain. Palpation assessment revealed scar tissue (see Fig. 9.1), that exceeded well beyond the incision line.

Gentle fascial/myofascial work was performed on her thigh, proximal to the surgical site/incision line on the knee.

During treatment the client kept asking, 'Aren't you going to work *on* my knee or my scar?'

After about 15 minutes of working on scar tissue on the affected leg, the client was asked to get up from the table, walk around and describe what she felt. She was amazed at how little back and knee pain she had and commented on how she felt increased blood flow around her knee and noticed the edema had lessened.

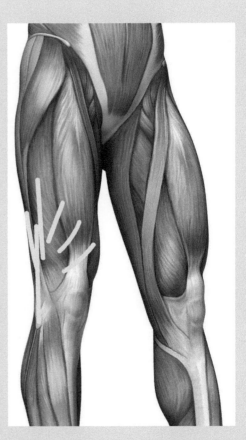

Fig 9.1
Yellow lines represent palpable scarring.

inclusive in the continuity from component to component.

Client-relayed fascial/myofascial indicators

Having the client describe the character and quality of what they feel can provide valuable information. Certain characteristics and qualities are commonly associated with CT and fascial distress. Additionally, certain indicators are useful for differential assessment:

- Stiffness – as stiffening is a physiological property of CT and fascia, consider stiffness a primary indicator of CT/fascial distress

- Burning, prickling or tingling sensation when tissue is manually loaded – due to drag on stuck or restricted tissue

- Compression, pulling or tugging sensation with or without movement or manual challenge – due to dense and/or stuck tissue

- Muscle weakness and fatigue not associated with muscle atrophy or motor dysfunction – restricted fascia can impair muscle contraction and force transmission capabilities

- Tension or tightness that does not resolve with linear stretching or other muscle targeted forms of therapy/treatment

- Tension or tightness that is non-responsive to muscle relaxants

- Muscular focused manual therapy techniques have produced non-satisfactory results or results are short lived

- Joint instability or feeling of *giving-out* with no mechanical laxity of joint associated tissues – associated with dense or restricted CT/fascia mediated proprioceptive dysfunction – see Sensory amnesia and proprioceptive disinformation example in Box 9.10 (p. 217)

- Pain referral pattern not associated with a neural path or pattern.

Clinical Consideration

Application to deform (change the shape) and stretch the soft tissue has an effect on the electrical and mechanical activities of muscles that are not being massaged but that are indirectly connected to the massaged tissue. MT appears to influence muscle motor tone not only through direct massage of the tissue but also through indirect effects on another distant soft tissue structure (Kassolik et al. 2009, Fritz 2013).

Pathophysiological Consideration

To clarify, fibrosis associated with pathophysiological scars is essentially aberrant collagen architecture in denser presentations of CT and fascia, whereas Stecco's defined densification occurs in the loose CT layers that are found inside and around denser CT and fascia. The loose/sliding layers are rich in water and other substances, such as adipose cells, glycosaminoglycans (GAGs) and hyaluronic acid (HA), which can affect CT and fascia's biomechanical properties. In healthy tissue, HA, which is highly hydrophilic, supports frictionless sliding, whereas over-use injury causes HA chains to fragment, aggregate and entangle, impacting CT and fascia's hydrodynamic and normal viscoelastic properties. Densification (increased viscosity) can impact normal sliding between adjacent tissues and/or structures, such as between the DF and underlying muscle, and between the muscle bundles and fibers. Stecco and colleagues suggest that the entangled chains of HA may be a cause of soft tissue restriction and myofascial pain (Stecco et al. 2013, Hammer 2013). The authors propose that over-use type impairments, and subsequent HA changes, are a common consequent of chronic scars.

Pathophysiological Consideration

Mechanoreceptors housed in densified spaces tend to be hyper-responsive to stretch, and upon stretch can elicit the transmission of pain messages. Muscle spindles embedded in densified epi- and perimysium may send aberrant feedback to the central nervous system (CNS), resulting in incoordination (Stecco et al. 2013, Hammer 2013).

Clinical Consideration

It is suggested that HA is the substance responding to manually applied mechanical load, resulting in a decrease in viscosity or density in the sliding layers. Normalization of viscosity/density supports a return to pain-free function by improving sliding between tissue layers and restoring normal proprioceptive function. Normalizing/disaggregation of pathological HA chains can be achieved by, increasing local tissue temperature, local alkalization, deep massage or physical therapies (Stecco & Stecco 2009, Stecco 2013).

Clinical Consideration

Stecco and colleagues assert that random treatment of densified points may not fully resolve the patient's pain and/or dysfunction and that lagging treatment effectiveness using manual load may be due to the fact that the correct combination of points/areas are not treated (Stecco & Stecco 2009, Stecco et al. 2013, Hammer 2013).

Pain

As noted, outcomes measured should be client-important and this includes gathering information about the client's pain. Various, *universal*, scales for assessing and documenting pain exist.

Three common scales used in MT to assess pain and its changes include the Verbal Rating Scale (VRS), Visual Analog Scale (VAS) and the numeric rating scale (NRS) (Gowan-Moody 2011). Examples of these can be readily accessed via the internet.

As outcome measures, all pain intensity rating strategies are used by care providers to establish a baseline, create a record of the client's pain experience, and to track any changes in pain over time (Gowan-Moody 2011).

It is important to note:

- The client's (current) self-reported pain intensity

- What the client's average pain intensity was over the past week (or other defined time period)

- The least/worse pain intensity the client experienced.

Treatment Protocol

The therapist's clinical reasoning skills, scope of practice, training and experience, in addition to the interests, concerns and informed consent of the client, influence the planning process. An integrated treatment planning process may involve working with a healthcare team to ensure that all care providers for a particular client understand each other's treatment focus and approach and that these are complementary (Fritz 2013).

Prior chapters have provided in-depth information on the various systems involved in the wound-healing process and those potentially harmed by a traumatic event, considerations pertaining to the client's emotional state, and establishing a solid therapeutic relationship. This information is intended to serve as a reference guide to assist with making informed treatment protocol decisions. The aim of this next section is to provide further guidelines for developing a safe, effective, evidenced informed, client-centered, treatment plan.

Establishing obtainable outcomes for each session or group of sessions is an important part of treatment planning. Each session will require the MT to make protocol decisions based on how the scar, surrounding area and other areas of concern currently present and, most importantly, the pain tolerance and comfort of the client during treatment.

If you are working with a recently acquired scar, please remember that scar maturation may take from a few months to several years. You will see many changes to the scar over this time. Adjustments in the tissue and progress in the wound-healing process require constant modification of your treatment plan (Kania 2012).

Safety First

MT appears to have few risks if utilized appropriately and is provided by a properly trained MT professional (NIH 2015).

Life-threatening or serious side-effects, such as dislodging a blood clot or implanted device, are rare. Adverse effects associated with MT techniques are almost exclusively attributed to aggressive application of (deep) techniques or massage provided by untrained or under-trained individuals.

As the treatment of traumatic scars in the later stages of healing or when working with mature scars can involve CT and fascial techniques, the authors advise that all necessary measures are taken to do no harm. Most MT entry-to-practice educational programs do not include intermediate or advanced levels of CT and fascial work. This book will provide some basic instruction for the application of CT and fascial techniques;

however, the authors' suggest that further training is acquired. The authors make the same recommendation for lymphatic work.

Contraindications (CIs) and Precautions

Within the profession it is commonly viewed that massage therapists should not rely on lists of specific CIs, but rather should use a set of medical and therapeutic guidelines pertinent to clinical applications and recent research developments. CIs are unique to each client and to each region of the body. The ability to reason clinically is essential to making appropriate decisions about the advisability of, modifications to, or avoidance of massage interventions (Fritz 2013).

The authors recommend researching each client's unique presentations. As professional healthcare providers, MTs must employ their training and best judgment when deciding whether or not to proceed with treatment. Due diligence on the part of the therapist will result in the best possible results for client-centered care.

General CIs and precautions for traumatic scar tissue clients are the same as with any client; however, some considerations are more common and therefore warrant note. Basic universal precautions include:

- Be mindful when working with those who are touch sensitive – physically and psychologically

- Fragile tissue such as newly grafted tissue and wounds in the early stages of healing – tread lightly or stay away completely

- Open wounds – if it's open and oozing and not yours, don't touch it.

Deep work

The deep techniques noted in this book are not appropriate for the following situations: acute neural distress and hard nerve pain; when a client is in emotional distress (to the degree that deeper work would elevate their anxiety or distress); osteoporosis; vascular pathologies; and cervical rheumatoid arthritis. Use sound judgment and proceed with appropriate consideration in such cases.

Some other general and local CI considerations for forceful and deep techniques include:

- Bone fractures or acute soft tissue injuries: wait for full healing (6 weeks – 3 months) – local

- Cortisone injections: local/2–3 months

- Inflammation: local/during acute stage

- Phlebitis, embolism, thrombus – local

- Newly forming scar tissue (including surgeries) – local/wait until the tissue is stable (about 6–7 weeks)

- Patients who have low blood platelet counts (e.g. as seen with splenomegaly, leukemia, chemotherapy), who are taking anticoagulant medications such as heparin or warfarin, or who have locally any potentially weak area of the skin such as near wounds (NIH 2015).

Additionally, acute inflammatory flare-ups may present with flu-like symptoms (malaise, unwell) which may be contraindicatory if treatment seems too overwhelming for the client that day.

Postsurgical and other intervention considerations

- Mastectomy: check with doctor whether massage in the area (anterior and posterior shoulder girdle and arm) is indicated. Sometimes it is not advisable to increase the lymphatic flow in that area.

- Pain medication: use caution regarding reduced sensation and greater possibility of tissue or nerve damage.

- Radiated tissue: take extreme care as tissue is delicate and easily damaged, avoid causing further pain and tissue irritation or damage.

- Cancer treatment: the National Cancer Institute urges MTs to take specific precautions with cancer patients and avoid massaging directly over:

  - the tumor site

  - open wounds

  - bruises

  - areas with skin breakdown

  - areas with a blood clot in a vein, and

  - sensitive areas following radiation therapy.

Psychological considerations

It is well documented that one of the benefits of receiving MT treatment is the general relaxation effect. For those who experience mental illness (e.g. stress disorders), finding ways to relax and stay in the present may perhaps offer a substantial benefit (Fitch 2014). However, as covered in Chapter 7, it is important for massage therapists working with traumatic scar clients to recognize certain behaviors that may require a need for concurrent psychological care. Numerous types of mental illness include symptoms of psychosis, delusions or profound mood swings (Fitch 2014).

Caution is advised for those diagnosed as *borderline*, the intermediary of neurosis and full psychosis, as there have been reports (although very few) about deep work triggering a psychotic episode. In a state of psychosis, the individual may not be able to understand or appreciate the nature of MT, and therefore MT will likely not provide significant benefit, or in some cases may make things worse. It cannot be emphasized enough that unless your client is receiving proper medical care for his or her condition, MT may exacerbate the symptoms and possibly put both therapist and client at risk.

In 2012, an estimated 9.6 million adults in the US experienced a serious mental illness in the past year, representing 4.1% of all US adults (NIMH 2015). It is imperative that massage therapists recognize potential indictor signs and symptoms before implementing treamtent. Traumatic scar tissue clients may exhibit significant mood disturbances, psychosis, hypermania or post-traumatic stress disorder (PTSD). Some clients may experience touch triggered responses when receiving bodywork. Medications that are prescribed for some of the above mentioned conditions can alter a client's ability to perceive reality, dull the senses or can enhance a clients delusion. When you encounter disturbing or out of the ordinary client behavior, you should refer the client for psychological care. If the client is currently in treatment, with the client's consent, contact with the mental health professional to discuss client-centered considerations and appropriate treatment can be of benefit to the client and lower therapist risk.

Dosage

Arguably, one of the most complex aspects of MT treatment planning is determining optimal dosage. This is certainly true when working with those with traumatic scars.

The multifactorial complexity of traumatic scars and the person will require individual consideration when determining dosage; frequency, duration, and number of treatments.

The stage of wound/tissue healing is the predominant component that guides clinical reasoning and decision-making with respect to what, when, how much and how to deliver safe and effective MT. Understanding what is happening during each stage and what outcomes are beneficial will drive the selection of technique type, duration and location of technique application and duration and frequency of treatment. Additionally, other client-centered considerations, such as frequency and duration based on what the client can afford and ability to travel to your clinic, are important factors in determining dosage.

Dosage considerations for stage of healing and specific techniques will be covered in more detail further on.

Clinical Consideration

MT dosage and desired outcomes

In a study conducted by Rapaport et al. (2012):

> ... pilot data suggest that there are sustained cumulative biologic effects of repeated massage on neuroendocrine and immune parameters in healthy volunteers, but these differ by dosage. Weekly massage increased circulating lymphocytes and decreased cytokine production with a minimal effect on HPA function. Whereas, twice weekly massage appears to potentiate neuroendocrine differences.

Although there is still much to be determined about MT dosage, mechanisms of action, effects and considerations for special populations, this preliminary data identifies that dosage makes a difference. This data suggests particular dosage relevance to scar tissue clients; weekly treatment may best address immune and inflammatory concerns whereas twice weekly may better address neruroendocrine factors that influence the HPA and subsequently, SNS hyperarousal. As discussed in Chapter 7, SNS hyperarousal can drive chronic inflammation which in turn can lead to pathophysiological scars. SNS hyperarousal is also linked to chronic stress.

Clinical Consideration

A recent study found that a 60-minute 'dose' of Swedish MT delivered once a week for pain due to osteoarthritis of the knee was both optimal and practical, establishing a standard for use in future research (Perlman et al. 2012). Sherman and colleagues (2014) showed that multiple 60-minute massage treatments per week (x 2–3) were more effective than fewer or shorter sessions for people with chronic neck pain, suggesting that several hour-long massage treatments per week may be the best 'dose' for people with this condition (Sherman et al. 2014).

Treatment Planning: Goal Setting and Intended Outcomes

By implementing the appropriate technique at the correct intensity and time, MT can facilitate inflammation, repair and remodeling.

Excessive inflammatory response, undue mechanical tension and delayed healing time are primary factors in pathophysiological scar formation. In brief, early scar management can help facilitate the healing process and guide the new tissue in its ability to attain normal collagen architecture, culminating in a scar capable of transmitting *normal* mechanical signals and force transmission. When addressing chronic presentations, mobilizing techniques can be utilized to address any adhesion and fibrosis driven impairments/dysfunctions with the ultimate outcome being restoration of function and ability to engage in all activities of daily living with minimal or no pain, discomfort or limitations (Fourie 2012, Rodríguez & del Río 2013).

First and foremost, the client's expressed goals are of utmost importance and will drive treatment planning. If the client's stated goal is complex, break this down into a series of smaller or more attainable goals.

In consideration of the client's expressed goals, and the process that is unfolding during each stage of healing, the therapist will draw on his/her professional expertise to identify specific intended outcomes for each session and for the long-term.

Developing a sound treatment strategy includes selecting and administering the appropriate interventions, namely MT techniques, that will achieve the client's expressed goals and therapist's intended outcomes – technique effects and application considerations are covered in more detail later in this chapter. Hot and cold therapy will not be covered in any great detail in this book with the exception of some client self- and/or home care recommendations which are provided in Chapter 10.

Ongoing documentation and periodic reassessment will be necessary. If results are not forthcoming in a reasonable amount of time, it may be necessary to re-evaluate your assessment and/or treatment approach. If this proves unsuccessful, another modality or practitioner may be the answer. It is imperative to make the client's well-being the number one priority.

Early stages of Wound Healing: Inflammation and Proliferation

Although treatment during the early stages of healing may prevent or reduce pathophysiological scarring, care and caution is advised. Although motion, including manual mobilization of tissue, plays an important role in collagen regeneration, excessive stretch of newly forming tissue /repeat wound trauma can interfere with healing.

Generally, manual manipulation is not indicated in the first 48–72 hours post-trauma, allowing fractured tissue fibers time to reunite and achieve sufficient strength needed to avoid subsequent separation (Kaariainen et al. 2001). Good wound closure is an important component in achieving physiological scars. Once epithelium has covered the wound, MFBs normally disappear by apoptosis and the granulation tissue eventually evolves into a scar containing few cells. Under pathological conditions, including poor wound closure and conditions that lead to fibrosis; however, the MFBs do not undergo apoptosis but instead proliferate and overproduce extracellular matrix (ECM) (Desmouliere et al. 1993, Ng et al. 2005).

Early treatment is generally directed at tissue peripheral to the scar or other areas of the body. Direct manipulation of scar tissue typically begins no sooner than 2 weeks post-trauma and during the first few weeks, tread lightly. It is important to avoid aggressive manipulation so as not to disrupt the healing tissue and prolong or instigate inflammation, which can result in exacerbating fibrosis and adhesion formation (Fourie 2012).

Recall from Chapter 5: the inflammation stage typically lasts 1–4 days and the proliferation stage typically 4–21 days, but may last for up to 6 weeks. In some cases edema, elevated temperature around the wound and pain may still be present throughout the proliferation stage.

Treatment outcomes

Essentially, early intervention focuses on pain management, attenuating stress and anxiety, attenuating inflammation and managing undue tissue tension as a means to facilitate client comfort and reduce or preventing undue adhesions and pathophysiological scar formation. In the latter days of proliferation, movement/mobilization of tissue supports improved tissue hydration and the state of ground substance (GS), facilitation of venous and lymphatic drainage, regulation of fibrin production, good fiber

orientation and sufficient strength of the newly forming scar.

Techniques

Techniques commonly employed are superficial fluid techniques and neural sedation. Judicious use of gentle CT and fascial techniques, in the form of brief, light-cyclical stretch/loading, are also indicated. Barrier should not be engaged near or around the injury site.

Dosage considerations

The presence of pain and inflammation are the primary indicators for treatment. The client's tolerance level may indicate a shorter duration treatment of 30 minutes, otherwise the typical duration of 60 minutes is indicated. Frequency of 1–3 treatments per week is a general guideline. Early stage care will typically be implemented for 6–12 weeks, followed by the transition to later stage care.

Clinical Consideration

A correlation between stress, anxiety, depression and pain has been identified, meaning that a relationship exists between these elements. Although stress, anxiety, depression and pain often are found together, whether any one of them causes any of the others is unclear. Regardless, the four conditions often respond to the same applications of massage (Fritz 2013).

Clinical Consideration

Numerous systematic reviews and clinical studies have suggested that, at least for the short-term, MT for cancer patients may reduce pain, promote relaxation and boost mood. Dryden and Moyer (2012) suggest that MT may induce neuroendocrine-mediated

Clinical Consideration (Cont.)

secretion of neurotransmitters and hormones, such as serotonin, dopamine, norepinephrine and oxytocin, producing an analgesic effect.

Clinical Consideration

A meta-analysis of 17 clinical trials concluded that MT may help to reduce depression (Hou et al. 2010).

Clinical Consideration

Heat in the therapeutic range, induces viscoelastic changes that improve tissue mobility. Mild heating can also have the effect of reducing pain and muscle spasm and promoting healing.

Clinical Consideration

Under physiological conditions, inflammation is an adaptive response aimed at restoring tissue integrity and functionality. The autonomic nervous system (ANS) plays an important role in modulating inflammatory responses. Physiologically, both the SNS and PSNS (parasympathetic nervous system) act synergistically to keep the inflammatory reaction circumscribed. SNS/PSNS imbalance can drive unabated or chronic inflammation, which in turn can drive processes that may lead to multiple complications including pathophysiological scars. Multiple complementary and alternative medicine interventions, including MT, have demonstrated a solid capacity to rebalance ANS function back to homeostasis and therefore may be an effective intervention for reducing or preventing pathophysiological scars (Moyer et al. 2004, Beider et al. 2007, Collet et al. 2014, Guan et al. 2014).

Clinical Consideration

Best and co-workers theorize that MT mediated mechanical stimulation of the mechanotransduction system results in the removal of cellular waste, reduction of edema, increased angiogenesis and attenuation of fibrosis (Best et al. 2013).

Clinical Consideration

Recall from Chapter 4: lateral or tangential forces appear to have a more notable impact on Ruffini endings, which are known to interface with the ANS. SNS activation tends to activate transforming growth factor beta-1 (TGF-β1) expression (and likely other cytokines), which has a stimulatory effect on MFB contraction, increasing fascial tone and stiffness. In addition, shifts in the ANS state can induce changes in pH, which also affects MFB contraction. Skillful, manual stimulation of mechanoreceptors in fascia, particularly of Ruffini or free nerve endings, can induce favorable changes in ANS tone (Chaitow 2014).

Pathophysiological consideration

Compromised vascularity, local ischemia and resultant hypoxia are primary factors in poor wound healing. Oxygen plays a key role in every healing phase including epithelialization, angiogenesis, collagen deposition, inflammation and bactericidal activity. Fibroblasts require a partial pressure of oxygen of 30–40 mmHg to synthesize collagen and enzymatic remodeling of collagen occurs between 20 and 200 mmHg. In comparison, chronic wounds have been measured to have a partial pressure of oxygen of 5–20 mmHg (Sheffield 1988, Franz et al. 2007, Gordillo & Sen 2003, Schreml et al. 2010, Gantwerker & Hom 2012).

Pathophysiological Consideration

*A variety of operative and non-operative proce-
dures are performed to improve post burn scar
quality. These include various topical therapies
that all share a similar mechanism of action,
ablating the skin in an attempt to yield a more
homogenous surface. Such approaches destroy
the epidermis and the basement membrane.
Ablating the epidermis of already scarred skin
with subsequent protracted reepithelialization
may possibly cause additional dermal fibrosis
by initiating a prolonged inflammatory response.
The ideal scar improvement modality would
leave the epidermis intact and rather improve
epidermal thickness via the subsequent release
of cell and tissue derived factors that modulate
dermal structure and collagen deposition*

(Rennekampff et al. 2010).

Clinical Consideration

Timing is everything – in pediatric burn patients,
hypertrophic scarring appears to be related to healing
time, with a healing time of 21 days or less leading
to the best long-term scar outcomes for patients.
According to Kishikova et al. (2014):

*Thorough initial scar management, in the form of
proper wound dressing, and follow-up management, in
the form of prophylactic scar therapy interventions, can
reduce healing time. The use of (prophylactic) MT for
burns taking more than 14 days to heal, and pressure
garments in those over 21 days, may reduce the inherent risk of hypertrophic scarring posed by prolonged
healing times. MT and pressure garments, used in
proper timing, optimize healing time and improve scar
outcomes. At 2 weeks post-burn, if healing appears to
lag, MT is indicated as a preemptive strike.*

Clinical Consideration

Pruritus is more likely to occur during active hypertrophy (i.e. early stages of maturation). It is prudent
that the evolution of hypertrophic scars inform treatment protocol. Additionally, staging will impact short
and long-term outcomes (Cho et al. 2014).

Clinical Consideration

Evidence suggests that inflammation and undue
mechanical tension can initiate or contribute to
hypertrophic scar (HTS) formation, and minimizing
inflammatory responses and mechanical forces may
prevent or reduce the formation of HTSs (Aarabi et al.
2007, Wang et al. 2011, Tziotzios et al. 2012, Rabello
et al. 2014).

Clinical Consideration

Maximizing oxygen delivery preoperatively can prevent or curtail poor wound healing postoperatively
(Gantwerker & Hom 2012). It may be of parallel value
to reduce ischemia during the healing process. MT
techniques aimed at addressing factors that contribute to ischemia and improving local circulation will
likely yield better healing outcomes.

Clinical Consideration

Several studies show that fetal skin wound repair
differs from postnatal – most notably is outcome; virtually no discernable difference in the reconstructed
tissue. The fetal limited inflammatory stage appears
to have a significant impact on the near normal

Clinical Consideration (Cont.)

organization of the repaired collagen matrix. Suggesting that decreasing or attenuating the inflammatory response/stage is an important focus in scar tissue management.

Clinical Consideration

The ECM is a bioactive structure that controls cell behavior through chemical and mechanical signals. Multiple studies have revealed that ECM controls organ and tissue development and subsequent function through cell anchorage; integrin-mediated activation and signaling; transduction of mechanical forces; and the sequestering, release and activation of growth factors. A better understanding of how the ECM and its mechanical forces can affect cell invasion, growth and differentiation, and the ECM's capacity to manipulate and direct fundamental cell functions and to apply this knowledge to tissue growth and repair, will be a cornerstone for furthering the fields of wound care and scar management (Discher et al. 2009, Hynes 2009, Gilbert et al. 2010, Dupont et al. 2011, Eming et al. 2014).

Clinical Consideration

Preventive measures are a major priority and need to be applied before, during and immediately after wound closure. Reducing mechanical tension in and around the scar is a significant consideration in terms of prevention of contractures, hypertrophic and keloid scars. Medical treatment of pathophysiological scars includes removal of the bulky scar tissue by reconstructive surgical techniques and/or injection of substances, such as collagenase, that promote

Clinical Consideration (Cont.)

collagen breakdown (Monstrey et al. 2014). Recall from Chapter 5: during wound healing, continuous or cyclical loading (brief, light stretch or compression – lengthening <30%) of mechanosensitive tissues stimulates resident fibroblasts to secrete collagenase (Tortora et al. 2007) reducing the potential of excess collagen formation (fibrosis and pathological cross-linking). Cyclical stretch/compression – involving approximately 10% of available tissue elasticity – doubles collagenase production, whereas continuous stretching appears to be 50% less productive (Carano & Siciliani 1996, Langevin 2010). And repeated, low amplitude tissue stretch seems to elicit an anti-inflammatory response (Yang et al. 2005).

Pathophysiological Consideration

Increased cross-link density results in altered tissue mechanical behavior, leading to more brittle collagen fibrils, which negatively impacts tissue viability. In addition to impact on tissue mobility, increased cross-link density is linked to skin wrinkling, cartilage impairment and bone embrittlement, as is seen in osteoporosis (Bailey 2001, Buehler 2008, Saito & Marumo 2009, Uzel & Buehler 2011).

Later Stages of Wound Healing: Remodeling

Recall from Chapter 5: with a normal wound, once remodeling is complete there should be no residual pain experienced, no significant loss of function and the scar should exhibit a normal appearance. As long as the scar appears redder than normal, remodeling is still under way. Generally speaking, physiological scar maturation concludes in several weeks to several months depending upon a number of factors including tissue type (skin is fast, about 7 weeks to full strength), extent of injury, injury location. Under abnormal circumstances, the remodeling stage can continue for years (Table 9.2).

Pathophysiological Consideration

With wounds, it seems that the greater the destruction the poorer the reconstruction, and undifferentiated tissue can be present for up to several months post trauma. Skin remodels more quickly than deeper tissue, so on the surface tissue the scar can appear *normal* (in presentation and function) but below the surface there may be a thick, dense, irregular presentation, devoid of microvacuole bubbles/sliding layer, which impacts function (Guimberteau 2012). See also Fig. 2.2.

General treatment guidelines

When working with traumatic scar tissue, the following general guidelines are recommended:

- Work the outer edges of the scar tissue first. With keloids in particular the greatest degree of tissue tension occurs along the scar outer margins.

- Next, work toward the center of the scar tissue. Usually the thickest part of the scar is the center.

- Do not overwork tissue, know when to say *when*. Begin somewhat conservatively, as it is best to do less at first than more.

- Provide sufficient time between treatments for the tissue to integrate the post-treatment changes.

Techniques

Commonly employed techniques include:

- Superficial fluid (if edema is still present)
- Nerve sedating

Time frame	Goal
Preoperative	Address patient specific comorbidities (e.g. *stress, *anxiety, pathologies and other factors that impact wound healing, such as diabetes, smoking) Limit use of medications known to have a negative impact on the healing process (e.g. anti-inflammatories)
Postoperative	Address factors that contribute to poor wound healing (poor or inadequate nutrition, *prolonged/overt inflammation, *hypoxia, *pain) Prevent repeat trauma at scar site *Improve blood supply, * facilitate adequate circulation and *oxygenation Keep wound hydrated with proper wound dressing Prevent infection and *improve immune functioning *Maximize healing environment (cellular, neural and circulatory considerations) *Manage microenvironment of the wound (alteration of signaling molecules to promote healthy scar formation and prevent excessive scarring, reduce mechanical strain impact on inflammatory mediators, profibrotic cytokines and proliferation of MFBs) Address psychological *stress and *anxiety *Address tissue tension, and stress to attenuate collagen deposition

*Factors that may be improved by MT.
(Adapted from Gantwerker & Hom 2012).

Table 9.2

Principles to improve wound healing and minimize scars

- Various compression and kneading, and

- CT and fascial mobilization techniques.

Treatment outcomes

The later stages of healing primarily focus on improving tissue hydration and the state of GS, reducing or preventing undue adhesions and pathophysiological scar formation, and guiding the healing tissue in its ability to attain, as close as possible, normal collagen architecture and functional capabilities.

During the remodeling stage, MT may shorten the time needed to form a healthy, mature scar (Cho et al. 2014). As noted, timing is everything, so early intervention (no later than 2 weeks post-trauma) may be ideal for the purpose of preventing or reducing the risk of delayed healing and subsequent pathophysiological scar formation. Additionally, treatment in this time frame may prove beneficial in reducing pain and pruritus.

Myofibroblast (MFB) activity is an important part of wound healing, as the tension generated by MFBs facilitates wound gap closure and formation of a mechanically sound scar. However, excess MFB-driven tension can result in excess collagen deposition, and so attenuating undue tissue tension is an important scar management component.

Bove and Chapelle (2012) assert that *keeping things moving* during healing may reduce or prevent layers from getting adhered to one another. If left unchecked or immobile, collagen fibers will cross-link and adhere in ways that can restrict movement, visceral motility and negatively impact muscle force generating capacity. Movement/mobilization ensures that newly formed tissue fibers align in a manner that allows for unrestricted motion. Movement/mobilization also impacts GS in ways that ensure tissue slide capabilities and fiber

stability (Hertling & Kessler 2006, Meert 2012, Stecco et al. 2013).

Dosage considerations

The presence of pain, inflammation, signs of delayed healing, undue tissue tension and problematic adherences are the primary indicators for treatment. The typical duration of 60 minutes is indicated. Frequency of one treatment per week is a general guideline. Later stage care will typically be implemented for 6–12 weeks.

Clinical Considerations

Non-threatening movement and loading during the healing process are instrumental in decreasing the potential of functional loss. Movement ensures that newly formed collagen fibers align in a manner that allows for unrestricted motion, and loading stimulates the tissue to form in ways that will support healthy function (e.g. the ability to meet tensional or load-bearing demands). *For example*: with muscular injuries (following an appropriate rest period allowing the scar tissue to stabilize) the benefits of controlled loading include improved alignment of regenerating myotubes, faster and more complete regeneration, and minimization of atrophy of surrounding myotubes (Jarvinen et al. 2007). In studies conducted on tendon (considered a form of fascia), controlled loading type exercise resulted in a more normalized tendon structure, as gaged by thickness and by the reduction of hypoechoic areas (Ohberg et al. 2004, Boyer et al. 2005). Movement also helps to reduce the potential of undue adhesions that can impact not only local tissues but also associated tissues and/or structures. It is important to follow standard therapeutic movement and exercise protocols during the various stages of rehabilitation (e.g. passive, active assisted, active, non-weight bearing, weight bearing).

Clinical Considerations

The margins of keloid scars tend to pull outward (i.e. exhibit considerable peripheral tension) whereas the center of the scar is subjected to milder tension (Ogawa et al. 2011). Therefore, MT along the peripheral margins may be most helpful in terms of attenuating tissue tension.

Clinical Considerations

It has been identified that mechanical forces can induce changes in the expression of ECM proteins and proteases. In a study by Kanazawa et al. (2009) it was revealed that uniaxial, cyclical stretching of skin fibroblasts resulted in down-regulation of agents known to stimulate persistent collagen proliferation associated with fibrosis and abnormal scarring. In another in vitro model, human hypertrophic scar samples responded to mechanical loading by inducing apoptosis (Derderian et al. 2005). Although the exact mechanism remains to be determined, it is hypothesized that massage can impact cellular structural and signaling milieu, thereby inducing beneficial effects through the ability to affect fibroblast apoptosis and remodeling (Bhadal et al. 2008, Chan et al. 2010, Cho et al. 2014).

Clinical Considerations

Hypertrophic scarring typically persists for 6 to 12 months and tends to regress over a period of 18 to 24 months (Oliveria et al. 2005). Pruritus is more likely to occur during active hypertrophy. It is prudent that the evolution of hypertrophic scars – whether the burn scar is in the early or late states of maturation – inform treatment protocol. Additionally, staging will impact short and long-term outcomes (Cho et al. 2014).

Clinical Considerations

MT may be a viable modality for attenuating post-burn hypertrophic scar pain, pruritus and scar characteristics such as thickness, melanin deposition, erythema, transepidermal water loss, and elasticity/tissue mobility (Cho et al. 2014).

Clinical Considerations

Burn rehabilitation MT has been shown to be effective in improving pain, pruritus, depression and scar characteristics in hypertrophic scars in post-burn patients (Roh et al. 2007, Cho et al. 2014).

Pathophysiological Consideration

Under normal, physiological conditions, restoration of a functional epidermal barrier is highly efficient, whereas repair of the deeper layers is less so and can potentially result in a scar that causes substantial loss of original tissue structure and function. *Meaning*: what we see on the surface can be very different than what may be happening in underlying tissues, such as the dermis, various CT and fascial layers. In all soft tissues and organs comprising CT, the parenchymal tissue can be replaced by the deposition of new ECM. If new ECM deposition is excessive this can gradually lead to tissue fibrosis and, ultimately, to diminished or loss of function. In addition to initial damage, ongoing multiple acute or chronic stimuli, including autoimmune reactions, infections, or mechanical injury can delay and negatively impact the healing process, resulting in abnormal remodeling (Guimberteau 2012, Eming et al. 2014).

Pathophysiological Consideration

Immobilization

As noted in Chapter 5, immobilization can lead to the formation of pathological cross-links and microadhesions between the pre-existing or non-injured collagen fibers as well as newly forming fibers, which in turn can impact slide/glide potential between the tissue layers. Impaired sliding between layers can result in tissue strain and subsequent inflammation. Immobilization also has a negative impact on tissue hydration and fascia's viscoelastic capabilities (e.g. underhydrated and more viscous GS) and the resultant stiffness can further impact mobility. Immobilization has also been shown to cause a decrease in correlating gray matter and to negatively impact relative neuroplasticity (Granert et al. 2011). As tissues become more stuck, the potential for movement diminishes even further, constituting a vicious cycle. Cramer et al. (2010) confirmed that inactivity and immobilization result in the development of adhesions in the facet joints. Duration of immobility was shown to correlate with the size, and frequency of the adhesions – longer duration is linked to more extensive adhesions.

Clinical Considerations

In the early stages of injury pain, pain medications, seriousness of injuries, casting and other interventions may impact the patient's ability to move. The authors offer that manual mobilization of skin and fascia may provide a means to prevent or reduce pathological cross-link formation during the time when the patient is not able to move in ways that would support the retention of slide/glide between tissue layers. Additionally, fascia hydrodynamically

Clinical Consideration (Cont.)

responds to mechanically applied strain in ways that can positively impact tissue pliability, improve tissue hydration, reduce edema and stiffness and improve ease of movement. If the patient is able to move with greater ease and less pain, they are more likely to do so and therefore more likely to be compliant with rehabilitation programs and exercises to be done at home.

Clinical Considerations

Pain-instigated fear of movement leads to a cycle of decreased movement, pathophysiological CT remodeling, inflammation and nervous system sensitization, all of which result in a further decrease in mobility. The mechanisms of a variety of treatments, including MT, may reverse these abnormalities by applying mechanical forces to soft tissues (Langevin & Sherman 2007, Fritz 2013).

Clinical Considerations

As the remodeling stage of wound healing is in great part driven by MFB-mediated mechanical tension, an important treatment focus is to shift tissue from a high-tension state, to a low-tension state, hypothetically, to induce MFB apoptosis, or to halt the transformation of fibroblasts to MFB. Manually applied techniques that can shift the ECM to a low-tension state might be able to inhibit excess pathological cross-links, which distort mobility between the fascial interfaces and, ultimately, would lead to pathophysiological scars (Hinz 2007, Rodríguez & del Río 2013).

Pathophysiological consideration

In addition to stimulating the differentiation of fibroblasts into MFBs, TGF-β1 can also induce the differentiation of myogenic cells into fibrotic cells in injured skeletal muscle, leading to fibrosis (Li et al. 2004, Cencetti et al. 2010, Rodríguez & del Río 2013).

Long-Standing/Mature Scars and Impairments

When working with long-standing or mature scars, treatment often shifts away from the scar itself and focuses more on the dysfunctions or impairments that develop as a result of the scar. These pathophysiological scars can be visibly evident on the surface in the form of skin contractures, hypertrophic and keloid scars or less visibly evident under the surface in the form of adhesions, fibrosis, CT and fascial contractures.

In some cases scars will become strongly fixed and may require surgical release, in which case, postsurgical MT care will be indicated.

Treatment outcomes

Essentially, the restoration of pain-free functional capabilities reigns supreme. It is in this stage that aberrant movement patterns may present and so myofascial chains/meridian considerations apply. It is also when chronic stress and chronic pain must be considered.

Treatment will primarily focus on mechanical cleavage of pathological cross-links and microadhesions, decreasing tissue density/GS viscosity and balancing SNS/PNS tone.

Techniques

Techniques commonly employed include:

- Superficial fluid (if edema is still present)

- Nerve sedating

- Various compression and kneading, and

- CT and fascial mobilization techniques.

Dosage considerations

The presence of chronic pain, chronic stress, undue tissue tension and problematic adherences are the primary indicators for treatment. The typical duration of 60 minutes is indicated. Frequency of one treatment per week is a general guideline and treatment can be ongoing indefinitely.

Depth and Pressure Grading

The sensitivity and acuity of our hands are our most powerful clinical tools. During scar assessment, evaluation and treatment, depth and pressure grading are important considerations. An expert understanding of how to gauge depth and pressure factors into client safety and enhances both the intake of important assessment/evaluation information and the effectiveness of treatment.

Various factors are to be considered in determining *how much* pressure is appropriate, including stage of healing, tissue type and location, technique type and desired outcome and, most importantly, client comfort (Fourie 2014).

Two measures of pressure grading are provided. Walton's (2011) five massage pressure levels are used most commonly with fluid movement, neural sedating and muscular techniques (e.g. Swedish and lymphatic techniques; see Box 9.7). Fourie and Robb's (2009) depth and grading of touch scale is used most commonly with CT and fascial/myofascial techniques (e.g. skin rolling and various loading techniques; see Box 9.8).

Techniques

Any carpenter will tell you that using the right tool for the job is a hugely important factor in efficiency and the quality of the outcome; the same applies to MT.

Box 9.7

Pressure levels

Pressure Level 1 – Very light pressure/ no lotion or small amount of lotion

No skin movement or movement of the most superficial layer of skin only.

Use of arms and hands, no leaning body mechanics or strength required. Applying massage lubricant and distributing on the skin. This should be the maximum pressure used for clients who have new skin grafts and/or neuropathy. As previously noted, direct work on newly grafted skin is contraindicated.

Slow, intentional speed is required for proper scar depth assessment and to monitor pressure level and tolerance of the client. Full, firm contact is important to maintain, taking the shape of the client's tissues.

Pressure Level 2 – Light pressure/light to medium amount of lotion

Slight movement engages the SF layer, where most adipose is found (if adipose tissue is present) and muscles.

Little hand strength needed, only for contouring. Use of arms and hands; no leaning body mechanics or strength required. Distributing massage lubricant over scar area if matured; around the scarred area if immature and showing signs of inflammation or edema modeling. This would be considered maximum pressure for most medically frail clients.

Pressure Level 3 – Medium pressure/light to medium amount of lotion

Some movement of medium layers of muscles, and adipose tissue, if present.

Slight movement of adjacent joints may occur if no underlying scar tissue has formed. Upper extremity strength or body mechanics necessary to introduce therapist body weight into this pressure; some hand strength is necessary for kneading the scarred area at this pressure. Maximum pressure for many clients experiencing illness or surgical recovery.

Pressure Level 4 – Strong pressure/light to medium amount of lotion

Movement of deep layers of muscle, fascia, tendon, adipose, blood vessels, if present.

Movement of adjacent joints is noticeable with this pressure if there is no scar tissue impeding movement. Significant upper body strength or good body mechanics may be necessary to introduce therapist body weight and deliver this pressure with the full hand. Caution is advised if the client has had scar release within the last 72 hours. Overworking a particular area could establish micro tears and inflammation in scar-released area. Squeezing tissue with fingers requires significant hand strength at this pressure. Therapists commonly switch from the full hand to smaller areas, such as the knuckles or forearms, in order to apply this pressure with less effort. Extreme caution is warranted if this pressure is used to release a scar mound that has encapsulated a nerve, artery, vein or more than one muscle group.

Pressure Level 5 – Deep pressure/light to medium amount of lotion

Movement of deepest layers of muscle, fascia, adipose, blood vessels, if present. Through the compressed soft tissue, the therapist engages the bones of the massage site with the bones of their hands (or elbow, forearm, or other

(Continued)

Box 9.7 (Continued)

massage surface), and the two move as a unit. Substantial upper body strength and excellent body mechanics, using the therapist's own weight, are needed to apply this pressure with the full hand; often one hand must be braced with the other to deliver this pressure. Used with healthy, robust clients preferring the deepest pressure. Extreme caution is warranted if this pressure is used to release scar mound that has encapsulated a nerve, artery, vein or more than one muscle group.

Adapted from Walton 2011.

Box 9.8

Depth and grading of touch

Grade 1–3

- Very light, mild, non-irritating
- Compared to moving an eyelid on the eyeball without irritating the eye
- Client experiences no discomfort
- Consistent with Walton's pressure levels 1 and 2.

Grade 4–6

- Moderate to firm
- Most MT techniques fall into this range
- Client may experience mild discomfort
- No tissue irritation or damage
- Consistent with Walton's pressure level 3 and 4.

Grade 7 and 8

- Firm, deep
- Trigger point work often falls into this range
- Client likely to experience some tolerable discomfort
- Possible post-treatment bruising
- Consistent with Walton's pressure level 4.

Grade 9 and 10

- Deep
- Client likely to experience extreme uncomfortableness and/or pain
- Strong potential for tissue damage and subsequent inflammation
- Deep transverse fractioning falls into this range
- Consistent with Walton's pressure level 5.

Adapted from Fourie & Robb 2009.

Identifying the target tissue/structure (e.g. lymph vessel, fascia, muscle), what the issue is (e.g. swelling, neural hypersensitivity, tissue adherence), and determining desired outcome (e.g. shift in fluid dynamics or volume, sedation, decreased tone) will guide selection of technique type and application, which includes dosage considerations and the area treated (e.g. the scar itself, tissue around the scar and scar-associated impairments in nearby or distant tissues). (See Table 9.3).

Basic techniques common to MTs worldwide will not be covered in this book (e.g. gliding, kneading and compressions with use of a lubricant).

As lymph, CT and fascia are key target tissues in scar tissue management, some detail will be provided for the safe and effective application of these tissue/issue specific techniques.

Influence fluid	Influence the CNS, PNS and integrins	Cleve microadhesions and pathological cross-links	Influence HA
Edema transport Local blood circulation ECM volume and concentration	Facilitate neural, physiological and mechanotransduction-mediated effects	Disengage or release stuck fibers and tissue	Normalize HA chains Increase HA
Attenuate edema-mediated hysteresis Dilute inflammatory milieu Neutralize pH Facilitate healing processes Shift GS viscosity Reduce: neural distress and pain Improve: hydration, fluid gap between fiber/layers, slide potential, viscoelasticity, pliability and mobility	Balance ANS Dampen or accelerate cellular activity (including MFBs) Reduce: neural distress, pain and undue tissue tension/tone Facilitate fluid shift (see fluid shift outcomes) Facilitate immune system activity	Reduce neural distress and pain Improve: slide potential, proprioception, mobility, and muscle contractile capabilities Normalization of movement patterns	Reduce: neural distress and pain Improve: fluid gap between fibers/layers, hydration, slide potential, proprioception viscoelasticity, pliability, mobility, and muscle contractile capabilities Normalization of movement patterns

Table 9.3

Summary of manually mediated outcomes

Manual Lymphatic Techniques

Early manual lymphatic work is credited to A.T. Still, dating back to the 1880s. Throughout the 1930s, E. Vodder, a clinical scientist, further developed treatment of various pathologies by manipulating the lymphatic system. The Vodder method is known as manual lymphatic drainage (MLD) (Chikly 2005, Zuther 2011).

In the late 20th century, Chickly developed lymph drainage therapy (LDT). His work has incorporated adapted techniques to `work the lymphatic system`. Both the Vodder and Chikly methods are taught extensively, with only slight variations in the techniques. In the authors' experience, both LDT and MLD effectively work with the lymphatic system.

Lymphatic technique protocol is quite complex and involves several levels of training. The explanation of techniques as follows is not to be misconstrued as a substitute for Lymphatic Certification. The technique guidance provided in this chapter is applicable for general swelling and mild edema associated with wound healing and mature scars. The authors emphasize that full certification in manual lymphatic work is warranted in order to better understand the application and protocol for the traumatic scar tissue client presenting with more serious lymphedema.

It is imperative the MT has proper training to recognize contraindications for performing lymphatic techniques on clients.

Basic Principle of Lymphatic Technique Application

Lymphatic techniques includes the manipulation of healthy lymph nodes and vessels located

- Establish a safe and productive intensity parameter with your client before beginning treatment. The authors recommend that an initial safe 'stop' point is 4 on the 0–10 numeric rating scale
- Consider treatment room temperature – a warmer environment is recommended
- Initiate contact with a slow, soft, yet somewhat firm, and confident touch
- Provide cycles of work interspersed with brief pauses and client feedback
- Be present, observe and appropriately respond to client verbal and non-verbal cues
- Specific to loading techniques:
  - Employ a layered approach
  - Engage CT and fascia/myofascia 3-dimensionally (e.g. lifting, torsion, bending)
  - Meet and match tissue resistance (rather than over-power/ force)
  - Apply a consistent/sustained force or pressure until barrier releases or apply consistent pressure while slowly moving along a line/vector – approximately 2–3 millimeters or ⅛ of an inch per client breath cycle
  - To achieve desirable viscoelastic deformation a fairly constant amount of manually applied force for up to 60 seconds is required
  - Generally 3–5 minutes of sustained tissue loading is required to shift GS viscosity (i.e. from viscous to more fluid)
  - Employ gapping type force to disengage problematic collagen cross-links and microadhesions (gapping within our scope of practice – for example lifting and bending type techniques)
  - It can be helpful to follow CT and fascial/myofascial work with superficial fluid and/or sedating techniques, and/or heat in the therapeutic range: 35–40°C or 99–104°F

Table 9.4

Treatment guideline summary

adjacent to the area with insuffienct lymph flow. This manipulation will result in lymphangiomotoricity in the areas (Zuther 2011).

Depending on the location of the edema, the thorax, ipsilateral and contralateral axillary, abdominal area, or inquinal lymph nodes may need to be activated.

If the lymphatic system is compromised in any way, techniques to engage the deeper nodes and the superficial nodes proximal to the scarred area are essential in removing the fluid. The lymph fluid is re-routed via tissue channels, anastomoses or collateral lymph vessels into more centrally located lymph vessels and nodes (Zuther 2011).

During Wound Healing

The goal of treatment during wound healing is to attenuate undue edema and to support tissue healing.

During the early stages of healing (day 2–6), edema is usually liquid, soft and easy to mobilize or move. Gentle lymphatic techniques (no more than PL3) applied proximal to the injury site can assist with lymph transport.

Scars, Adhesions and Edema

Scars and adhesions disrupt the network of lymph capillaries and hinder lymph drainage. This makes the treatment of edema in the affected area more difficult.

When performing lymphatic techniques, scars can interrupt the lymph flow. When there is a scar in the stroke pathway, it is recommended that you stroke around the scar and not through it because the transfer of fluid across a scar is usually ineffective.

Scars located perpendicular to lymph collectors can prevent lymphatic drainage, especially if the scar tissue adheres to the fascia or exceeds 3 mm in width (Zuther 2011).

Traumatic scarring can be a cause for post-traumatic secondary lymphedema. Physical trauma may cause a reduction of the transport capacity of the lymphatic system if the lymphatic system was healthy prior to the injury. Traumatic events, such as surgery and burns, result in inflammatory responses accompanied by high-protein edema (Zuther 2011).

Traumatic edema results in increased tissue pressure and extended diffusion distance between the blood capillaries and the tissue cells. This causes a lack of oxygen and nutrients to the traumatized area; disruption of drainage which results in the delay of healing; irritation of pain receptors and delay of scar healing or increase in scar formation (Zuther 2011).

Lymphatic techniques improves lymph vessel activity proximal to the traumatic scar tissue area. This reduction in swelling, along with the decrease in diffusion distance improves local oxygenation and nutrition. This action accelerates the drainage and elimation of waste products. Thus, tissue pressure is reduced along with the pain associated with the traumatic edema (Zuther 2011).

Clinical Consideration

Edema, excess fluid in the interstitial space, is part of the normal inflammatory process.

Undue and/or prolonged edema can compromise diffusion of cellular waste, a bi-product of activity or cell apoptosis, and nutrients between the blood capillaries and cells and subsequently can delay or impair healing, resulting in fibrosis.

Effective muscle contraction, diaphragmatic breathing and peristalsis have a positive impact on lymph transport. Manual lymphatic techniques are also hypothesized to improve lymphatic transport (Eisenhart et al. 2003, Korosec 2004, Knott et al. 2005, Hodge et al. 2007, Vairo et al. 2009, Chikly 2002, Földi 2012).

It is hypothesized that manual lymphatic therapy:

- Stimulates the lymphatic system via an increase in lymph circulation

Clinical Consideration (Cont.)

- Expedites the removal of biochemical wastes from body tissues

- Enhances body fluid dynamics, thereby facilitating edema reduction

- Balances SNS/PSNS tone, facilitating a homeostatic or relaxed state.

Basic Lymphatic Techniques (Adapted From Zuther 2011)

All basic lymphatic techniques are applied at pressure level 1 (see Box 9.7).

Half-moon or circles

Half-moon or circles technique comprises circle-shaped stretching of the SF with the palmar surface of the fingers. Consistent pressure is applied on the downward stroke of the circle using radial or ulnar deviation of the wrist. The MT's hand is always relaxed and maintains contact with the skin. This technique may be applied with both hands at the same time or alternating hands for manipulation of an area (Fig. 9.2).

For the sequence for clearing the head and neck (see Fig. 9.2): begin near the distal end of the sternocleidomastoid muscle (SCM) just proximal to the cervical lymph pathway terminus (yellow dot in Fig. 9.2A). Using the palmar surface of the fingers, apply level 1 pressure (loading/stretching the skin and SF) in a half-moon/circular motion (purple arrow) along the cervical lymphatic pathway (white line). In a half-moon/circular motion (with no loading or stretch of the skin or fascia) glide the fingers upward to a position slightly above where the previous stroke began (orange and yellow arrows) – then perform another half-moon/circular motion with the fingers. This technique is perfomed as

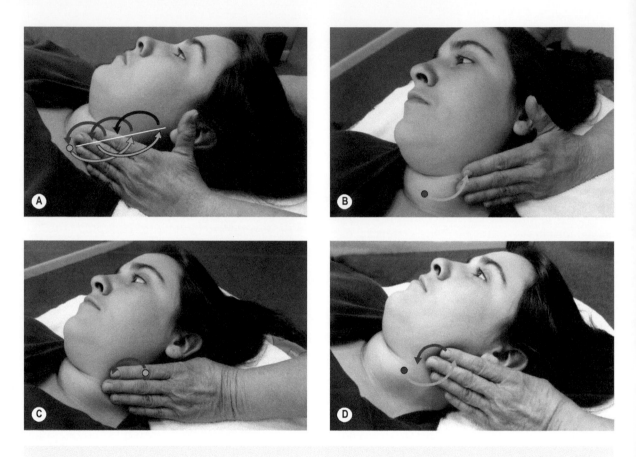

Figure 9.2

Half-moon/circles: clearing the head and neck. (**A**) Begin near the distal end of the SCM just proximal to the cervical lymph pathway terminus (yellow dot). Apply level 1 pressure in a half-moon/circular motion (purple arrow) along the cervical lymphatic pathway (white line). Glide the fingers upward to a position slightly above where the previous stroke began (orange and yellow arrows) then perform another half-moon/circular motion with the fingers. Perform in a continuous sequence (1–5) moving upward along the margin of the SCM/lymphatic pathway. (**B–D**) Purple arrow: downward/drainage stroke; yellow arrow: upward (pressure-less) glide; purple dot: end of previous downward stroke; yellow dot: end of previous upward stroke.

a continuous sequence (see Fig. 9.2 B–D) moving upward along the margin of the SCM/lymphatic pathway. Remember: pressure or push of the fluid is always toward the terminus on the downward stroke – ensuring drainage of lymph toward the terminus. This technique may be applied unilaterally, bilaterally or by alternating hands for treatment of a larger area. It is important to remember that lymph is a one-way system. Moving the fluid out of the efferent lymph vessels into the terminus is crucial to proper execution of lymphatic techniques. In any area of the body always begin the sequence just proximal to the terminus to ensure that the lymph pathway is cleared so excess fluid can drain into the terminus without becoming congested.

Pumping

Pumping technique is mainly used on the extremities and continues the use of the circle-shapted stretching of the skin. The MT may use their entire palm flat on the skin surface and may use one or both hands to achieve the result. The hand is in a palmar flexion with ulnar deviation and transitions into radial deviation and wrist extension at the end of the stroke (see Fig. 9.3).

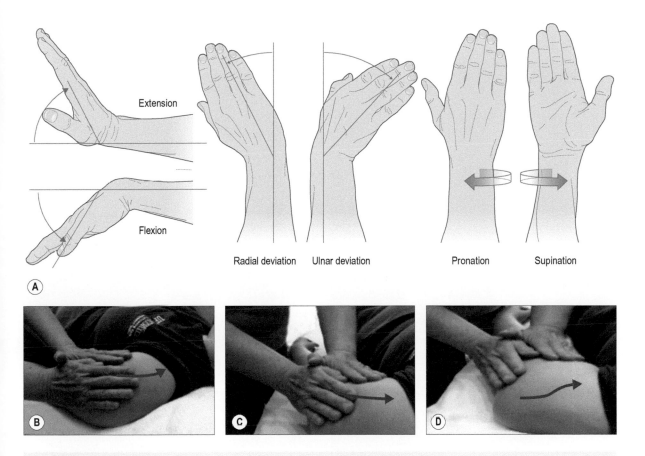

Extension

Flexion

Radial deviation   Ulnar deviation   Pronation   Supination

(A)

(B)   (C)   (D)

Figure 9.3

Pumping: clearing the extremities (right arm). Pumping is mainly used on the extremities and also involves circle-shaped stretching of the skin and SF. The MT may use their entire palm, flat on the skin surface and may use one or both hands to achieve the result. The hand is in wrist flexion with ulnar deviation and transitions into radial deviation and wrist extension at the end of the stroke. All strokes begin proximal to the terminus and move distal. (A) Directional movements of the hand/wrist; (B–D) arrows indicate the direction of lymph flow.

Scooping

Scooping technique is used only on the extremities. Again, using half circle movements, the MT transitions from palmar flexion and pronation into dorsal-flexion and supination and moving back to palmar flexion and pronation at the end of the stroke. The MT may use one hand or both (see Fig. 9.4).

Rotary

The rotary technique is commonly used on the thorax. Half circles are generated with the hand elevated, the thumb abducted, with the finger joints neutral and the fingertips in contact with the SF. The MT places the hand on the skin with the ulnar side without pressure, while the thumb goes into abduction. The SF is displaced with

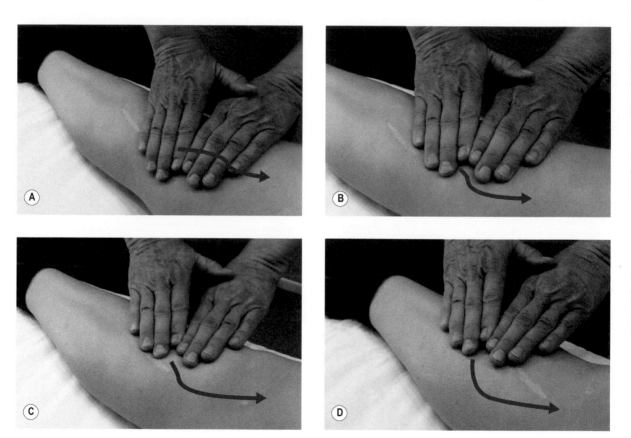

Figure 9.4

Scooping: clearing the extremities (lower leg). This technique is used only on the extremities. Again, using half-moon/circular movements, the MT transitions from palmar flexion and pronation into dorsal-flexion and supination and moving back to palmar flexion and pronation at the end of the stroke. The MT may used one hand or both. All strokes begin proximal to the terminus and move distal. (A–D) Red arrows indicate the direction of lymph flow.

increasing stretch toward the drainage area with the thumb moving to adduction at the end of the stroke. The MT then moves the hand to the next area to be manipulated and repeats the technique. The MT may use one or both hands (see Fig. 9.5).

Alternating pump and stationary circle technique

Alternating pump and stationary circle technique is commonly used on the side of the thorax and extremites. The efficacy of the lymphatic

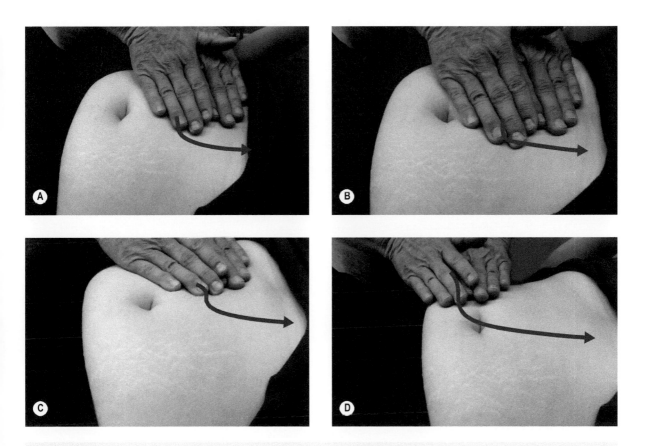

Figure 9.5

Rotary (thorax). Half-moon/circles are generated with the hand elevated, the thumb abducted, with the finger joints neutral and the fingertips in contact with the skin and SF. The MT places the hand on the skin with the ulnar side without pressure, while the thumb goes into abduction. The SF is displaced with increasing stretch toward the drainage area with the thumb moving to adduction at the end of the stroke. The MT then moves the hand to the next area to be manipulated and repeats the technique. The MT may use one or both hands. All strokes begin proximal to the terminus and move distal. (A–D) Red arrows indicate the direction of lymph flow.

system prior to the start of the specific scar tissue work will ensure a much healthier environment for the entire session. Through years of clinical experience the following protocol for clearing the lymphatic system prior to scar work has yielded solid results (see Fig. 9.6):

- Begin with clearing the head area first. Start proximal to distal on the SCM using half circles toward the terminus.

- Proceed with half circles proximal to distal along the mandible, masseter, temporalis, and the occipitofrontalis.

- Use pumping or scooping techniques on the upper extremites, one extremity at a time.

- For the thorax, use the rotary technique.

- Repeat pumping or scooping technique on the lower extremities, one extremity at a time.

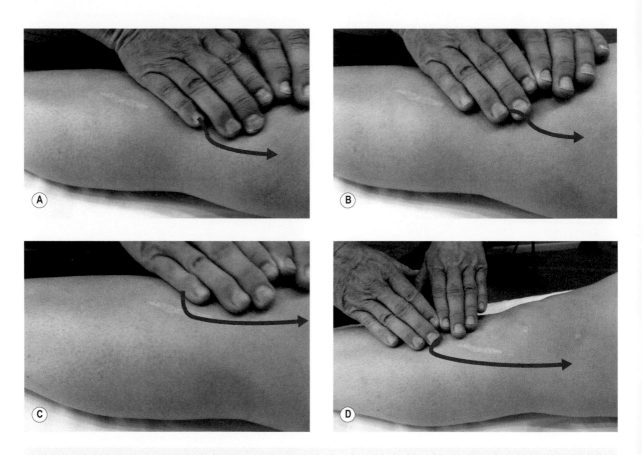

Figure 9.6

Alternating pump and stationary circle technique. This technique is used on the side of the thorax and extremites. The efficacy of the lymphatic system prior to the start of the specific scar tissue work will ensure a much healthier environment for the entire session. All strokes begin proximal to the terminus and move distal. (A–D) Red arrows indicate the direction of lymph flow.

If there is time available after you have completed other scar tissue work (e.g. CT and fascia/myofascial techniques), repeating the lymphatic techniques may prove helpful to removing waste products released by the tissue. It is imperative the MT has proper training to recognize contraindications for performing lymphatic techniques on clients.

Skin/CT and Fascia/Myofascial Techniques

MT affects fascia/myofascia through the same proposed biologically plausible mechanisms associated with other MT soft-tissue techniques that use manual force applied in various strain directions (Eagan et al. 2007, Simmonds et al. 2012, Fritz 2013).

There are various indirect and direct approaches to working with skin/CT and fascia. Four of the most commonly known direct approaches include; Rolfing© and Structural Integration (originating from the work of Ida P. Rolf and furthered by many, including Myers), Fascial Manipulation© (the work of the Steccos), fascial/myofascial therapy (covers a broad spectrum of methods, predominantly originating from osteopathy) and CT massage (originating from the work of E. Dicke and, later, M. Ebner).

The four identified approaches share similarities and differences in theory, principles and technique application. Although the authors have studied all four of these approaches, no specific training for any one identified approach will be provided; however, general guidance for the application of common direct therapeutic loading techniques known to achieve desirable scar and scar-related impairment outcomes will be supplied.

Basic Principles of CT and Fascial/Myofascial Technique Application

One of the most obvious differences between CT and fascial/myofascial techniques and other massage techniques is that a lubricant is generally not applied.

Lack of lubricant allows for engaging or hooking into CT and fascia and the ability to *load* the tissue and create *drag*. As tissue is therapeutically loaded and moved it will eventually encounter barrier and bind. Recall, barrier is the first-felt slight resistance to manually applied challenge, and bind is the point where tissue no longer moves freely/easily with mechanical force application.

Drag can be graded (Fritz 2013) (see Box 9.9). Generally speaking, when working with traumatic scar tissue, skin/CT and fascial/myofascial techniques are aimed at drag level 2–3.

As discussed throughout this book, pathophysiological scars are characterized by pathologically excessive dermal fibrosis and aberrant wound healing. During the wound-healing process, measures taken to prevent aberrant wound healing is to be considered a primary treatment focus, and this includes employing techniques designed to address undue tissue tension. As noted at the beginning of this chapter, employing techniques designed to interface with the tension/tone regulators, the nervous system (NS) and integrin system, will achieve the desired outcome.

When working with established traumatic scar tissue, skin/CT and fascial/myofascial

---

Box 9.9

Drag scale

- 0: no drag
- 1. moves the tissue but no bind occurs
- 2: moves the tissue to bind
- 3: maximum drag, moves the tissue beyond bind.

Adapted from Fritz 2013.

techniques are directed at releasing tissue restrictions or dense or stuck sliding layers that have been identified through assessment and evaluation.

Clinical Consideration

Various forms of thermotherapy (i.e. heat in the therapeutic range) can be utilized during and after treatment to produce a variety of results. In addition to commonly known circulatory and muscular effects and other effects noted in this chapter (e.g. the effect of heat on HA), it is suggested that an increase in local tissue temperature results in a shift in GS viscosity, which in turn improves tissue mobility and reduces stiffness and painful contractures associated with rigid collagenous fibers in fascia (Klingler 2012). Thermotherapy in the form of paraffin wax application can help render scar tissue softer and more pliable, resulting in decreased stiffness, improved collagen fiber extensibility and mobility (Sandqvist et al. 2004, Sinclair 2007). Utilizing a local paraffin bath application before working with scar tissue from a burn injury can yield significant, measurable increases in local freedom of movement (Sinclair 2007). Heating scar tissue, thus rendering the tissue more pliable, prior to applying myofascial techniques can facilitate technique productivity and reduce potential client discomfort during and post treatment.

When targeting tissue restrictions, techniques are generally applied just before or at barrier or the point of bind, at varying angles to the restriction. With some approaches pressure or force is sustained at a constant throughout application in a specific locale (Fritz 2013). Another approach employs slow drag or movement of tissue along a particular line or vector at the rate of approximately 2–3 mm or 1/8 of an inch per client breath cycle. This slow-movement approach is also recommended for self-treatment using a foam roller (Schleip & Baker 2015). Attempting to drag the tissue too quickly increases the incidence of injury.

The primary treatment focus is restoration of normal tissue barrier end-feel. A layer approach to treatment is typically applied, working from superficial to deep. Superficial restrictions are resolved before moving into deeper layers.

When working with long-standing/chronic scars, local concerns are typically addressed prior to global ones.

When working to improve tissue slide/glide, by impacting the state of HA in the sliding layer – resulting in increased HA lubrication potential – vertically applied vibration, tangential/laterally applied oscillation and shearing force application appear to achieve the best results (Day et al. 2012, Roman et al. 2013).

Skin, CT and Fascial/Myofascial Techniques

Different types of mechanical force-loading are used to treat various presentations in skin CT and fascia/myofascia and to achieve specific outcomes (Pilat 2003, Chaitow & DeLany 2008, Chaudhry et al. 2008, Fritz 2013, Fourie 2014, Chaitow 2014, Pilat 2014). The amount of force or pressure used will vary depending upon presentation and depth of target tissue.

Therapeutic Loading Techniques

These techniques are typically used to address CT and fascia.

CT and fascia respond biomechanically to compression and tension. Determining and engaging barrier are key elements in CT, fascial/myofascial loading techniques. When used in a treatment context, barrier is engaged and a consistent force or pressure is sustained until a release is felt. Release is commonly felt as a decrease in resistance or softening of tissue that renders the tissue more pliable and mobile. Release allows for the ability to move

Box 9.10

Sensory amnesia and proprioceptive disinformation example

KS is a burn survivor. Her injury was over 20 years old when she came to my clinic.

KS's scar tissue was adhered to multiple layers of muscle, bone and structures of the left lower extremity, including the deep rotators of the hip that all insert on or very near the greater trochanter of the femur and ischial tuberosity.

The scar tissue restrictions resulted in dysfunctional and undifferentiated movement patterns involving the pelvis and hip joint. Assessment showed that her left sacral iliac (SI) joint lacked mobility and there was abnormal activation of the deep rotators during hip extension.

Each session released another small section of scar tissue that led to changes in the pelvic, thoracic and lumbar regions.

During one session, we targeted scar tissue that adhered to the biceps femoris, quadratus femoris and the obturator muscles – near their collective attachments on/around the ischial tuberosity and greater trochanter.

Upon release of scarred tissue in these areas, KS reported immediate improved hip and pelvis mobility but also some soreness. And so it was suggested that KS take it easy that evening and the next day, to allow her body a chance to integrate the work and new found freedom. However, she decided to go to her tennis practice that night.

At practice, as she was moving backward for an overhead, KS fell. And fell again three times that evening at practice, each time while moving backward. At the next tennis practice she was a little hesitant but decided to try the overhead/backward movement again. This time she did not fall.

KS reported her experience at the next treatment session. What happened? The long-standing scar tissue had changed her movement pattern and these changes impacted her proprioception and muscle activation sequencing (i.e. timing and velocity of muscle contraction).

It was explained to KS that after the tissues bound by scar tissue are freed, it may take a while for proprioception to normalize. As various fibers and bundles of fibers have been inactive or underactive ... it is as if they are waking up from a deep sleep. These elements, previously in their state of *suspended animation,* can be proprioceptively confused or even in a state of amnesia until they become re-familiarized with a particular demand and newly available movement pattern. Basically, the muscles had to relearn their function when called into action.

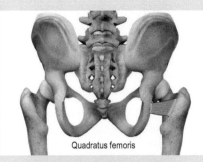
Quadratus femoris

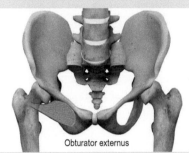
Obturator externus

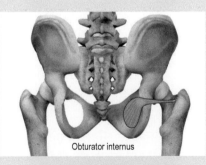
Obturator internus

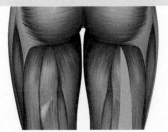
Biceps femoris

Fig 9.7
Traumatic scar formation

the tissue beyond the initial barrier without having to apply more pressure (Andrade 2013).

General application protocol:

- Engage at the edge of the first restriction barrier, and hold a constant force/pressure until a release is felt – typically 60–90 seconds

- There is no movement of tissue or therapist hands once barrier is engaged, until a release is felt

- Once release of the first barrier occurs, the therapist's hands follow the release to the next barrier

- The process is repeated through a possible 3–6 barriers, and subsequent barriers may take longer to release (3–5 minutes) and for the client's pain/discomfort to diminish

- The entire treatment process, in one general locale, may take up to 25–30 minutes

- Pressure grading can vary, but is typically applied in the 4–6 range (see Box 9.8).

As previously noted, another protocol includes the ultra-slow drag or movement of the therapist's hands/fingers/elbow/forearm along a particular vector. This approach is commonly employed when working with myofascial meridians and will not be covered in depth in this book. For a deeper understanding of this approach the authors recommend the study of *Anatomy Trains* (Myers 2013) or other Structural Integration/Rolf type methods.

Clinical Consideration

As all of the therapeutic loading techniques are application of mechanical strain, all have the potential to influence neurophysiological and integrin-mediated responses. Additionally, mechanical strain stretches tissue and generates heat, which in turn influence tissue pliability and mobility.

Tension technique

Tension technique is the tensile opposition of structures in the form traction, drag, glide, stretch, extension and elongation. The intended outcome is lengthening tissue and cleaving excessive/undue collagen cross-links and disengaging fine pathological cross-links, as illustrated in Figure 9.8.

Compression technique

Compression technique comprises downward-perpendicular pressure, or approximation of two structures in the form of squeezing, grasping to increase pressure. Intended outcomes include influencing fluid movement and endorphin release, as shown in Figure 9.9.

Bending

Bending technique combines compression and tension loading – one side of the tissue is

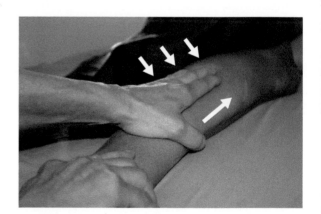

Figure 9.8

Tension. The lower leg is being anchored by the therapist's right hand, while the left hand engages the tissue by applying compression (begin at pressure grade 1–3 (see Box 9.8) and slowly increase until barrier is felt), then glide slowly, creating drag and tensioning in a proximal direction.

compressed as the other side is elongated, often performed cross-fiber. It is intended to influence tissue length, tissue glide and fluid movement, and mechanical cleavage/disengagement of undue cross-links (see Fig. 9.10a & b).

Shear

Oblique or laterally applied gliding type movement of one tissue or layer in reference to another. Intended outcome is to influence fluid dynamics (e.g. GS and HA changes: shift GS viscosity and increase the lubrication potential of HA in the sliding layers), generate heat and mechanical cleavage/disengagement of undue cross-links – culminating in improved tissue mobility and slide/glide capabilities (see Fig. 9.11a & b).

Torsion/rotation

Torsion/rotation is twisting-type loading; essentially, a combination of compression and tension where there is simultaneous compression of some fibers with elongation of others. Multiple

intended outcomes associated with compression and tension as noted above, as illustrated in Figure 9.12.

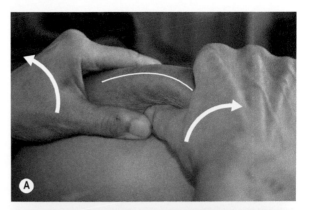

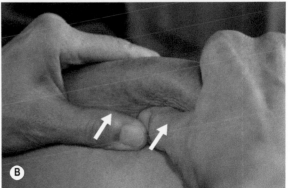

Figure 9.10

(A) **Bend**. Begin by grasping the bulk of tissue in an approximation–compression manner: simultaneously apply pressure into the tissue with the thumbs and deviate the wrists in an ulnar direction (arrows) to bend the tissue (begin at pressure grade 1–3 (see Box 9.8) and slowly increase until barrier/bind is felt). (B) **Combined bend and shear**. Once the tissue is grasped and bend is achieved (see A), slowly shear across (parallel to) the underlying tissues (white line). Bend combined with shearing achieves a skin rolling-type effect. Similarly, approximation–compression can be combined with shearing.

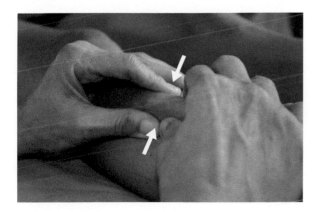

Figure 9.9

Approximation-compression. The therapist applies equal amount of pressure with the thumbs and fingers to achieve approximation-compression of the tissue (begin at pressure grade 1–3 (see Box 9.8), and slowly increase until barrier/bind is felt).

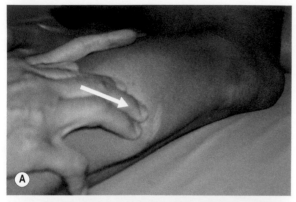

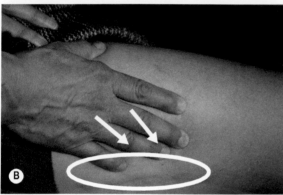

Figure 9.11

(A) **Shear**: begin by engaging the tissue with compression (begin at pressure grade 1–3 (see Box 9.8) and slowly increase until barrier is felt) – once barrier is engaged, slowly shear-glide in a lateral/angular direction. (A) The tissue is being sheared across the surface of the tibia. (B) **Using shearing for barrier/assessment**: often dimpling or puckering can be observed when shearing is applied near an area of stuck or adhered tissue – as noted in the circled area.

Other Techniques

Oscillations

Oscillation techniques, in the form of shaking, movement back and forth, and rocking, have

been found to be effective in mobilizing tissue layers, disengaging stuck tissue and increasing the lubrication potential of HA in the sliding layers. Oscillations are commonly applied in combination with compression or lifting. Oscillations can be used to address superficial and deeper layers of tissue. Barrier considerations apply.

Clinical Consideration

It is common to employ combinations of loading techniques. *Example*: combining compression with shearing/oscillation creates a heat generating and friction-like effect that impacts HA in ways that increase its lubrication potential and thereby improves tissue slide/glide capabilities (Roman et al. 2013).

Lifting techniques

The techniques in this category are aimed at lifting and separating one component away from another, such as muscle away from underlying bone or skin away from underlying SF. Lifting techniques can be combined with tension, bending, shear and torsion and can be utilized to address both superficial and deeper tissues/layers. Barrier considerations apply.

Vertical lifts

Vertical lifts, a form of tension loading, can be used to treat scars and/or tissue that can be gripped between the thumb and fingers. A vertical or perpendicular lift/stretch is applied and held until a release is felt, allowing for further stretch. The technique can be applied in sequence, with brief rest periods, until no further tissue mobilization or stretch can be elicited (Fourie 2014), as illustrated in Figure 9.13a & b.

Skin rolling

Skin that is stuck or adhered to SF can occur as a result of trauma and may suggest underlying

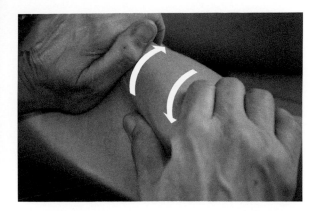

Figure 9.12

Torsion/rotation. Begin by grasping the tissue in an approximation-compression manner – then twist the tissue in opposing directions to achieve torsion/rotation (begin at pressure grade 1–3 (see Box 9.8), and slowly increase until barrier/bind is felt.

problems such as scarring that extends to deeper tissue.

Skin rolling, a combination of lifting, tension and shearing loading, is considered to be a form of CT massage and is commonly used in the treatment of postsurgical scarring and scars associated with burns (Kobesova et al. 2007, Pohl 2010, Fourie 2014). Skin rolling is not indicated for keloids (Fourie 2012).

Skin rolling can be used to address various layers of tissue and the technique can be graded (Holey & Dixon 2014):

- Grade 1: is the most superficial, engaging the layers of skin only

- Grade 2: engages the interface between the skin and underlying SF

- Grade 3: engages deeper layers (e.g. the interface between the superficial and DF and between the DF and underlying muscle).

The technique is aimed at lifting layers away from one another and mobilizing the stuck tissue. Skin rolling has been shown to modify collagen density – consistent with a desirable shift in fluid dynamics that results in improved tissue pliability (Pohl 2010) – illustrated in Figure 9.14. Skin rolling, at grade 3, has also been shown to sedate SNS hyperactivity and therefore can be useful for ANS rebalancing (Andrade 2013, Holey & Dixon 2014). Under certain circumstances skin rolling can be moderately to intensely uncomfortable or painful for the client, and so the authors recommend appropriate consideration of client comfort. Pushing into and through significant pain is not recommended. Skin rolling can be performed with or without the use of lotion/lubricant.

Alphabet Techniques

Most massage therapists will readily recognize the terms Cs, Ss and Js in reference to technique application. These techniques can be utilized to address both superficial and deeper tissues/layers. Barrier considerations apply (see Figs. 9.14–9.16):

- Cs (Fig. 9.15): a form of compression and bending loading – where one side of the tissue compresses and the other is tensioned – elicits both circulatory and lengthening effects, generally aimed at engaging deeper layers/tissue, although can be applied to engage the skin and SF layer Ss (Fig. 9.16), a multidirectional form of loading, similar to Cs.

- J-stroke (Fig. 9.17): combination of tension, compression and bending that elicits both circulatory and lengthening effects, generally aimed at engaging more superficial layers/tissue. Like gentle circles, this technique can be used in the earlier stages of healing, once the scar is stable (i.e. no risk of dehiscence). Typically, pressure grades 1–4 (see Box 9.8) are used when applying this technique. J-stroke can be performed with or without the use of lotion/lubricant.

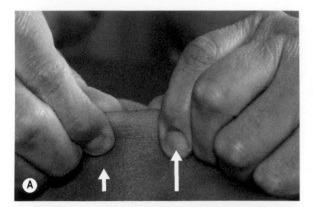

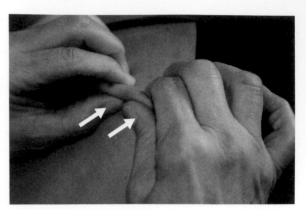

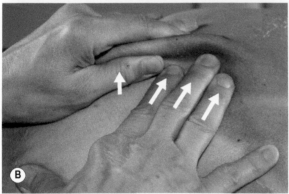

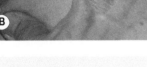

Figure 9.14

Skin rolling. Begin by applying approximation-compression (as described in Fig. 9.9) then glide/roll the tissue between the thumbs and fingers, parallel to the surface of the body (arrows). The bulk of and depth with which the tissue is grasped will determine the layer of tissue impacted (e.g. epidermis, dermis and SF/CT – see the Holey and Dixon Grading Scale, p. 221). Grade 2 is demonstrated in this illustration.

Figure 9.13

Lifting. Begin by grasping the tissue in an approximation-compression manner (apply enough pressure to be able to securely hold onto the tissue), then lift the tissue away from underlying structures. This technique can be used near and directly over scars (in the appropriate stage of healing). Lifting can be combined with shearing (see B) and oscillations – with oscillations the tissue is lifted and then sheared in a back and forth manner. (B) **Lift and shear**. As in (A), the therapist's left hand grasps the tissue in an approximation-compression manner and lifts the tissue – simultaneously, the right hand shears underneath the lifted tissue. This technique application achieves a skin rolling-type effect.

Gross stretch

Gross stretch technique is a combination of tension and compression, and is utilized to engage broader areas of tissue. Gross stretch can be used when more intense, isolating or deeper techniques, such as skin rolling or shear, are uncomfortable for the client to receive. Gross stretch can also be used to pre-warm and soften tissue prior to applying more intense type of techniques. This technique can be used to address either superficial or deeper tissue layers. Pressure can vary from very light (grade 1–3 – see Box 9.8) to moderate (grade 4–6). Barrier considerations apply.

Gentle circles

Gentle circle technique, a combination of tension and compression, is used to target superficial

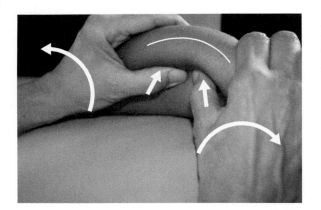

Figure 9.15

'Cs'. Begin as noted in Fig. 9.10 – grasp the bulk of tissue in an approximation-compression manner. Simultaneously apply pressure into the tissue with the thumbs and deviate the wrists in an ulnar direction (curved arrows), bending the tissue into the letter 'C' until barrier/bind is felt.

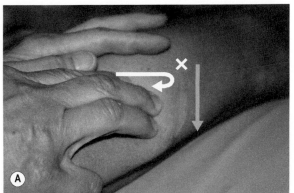

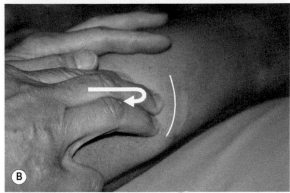

Figure 9.17

J-stroke. Begin at one end of the scar (X), apply compression (pressure grading can vary depending upon the stage of healing and client comfort) then slowly glide in to the scar margin and circularly glide back away from the scar (white arrow), making a letter 'J'. This technique can be applied along the entire length of the scar (yellow arrow). (B) **J-stroke – compression, tension and bending**. As noted in (A), glide into the scar margin, bending the scar tissue (white line) and then circularly glide back.

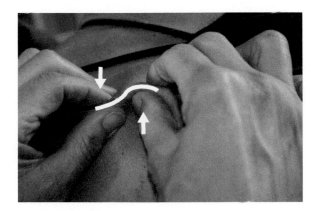

Figure 9.16

'Ss'. Begin by grasping the tissue in an approximation-compression manner, then apply pressure into the tissue with the thumbs and fingers in opposing directions, bending the tissue into the letter 'S' (begin at pressure grade 1–3 (see Box 9.8), and slowly increase until barrier/bind is felt).

tissue layers. Like J-strokes, gentle circles can be used in the earlier stages of healing, once the scar is stable (i.e. no risk of dehiscence). Typically, pressure grades 1–4 (see Box 9.8) are used when applying this technique. This technique is also commonly used as a form of client self-massage. Lotion/lubricant is typically used to perform this technique.

Clinical Consideration

Some of the benefits of myofascial techniques may be due to neurophysiological effects (Cantu & Grodin 2001). According to Schleip (2003), fascial/myofascial techniques impact the NS in ways that lead to a global decrease in SNS tone, which in its turn produces a vasomotor response that results in short-term changes in fascial viscoelasticity, thus improving slide/glide between tissue layers. Others suggest myofascial techniques may result in structural changes, such as the cleavage of collagen cross-links or collagen fibril microfailure (Threlkeld 1992, Simmonds et al. 2012, Tozzi 2012).

Clinical Consideration

Irritated nerves do not like to be stretched. When you are working with nerves inside scar tissue, work the outer edges of the scar first. If working with scars near a large nerve branch area, such as the lumbar, brachial plexuses, let your client know that they may experience some discomfort following treatment. If using more forceful techniques, like transverse frictions, some post-treatment may occur. Instruct your client to employ anti-inflammatory measures, such as ice application, following treatment.

Clinical Consideration

It is important to note that eliciting paresthesia sensations may indicate neural distress. Exercise caution if strong paresthesia sensations are elicited when

Clinical Consideration (Cont.)

the barrier is challenged as too much strain/pulling or compression of sensitive neural structures may exacerbate the client's symptoms and/or drive SNS hyperarousal. The authors discourage the application of too strong or forceful barrier challenge, both during assessment and treatment, as this tends to prove counterproductive.

Pathophysiological Consideration

Changes in the skin and SF often mirror changes in deeper fascia. Skin folds or creases in the neck have been correlated with cervical joint dysfunction (Gunn & Milbrandt 1978). It has been shown that the skin and SF are more adherent and resistant to skin rolling techniques over spinal levels which are dysfunctional (Taylor et al. 1990). The same applies in the reverse, because the layers are interconnected, distortions or restrictions in DF are often reflected in the skin and SF.

Clinical Consideration

Manual therapy techniques treat the fascial layers by altering density, tonus, viscosity, and the arrangement of fascia (Findley et al. 2012).

Clinical Consideration

As the mechanophysiological conditions of injured skin greatly influence the degree of scar formation, scar contracture and abnormal scar progression/generation, Ogawa et al. (2011) suggests the use of

Clinical Consideration (Cont.)

strategies for scar prevention and treatment include those that influence receptors sensitive to mechanical forces. Mechanical forces such as stretching tension, shear force, scratch, compression, hydrostatic pressure, and osmotic pressure can be perceived by integrins and various sensory nerve receptors. Different forms of manual loading and mechanical strain result in mechanotransduction-mediated effects that exert a positive influence on remodeling and healthy scar formation (Chaitow 2014).

General Treatment and Technique Safety Considerations

It is not productive to 'over-power', plough through or force tissue release – this will result in undue client discomfort and other undesirable outcomes.

Minimize the potential of client post-treatment soreness and/or bruising by working slowly. Primary causes of adverse reactions are attempting to push too fast and being too forceful or aggressive with the tissue. The general idea is to coax and encourage a release.

If there feels like too much resistance in the client's tissue, pause, ease up and/or slow down. If the client's tissues do not seem to be favorably responsive, pause treatment and re-evaluate. Sometimes a simple change like easing up, slowing down or changing technique and/or the angle or direction of technique application will prove productive.

Avoid over-treating. Initially 5–15 minutes in a particular area is relatively safe. As your skill and confidence levels evolve, longer periods of time can be spent in a particular area, allowing for progression into deeper layers of tissue. Progress at a rate that is congruent with the development of your skill level.

When employing deeper techniques and when working with traumatic scar tissue clients, it is important to appreciate the difference between the work occurring as intense verses invasive and distressing.

It is the nature of this work to be intense at times. 'Intense' is described as a focused, tolerable level of discomfort which does not adversely affect the client's sense of comfort, feeling of safety or relaxed breathing. Although treatment may at times feel intense, the client is able to detect an undercurrent of productivity.

Whereas 'invasive' can be described as that which manifests to the client as unproductive or overwhelming pain or discomfort, feeling like their body or tissues are being forced or over-powered. Anything that is perceived by the client as invasive or alarming may excite a protective response from the SNS. Such a response is considered counterproductive.

The authors subscribe to a non-invasive, non-alarming approach. As noted, during treatment the client may experience some discomfort (some) but there ought to be a simultaneous undercurrent of productivity. Following treatment the client may feel some mild discomfort that ought to resolve within 24 hours post-treatment. With the exception of transverse frictions (not covered in this book), the client should not experience any inflammation, bruising or any moderate to severe pain attributable to the techniques.

Clinical Consideration

In various studies conducted excessive force was not required in order to elicit a positive response – this work does not have to be painful to be productive. **This cannot be emphasized enough!**

Remember that everyone has different levels of sensitivity to touch – use sound judgment and proceed accordingly. Also be mindful of ANS response and emotional release considerations – a discussion with your client, prior to treatment, may be appropriate.

If you cannot seem to find a position that feels comfortable to your body, pause treatment, and change your position, or you may need to ask the client to change position. Be ever mindful of your body positioning. At no time should you compromise your comfort or well-being – therapist self care considerations will be covered in more detail in Chapter 10.

Post-Treatment Recommendations

The authors advise three general post-treatment selfcare measures for clients, to facilitate the

work further and help reduce the incidence of post-treatment soreness:

- Heat application – as the authors employ the techniques in a manner that does not instigate inflammation, heat in the therapeutic range (35–40°C or 99–104°F) is indicated. In general, moist-heat application is favored as it seems to penetrate the tissues better.

- Hydration – suggest the client drink 2–3 glasses of water.

- Gentle movement – now that the tissue moves/slides more freely, it is important to keep it moving.

Client self care will be covered in more detail in Chapter 10.

References

Aarabi S, Bhatt KA, Shi Y et al (2007) Mechanical load initiates hypertrophic scar formation through decreased cellular apoptosis. FASEB J 21(12): 3250–61.

Alder S (2015) Available at: http://www.goodreads.com/quotes/633610-the-most-important-thing-in-communication-is-hearing-what-isn-t [Accessed 27 March 2015].

Andrade CK (2013) Outcome-based massage: putting evidence into practice. Baltimore: Lippincott Williams & Wilkins.

Andrade CK, Clifford P (2008) Outcome-based massage: from evidence to practice. Baltimore: Lippincott Williams and Wilkins.

ASRM Committee (2013) Pathogenesis, consequences, and control of peritoneal adhesions in gynecology surgery: a committee opinion. Fertility and Sterility 99:1550. Doi:10.1016/j.fern-stert.2013.02.031.

Bailey AJ (2001) Molecular mechanisms of ageing in connective tissues. Mechanisms of Ageing and Development 122(7): 735–755.

Beider S, Mahrer NE, Gold JI (2007) Pediatric massage therapy: an overview for clinicians. Pediatric Clinics of North America 54 (6): 1025–1041.

Best TM, Gharaibeh B, Huard J (2013) Stem cells, angiogenesis and muscle healing: a potential role in massage therapies? British Journal of Sports Medicine 47: 556–560.

Bhadal N, Wall IB, Porter SR et al (2008) The effect of mechanical strain on protease production by keratinocytes. British Journal of Dermatology 158(2): 396–8.

Bouffard NA, Cutroneo KR, Badger GJ et al (2008) Tissue stretch decreases soluble TGF-β and type I procollagen in mouse subcutaneous connective tissue: Evidence from ex vivo and in vivo models. Journal of Cell Physiology 214: 389–395.

Bove G, Chapelle S (2010) Lessons from the Conference: 'Highlighting massage therapy in complimentary and integrative medicine'. Journal of Bodywork and Movement Therapies 14: 312–414.

Bove GM, Chapelle SL (2012) Visceral mobilization can lyse and prevent peritoneal adhesions in a rat model. Journal of Bodywork and Movement Therapies 16(1): 76–82.

Boyer MI, Goldfarb CA, Gelberman RH (2005) Recent progress in flexor tendon healing. The modulation of tendon healing with rehabilitation variables. Journal of Hand Therapy 18: 80–5; quiz 86.

Buehler MJ (2008) Nanomechanics of collagen fibrils under varying cross-link densities: Atomistic and continuum studies. Journal of the Mechanical Behavior of Biomedical Materials 1(1): 59–67.

Cantu RI, Grodin AJ (2001) Myofascial manipulation: theory and clinical application. Austin: Pro-Ed.

Carano A, Siciliani G (1996) Effects of continuous and intermittent forces on human fibroblasts in vitro. European Journal of Orthodontics 18(1): 19–26.

Cencetti F, Bernacchioni C, Nincheri P et al (2010) Transforming growth factor-beta1 induces transdifferentiation of myoblasts into myofibroblasts via upregulation of sphingosine kinase-1/S1P3 axis. Molecular Biology of the Cell 21(6): 1111–1124.

Chaitow (2014) Fascial dysfunction – manual therapy approaches. Pencaitland, UK: Handspring Publishing.

Chaitow L, DeLany J (2008) Clinical application of neuromuscular techniques, 2nd edn. Edinburgh: Churchill Livingstone Elsevier.

Chan MW, Hinz B, McCulloch CA (2010) Mechanical induction of gene expression in connective tissue cells. Methods in Cell Bioliology 98: 178–205.

Chaudhry H, Schleip R, Ji Z et al (2008) Three-dimensional mathematical model for deformation of human fasciae in manual therapy. JAOA: Journal of the American Osteopathic Association 108(8): 379–390.

Chikly BJ (2002) Silent Waves: theory and practice of lymph drainage therapy: with applications for lymphedema, chronic pain, and inflammation. Scottsdale, AZ: IHH Publishing.

Chikly BJ (2005) Manual techniques addressing the lymphatic system: origins and development. Journal of the American Osteopathic Association 105: 457–474.

Cho Y, Jeon J, Hong A et al (2014) The effect of burn rehabilitation massage therapy on hypertrophic scar after burn: a randomized controlled trial. Burns: Journal of the International Society for Burn Injuries 12/2014; DOI: 10.1016/j.burns.2014.02.005.

Clark ME, Gironda RJ (2002) Practical utility of outcome measurement. In: Weiner RS (ed). Pain management: a practical guide for clinicians, 6th edn. Boca Raton: CRC Press.

Cohen DB, Kawamura S, Ehteshami JR, Rodeo SA (2006) Indomethacin and celecoxib impair rotator cuff tendon-to-bonehealing. American Journal of Sports Medicine 34: 362–369.

Collet JP, Fazeli M, Guan L (2014) Research talks – a comprehensive model of stress, inflammation and health to support, evaluate and guide personalized complementary and alternative interventions. In: CAM Research Symposium, November, Calgary, Canada.

Cramer GD, Henderson CN, Little JW et al (2010) Zygapophyseal joint adhesions after induced hypomobility.

Journal of Manipulative and Physiological Therapeutics 33(7): 508–518.

Day JA, Copetti L, Rucli G (2012) From clinical experience to a model for the human fascial system. Journal of Bodywork and Movement Therapies 16(3): 372–380.

Derderian CA, Bastidas N, Lerman OZ et al (2005) Mechanical strain alters gene expression in an in vitro model of hypertrophic scarring. Annals of Plastic Surgery 55(1): 69–75.

Desmouliere A, Geinoz A, Gabbiani F, Gabbiani FT (1993) Transforming growth factor-beta 1 induces alpha-smooth muscle actin expression in granulation tissue myofibroblasts and in quiescent and growing cultured fibroblasts. The Journal of Cell Biology 122: 103e111.

Discher DE, Mooney DJ, Zandstra PW (2009) Growth factors, matrices, and forces combine and control stem cells. Science 324: 1673–1677.

Dryden T, Moyer CA (eds) (2012) Massage therapy: integrating research and practice. Champaign, Ill: Human Kinetics.

Dupont S, Morsut L, Aragona M et al (2011) Role of YAP/TAZ in mechanotransduction. Nature 474: 179–183.

Eagan TS, Meltzer KR, Standley PR (2007) Importance of strain direction in regulating human fibroblast proliferation and cytokine secretion: a useful in vitro model for soft tissue injury and manual medicine treatments. Journal of Manipulative and Physiological Therapeutics 30(8): 584–592.

Eisenhart AW, Gaeta TJ, Yens DP (2003) Osteopathic manipulative treatment in the emergency department for patients with acute ankle sprains. Journal of American Osteopathic Association 103: 417–421.

Eming S, Martin P, Tomic-Canic M (2014) Wound repair and regeneration: mechanisms, signaling, and translation. Science Translational Medicine [serial online]. 6(265): 265sr6.

Eti AF editor (2006) Ağrı Doğası ve Kontrolü, 1st edn. Istanbul: Bilim Yayınları, pp 135–47.

Ezzo J (2007) What can be learned from Cochrane Systematic Reviews of massage that can guide future research. Journal of Alternative and Complementary Medicine 13(2): 291–295.

Fearmonti R, Bond J, Erdmann D, Levinson H (2010) A review of scar scales and scar measuring devices. Journal of Plastic Surgery 10: 354–363.

Findley T, Chaudhry H, Stecco A, Roman M (2012) Fascia research – a narrative review. Journal of Bodywork and Movement Therapies 16(1): 67–75.

Fitch P (2014) Talking body, listening hands: a guide to professionalism, communication and the therapeutic relationship. Upper Saddle River, NJ:Prentice Hall.

Földi M (2012) Foeldi's textbook of lymphology: For Physicians and Lymphedema therapists, 3rd edn. St Louis, MO: Mosby.

Fourie W (2012) In: Schleip R, Findley T, Chaitow L, Huijing P (eds) Fascia: the tensional network of the human body. Edinburgh: Churchill Livingstone Elsevier.

Fourie W (2014) Management of scars and adhesions. In: Chaitow L, ed. Fascial dysfunction: manual therapy approaches. Ch. 18. Pencaitland, UK: Handspring Publishing.

Fourie WJ, Robb KA (2009) Physiotherapy management of axillary web syndrome following breast cancer treatment: discussing the use of soft tissue techniques. Physiotherapy 95(4): 314–320.

Franz MG, Steed DL, Robson MC (2007) Optimizing healing of the acute wound by minimizing complications. Current Problems in Surgery 14: 691–763.

Fritz S (2013) Mosby's Fundamentals of therapeutic massage, 5th edn. Maryland Heights, MA: Elsevier Mosby.

Gantwerker E, Hom D (2012) Principles to minimize scars. Facial Plastic Surgery: FPS [serial online]. October 28(5): 473–486.

Geiersperger K (2009) Wundheilung und Ernahrung. Master Theisis fur der Universitatslehrgang fur sports physiotherapy. Paris Lodron Universitat – Abteilung Sportwissenschaften.

Gilbert PM, Havenstrite KL, Magnusson KE et al (2010) Substrate elasticity regulates skeletal muscle stem cell self-renewal in culture. Science 329: 1078–1081.

Gordillo GM, Sen CK (2003) Revisiting the essential role of oxygen in wound healing. American Journal of Surgery 186: 259–263.

Goutos I, Dziewulski P, Richardson PM (2009) Pruritus in burns: review article. Journal of Burn Care and Research 30: 221–8.

Gowan-Moody D (2011) The use of pain rating scales - a low back pain model. TouchU.ca online course. Available at: www.touchu.ca [Accessed 18 February 2015].

Granert O, Peller M, Gaser C et al (2011) Manual activity shapes structure and function in contralateral human motor hand area. NeuroImage 54(1): 32–41.

Guan L, Collet JP, Yuskiv N et al (2014) The effect of massage therapy on autonomic activity in critically ill children. Evidence-based Complementary and Alternative Medicine: eCAM, 2014, 656750.

Guimberteau (2012) Scars and Adhesions Panel - Lecture notes from The 3rd International Fascia Research Congress, Vancouver, 28–30 March.

Gunn CC, Milbrandt WE (1978) Early and subtle signs in low-back sprain. Spine 3(3): 267–281.

Gürol AP, Polat S, Akçay MN (2010) Itching, pain, and anxiety levels are reduced with massage therapy in burned adolescents. Journal of Burn Care & Research 31(3): 429–432.

Hammer W (2013) Dynamic Chiropractic Canada – October 1, Vol 06, Issue 10. Available at: http://www.dynamicchiropractic.ca/mpacms/dc_ca/article.php?id=56688 [Accessed 24 February 2015].

Hertling D, Kessler RM (2006) Management of common musculoskeletal disorders: physical therapy principles and methods. Philadelphia: Lippincott Williams & Wilkins.

Hinz B (2007) Formation and function of the myofibroblast during tissue repair. Journal of Investigative Dermatology 127, 526–537.

Hinz B (2009) Tissue stiffness, latent TGF-beta1 activation, and mechanical signal transduction: implications for the pathogenesis and treatment of fibrosis. Current Rheumatology Reports 11(2), 120e126.

Hodge LM, King HH, Williams AG et al (2007) Abdominal lymphatic pump treatment increases leukocyte count flux in thoracic duct lymph. Lymphatic Research and Biology 5: 127–134.

Holey EA, Dixon J (2014) Connective tissue manipulation and skin rolling. In: Chaitow L (ed) Fascial dysfunction: manual therapy approaches. Pencaitland, UK: Handspring Publishing, Ch. 7.

Hou WH, Chiang PT, Hsu TY et al (2010) Treatment effects of massage therapy in depressed people: a meta-analysis. Journal of Clinical Psychiatry 71: 894–901. Doi:10.4088/JCP.09r05009blu.

Hynes RO (2009) The extracellular matrix: not just pretty fibrils. Science 326: 1216–1219.

Jarvinen TA, Jarvinen TL, Kaariainen M et al (2007) Muscle injuries: optimizing recovery. Best Practice and Research Clinical Rheumatology 21: 317–31.

Kaariainen M, Liljamo T, Pelto-Huikko M et al (2001) Regulation of alpha-7 integrin by mechanical stress during skeletal muscle regeneration. Neuromuscular Disorders 11: 360–69.

Kanazawa Y, Nomura J, Yoshimoto S et al (2009) Cyclical cell stretching of skin-derived fibroblasts downregulates connective tissue growth factor (CTGF). Connective Tissue Research 50: 323.

Kania (2012) Scars. Ch 15. In: Dryden T, Moyer C (eds) Massage therapy: integrating research and practice. Champaign, Il:Human Kinetics.

Kassolik K et al (2009) Tensegrity principle in massage demonstrated by electro and mechanomyography. Journal of Bodywork and Movement Therapy 13: 164.

Kishikova L, Smith MD, Cubison T (2014) Evidence based management for paediatric burn: new approaches and improved scar outcomes. Burns 40(8): 1530–1537.

Klingler W (2012) In: Schleip R, Findley T, Chaitow L, Huijing P (eds) Fascia: the tensional network of the human body. Edinburgh: Churchill Livingstone Elsevier, ch 7.18, pp 421–424.

Knott EM, Tune JD, Stoll ST, Downey HF (2005) Increased lymphatic flow in the thoracic duct during manipulative intervention. Journal of American Osteopathic Association 105: 447–456.

Kobesova A et al (2007) Twenty-year-old pathogenic 'active' postsurgical scar: a case study of a patient with persistent right lower quadrant pain. Journal of Manipulative and Physiological Therapeutics 30(3): 234–238.

Korosec BJ (2004) Manual lymphatic drainage therapy. Home Health Care Management and Practice 17: 499–511.

Langevin H (2010) Presentation: ultrasound imaging of connective tissue pathology associated with chronic low back pain. 7th Interdisciplinary Congress on Low Back and Pelvic Pain, Los Angeles.

Langevin HM, Sherman KJ (2007) Pathophysiological model for chronic low back pain integrating connective tissue and nervous system mechanisms. Medical Hypotheses 68: 74.

Lee, TS, Kilbreath SL, Refshauge KM et al (2008) Prognosis of the upper limb following surgery and radiation for breast cancer. Breast Cancer Research and Treatment 110: 19–37.

Lewis C (2015) Instructors on the front line-observation. Available at: http://www.abmp.com/instructors_on_the_front_lines/IFL_Topic_4.php [Accessed 4 June 2015].

Lewit K, Olsanska S (2004) Clinical importance of active scars: abnormal scars as a cause of myofascial pain. Journal of Manipulative and Physiological Therapeutics 27(6): 399–402.

Li Y, Foster W, Deasy BM et al (2004) Transforming growth factor-beta1 induces the differentiation of myogenic cells into fibrotic cells in injured skeletal muscle: a key event in muscle fibrogenesis. American Journal of Pathology 164 (3): 1007e1019.

Magra M, Maffulli N (2006) Nonsteroidal antiinflammatory drugs in tendinopathy: friend or foe. Clinical Journal of Sports Medicine 16: 1–3.

Meert GF (2012) Fluid dynamics in fascial tissues. pp 177–182. In Schleip R, Findley T, Chaitow L, Huijing P (eds) (2012) Fascia. The tensional network of the human body. Edinburgh: Churchill Livingstone Edinburgh.

Monstrey S, Middelkoop E, Vranckx JJ et al (2014) Updated scar management practical guidelines: non-invasive and invasive measures. Journal of Plastic, Reconstructive and Aesthetic Surgery 67(8): 1017–1025.

Moyer CA, Rounds J, Hannum JW (2004) A meta-analysis of massage therapy research. Psychological Bulletin 130 (1): 3–18.

Moyer CA, Dryden T, Shipwright S (2009) Directions and dilemmas in massage therapy research: a workshop report from the 2009 North American Research Conference on Complementary and Integrative Medicine. International Journal of Therapeutic Massage and Bodywork 2(2): 15.

MSKTC (2011) Wound Care and Scar Management after Burn Injury – 2011 Model Systems Knowledge Translation Center (MSKTC). Based on research by Burn Injury Model Systems. Available at: http://www.phoenix-society.org/resources/entry/burn-wound-care [Accessed 17 January 2015].

Myers TW (2013) Anatomy trains: myofascial meridians for manual and movement therapists, 3e. Edinburgh: Churchill Livingstone Elsevier.

Ng CP, Hinz B, Swartz MA (2005) Interstitial fluid flow induces myofibroblast differentiation and collagen alignment in vitro. Journal of Cell Science 118(20): 4731–4739.

NIH (2015) Massage therapy for health purposes: what the science says. Available at: https://nccih.nih.gov/health/providers/digest/massage-science [Accessed 21 February 2015].

NIMH (2015) Serious mental illness (SMI) among U.S. adults. Available at: http://www.nimh.nih.gov/health/statistics/prevalence/serious-mental-illness-smi-among-us-adults.shtml [Accessed 26 February 2015].

Ogawa R, Akaishi S, Huang C et al (2011) Clinical applications of basic research that shows reducing skin tension could prevent and treat abnormal scarring: the importance of fascial/subcutaneous tensile reduction sutures and flap surgery for keloid and hypertrophic scar reconstruction. Journal of Nippon Medical School 78(2): 68–76.

Ohberg L, Lorentzon R, Alfredson H (2004) Eccentric training in patients with chronic Achilles tendinosis: normalised tendon structure and decreased thickness at follow up. British Journal of Sports Medicine 38: 8–11; discussion 11.

Oliveira GV, Chinkes D, Mitchell C, Oliveras G, Hawkins HK, Herdon DN (2005) Objective assessment of burn scar vascularity, erythema, thickness, and planimetry. Dermatologic Surgery 31(1): 48–58.

Perlman AI, Ali A, Njike VY et al (2012) Massage therapy for osteoarthritis of the knee: a randomized dose-finding trial. PLOS One 7(2): e30248.

Philadelphia Panel (2001) Evidence-based clinical practice guidelines on selected rehabilitation interventions for low back pain. Physical Therapy 81: 1641–1674.

Pilat A (2003) Myofascial therapies: myofascial induction. Madrid: Mc-Graw-Hill Interamericana.

Pilat A (2014) MIT. In: Chaitow L (ed) Fascial dysfunction: manual therapy approaches. Pencaitland, UK: Handspring Publishing, Ch. 14.

Pohl H (2010) Changes in structure of collagen distribution in the skin caused by a manual technique Journal of Bodywork and Movement Therapies 14(1): 27–34.

POSAS Group (2015) Available at: http://www.posas.org/ [Accessed 10 April 2015].

Post-White J, Kinney ME, Savik K et al (2003) Therapeutic massage and healing touch improve symptoms in cancer. Integrative Cancer Therapies 2: 332–344.

Prendergast SA, Rummer EH (2012) Connective tissue manipulation. Schleip R, Findley T, Chaitow L, Huijing P (eds) Fascia: the tensional network of the human body. Edinburgh: Churchill Livingstone Elsevier, Ch 7.6, pp 328–334.

Rabello FB, Souza CD, Farina Júnior JA (2014) Update on hypertrophic scar treatment. Clinics 69(8): 565–573.

Rapaport MH, Schettler P, Bresee C (2012) A preliminary study of the effects of repeated massage on hypothalamic–pituitary–adrenal and immune function in healthy individuals: a study of mechanisms of action and dosage. The Journal of Alternative and Complementary Medicine 18(8): 789–797.

Rennekampff HO, Aust M, Vogt PM (2010) Medical needling. In: Color Atlas of Burn Reconstructive Surgery. Berlin Heidelberg: Springer-Verlag, pp 72–75.

Rodríguez RM, del Río FG (2013) Mechanistic basis of manual therapy in myofascial injuries. Sonoelastographic evolution control. Journal of Bodywork and Movement Therapies 17(2): 221–234.

Roh YS, Cho H, Oh JO, Yoon CJ (2007) Effects of skin rehabilitation massage therapy on pruritus, skin status, and depression in burn survivors. Taehan Kanho Hakhoe Chi 37: 221–6.

Roman M, Chaudhry H, Bukie B et al (2013) Mathematical analysis of the flow of hyaluronic acid around fascia during manual therapy motions. JAOA: Journal of the American Osteopathic Association, 113(8): 600–610.

Ryan C (2013) Slide matters – and other fascial significant [paradigm shifting] considerations. Interview with Antonio Stecco MD. Massage Matters Canada – A journal for registered massage therapists. Spring.

Sackett D, Straus S, Richardson WS et al (2000) Evidence-based medicine: how to practice and teach EBM, 2nd edn. Edinburgh: Churchill Livingstone.

Saito M, Marumo K (2009) Collagen cross-links as a determinant of bone quality: a possible explanation for bone fragility in aging, osteoporosis, and diabetes mellitus. Osteoporosis International 21(2): 195–214.

Sandqvist G, Akesson A, Eklund M (2004) Evaluation of paraffin bath treatment in patients with systemic sclerosis. Disability and Rehabilitation 26(16): 981–987.

Schleip R (2003) Fascial plasticity 1. A new neurobiological explanation. Journal of Bodywork and Movement Therapies 7:11e19.

Schleip R, Baker A (2015) Fascia in sport and movement. Pencaitland, UK: Handspring Publishing.

Schreml S, Szeimies RM, Prantl L et al (2010) Oxygen in acute and chronic wound healing. British Journal of Dermatology 163: 257–268.

Sheffield PJ (1988) Tissue oxygen measurements. In: Davis JC, Hunt TK, eds. Problem wounds: the role of oxygen. New York: Elsevier.

Sherman KJ, Cook AJ, Wellman RD et al (2014) Five-week outcomes from a dosing trial of therapeutic massage for chronic neck pain. Annals of Family Medicine 12(2): 112–120.

Simmonds N, Miller P, Gemmell H (2012) A theoretical framework for the role of fascia in manual therapy. Journal of Bodywork and Movement Therapies 16(1): 83–93.

Sinclair M (2007) Modern hydrotherapy for the massage therapist. Baltimore: Lippincott Williams and Wilkins.

Stecco L, Stecco C (2009) Fascial manipulation for musculoskeletal pain and fascial manipulation - the practical part. Padova: Piccin.

Stecco A, Gesi M, Stecco C, Stern R (2013) Fascial components of the myofascial pain syndrome. Current Pain and Headache Reports 17:352.

Tappan F, Benjamin P (1998) General principles for giving massage. In: Tappan's Handbook of healing massage techniques; classic, holistic and emerging methods, 3rd edn. Upper Saddle River: Prentice Hall, pp 72–75.

Taylor P, Tole G, Vernon H (1990) Skin rolling technique as an indicator of spinal joint dysfunction. The Journal of the Canadian Chiropractic Association 34(2): 82.

Threlkeld AJ (1992) The effects of manual therapy on connective tissue. Physical Therapy 72: 893e902.

Tortland PD (2007) Sport injuries and nonsteroidal anti-inflammatory drug (NSAID) use. Connecticut Sport Medicine, Winter:13–14.

Tortora GJ, Funke BR, Case CL (2007) Introduction to microbiology. San Francisco: Pearson Benjamin Cummings.

Tozzi P (2012) Selected fascial aspects of osteopathic practice. Journal of Bodywork and Movement Therapies 16 (4): 503e519.

Tziotzios C, Profyris C, Sterling J (2012) Cutaneous scarring: pathophysiology, molecular mechanisms and scar reduction therapeutics Part II. Strategies to reduce scar formation after dermatologic procedures. Journal of the American Academy of Dermatology 66(1): 13–24.

Uzel SG, Buehler MJ (2011) Molecular structure, mechanical behavior and failure mechanism of the C-terminal cross-link domain in type I collagen. Journal of the Mechanical Behavior of Biomedical Materials 4(2): 153–161.

Vairo GL, Miller SJ, Rier NCI, Uckley WI (2009) Systematic review of efficacy for manual lymphatic drainage techniques in sports medicine and rehabilitation: an evidence-based practice approach. Journal of Manual and Manipulative Therapy 17(3): 80E–89E.

Van den Berg F (2010) Angewandte physiologie – Band 1: Das bindegewebe des bewegunfsapparates; verstehen und beeinflussen [applied physiology – vol. 1; The connective tissue of the locomotor apparatus; understanding and influencing]. Stuttgart: Thieme Verlag.

Van den Berg F (2012) In: Schleip R, Findley T, Chaitow L, Huijing P (Eds) Fascia: the tensional network of the human body. Edinburgh: Churchill Livingstone Elsevier, pp 149–155.

van der Wal MB, Tuinebreijer WE, Bloemen MC et al (2012) Rasch analysis of the Patient and Observer Scar Assessment Scale (POSAS) in burn scars. Quality of Life Research 21(1): 13–23.

Wang J, Hori K, Ding J et al (2011) Toll-like receptors expressed by dermal fibroblasts contribute to hypertrophic scarring. Journal of Cell Physiology 226(5): 1265–73.

Walton T (2011) Medical conditions and massage therapy; a decision tree approach. Baltimore: Lippincott Williams and Wilkins.

Yang G, Im HJ, Wang JHC (2005) Repetitive mechanical stretching modulates IL-1β induced COX-2, MMP-1 expression, and PGE 2 production in human patellar tendon fibroblasts. Gene 363: 166–172.

Zuther JE (2011) Lymphedema management: the comprehensive guide for practitioners. Stuttgart: Thieme.

Resources and Further Reading

Marieb E (2012) Essentials of human anatomy and physiology, 7th edn. San Francisco: Pearson Publishing Benjamin Cummings.

Nelson D (2013) The mystery of pain. Philadelphia: Singing Dragon.

Werner R (2012) A massage therapist's guide to pathology. Philadelphia: Lippincott Williams & Wilkins.

Comparison of before and after treatment

Massage therapists can play an active role in a client's healing and recovery. By implementing the appropriate technique at the correct intensity and time, massage therapy can facilitate the healing process and minimize the aesthetic/cosmetic, emotional and functional impact on the patient. Clients with long-standing mature scars can also benefit from treatment.

This series of comparative photos (pre/post-treatment) illustrates some of the potential changes facilitated by safe and effective treatment.

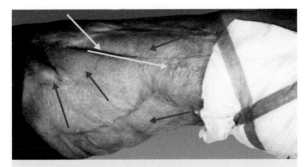

Figure A.1 Pre-treatment

Medial thigh 4th degree skin grafts from a de-gloving injury. Initial insult was in 1986. First specific work began in Winter 2009.

Note bandaged posterior popliteal fascia ulceration. This was a condition due to the lack of pliability of the scar tissue from the hamstrings and quads.

Yellow lines indicate scar keloid that is adhered to the muscle.

Red lines indicate scarred pockets of edema.

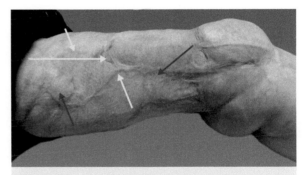

Figure A. 2 Post-treatment

Medial thigh 4th degree keloid and hypertrophic scar release, Sring 2015.

Note popliteal fossa is no longer bandaged due to the scar releases. Note the leather look of the grafted skin. Due to the lack of a dermis in the 4th degree insult, keeping the scar tissue moisturized is a high priority for home care treatment.

Notice the yellow and red lines indicating scar release and release of edema pockets in the leg. Also worthy of attention is the pallor of the skin and muscle development of the area from Figure A-1.

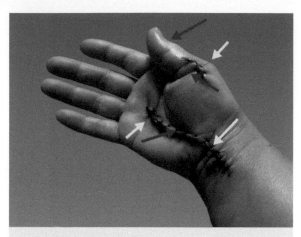

Figure B.1 Pre-treatment

Open carpal tunnel and Camitz opponensplasty surgery, June 2014.

Yellow lines indicate scar keloid that is adhered to the muscle.

Red lines indicate scarred pockets of edema.

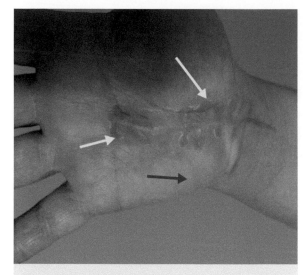

Figure B.2 Post-treatment

Surgical scar after months of scar management therapy, August 2014.

Note keloid scar has changed in pallor, depth and pliability. Notice pockets of edema have subsided substantially and keloid is beginning to flatten.

Yellow lines indicate scar keloid that is adhered to the muscle.

Red lines indicate scarred pockets of edema.

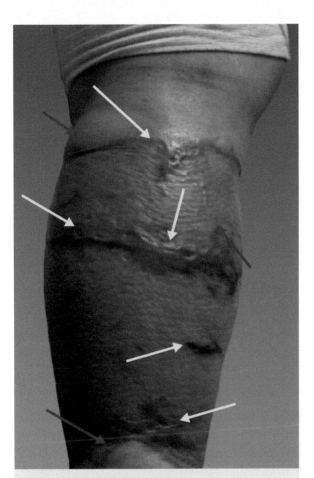

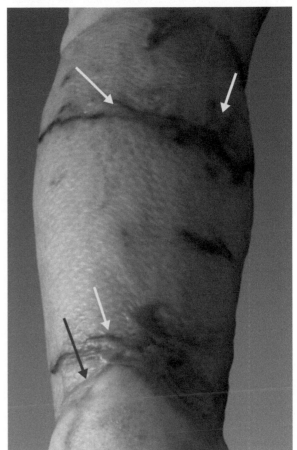

Figure C.1 Pre-treatment

De-gloving injury of left calf with 3rd degree scars. First seen August 2014.

Note how thick and red the keloids are on the grafting lines. Notice the pull of the tissue surrounding the scar and the edema pockets at the base of gastroc and soleus into the Achilles tendon.

Yellow lines indicate scar keloid that is adhered to the muscle.

Red lines indicate scarred pockets of edema.

Figure C.2 Post-treatment

2 December 2014, after bi-monthly 30-minute scar management sessions.

Note the keloid scarring has started to flatten and change pallor. Pockets of edema are diminished as scars are released. Edema modeling is still present at the graft line of the lower keloid at the gastroc, soleus and Achilles tendon. Due to the lymphatic system being compromised, the client was advised to seek manual lymphatic drainage and scar management as maintenance work every 4–6 weeks.

Yellow lines indicate scar keloid that is adhered to the muscle.

Red lines indicate scarred pockets of edema.

Client and therapist self care

Self care is health care

Health is a dynamic, subjective process that is experienced uniquely among individuals. Self care is defined as a process of maintaining health through health promoting practices and managing illness or injury (Riegel et al. 2012).

General self care (e.g. personal hygiene and nutritional practices) and illness or injury-specific self care differ. General self care measures are typically influenced by age, gender, culture, education and socioeconomic status. When in association with illness or injury, self care measures are often influenced by the healthcare provider.

In the massage therapy (MT) practice context, client self care includes an array of activities, such as therapist-recommended post-treatment homecare (e.g. heat application and stretch exercise). The trauma experienced by individuals varies greatly, as do issues that arise during acute care, rehabilitation, and throughout the remainder of life. And so, client self/homecare measures will not be the same for all clients and will likely not be consistent over time (Dahl et al. 2012, Riegel et al. 2012).

The practice and performance of activities by the client, on their own behalf, to support and maintain life, health and wellbeing is an essential part of the post-trauma recovery process (Orem 1991, Riegel et al. 2012). Client self-investment is crucial, as self care is considered essential in the management of chronic presentations, such as mature traumatic scar tissue.

As professional healthcare providers, when we interact with clients, our intention is that the partnership we form will serve to motivate them to engage in self care and to be consistent with any selfcare recommendations.

In the many articles on self care for therapist found in professional journals, a common theme prevails. The bottom line in any caregiving situation is, the very best thing we can do for those who depend on us is to take care of ourselves.

Being a MT practitioner is challenging on many levels. The physicality of the work along with empathetic demands can take a toll. Solid selfcare practices are a must for career longevity. Empathy strain, burnout, compassion fatigue and indirect trauma can be inevitable byproducts our professional demands and certainly so when working with trauma survivors. Effective therapist selfcare strategies are essential to support the therapist who will be in the presence of and touching the pain of others.

The aim of this chapter is to provide information to help guide the development and implementation of effective client and therapist selfcare/homecare strategies.

Self Care

Self care as an all-encompassing term captures those practices and activities we engage in:

- When healthy, as a means to prevent illness and reap all the benefits of living a healthy lifestyle
- During acute illness/injury, to speed the healing process and decrease the incidence of complications or recurrence
- During chronic illness/injury, to help manage and minimize the impact and support good quality of life.

Generally, with recently acquired/acute injuries, the client may be *inexperienced*, whereas health professionals are more experienced or well-versed in the acute presentation, requiring the professional to guide the client (Holman & Lorig 2004). Assisting the client to become more knowledgeable and skilled will impact the effectiveness of their selfcare measures.

With chronic presentations, however, those roles may no longer apply. Often the client is accustomed to their circumstances, living in their body each and every day; therefore, the client needs to be engaged as a more active partner, applying his or her knowledge to the process of developing sound selfcare strategies – although, initially, the client may need assistance with how to engage as an effective participant (Holman & Lorig 2004).

Important outcomes of self care include the maintenance of good health and wellbeing; illness/injury management; and improved quality of life. Additionally, an increase in the client's perceived control over the illness or injury and a decrease in the anxiety, often associated with chronic presentations, is also desirable. Such patient-centered outcomes are of primary importance and ought to be the primary goal in all forms of health care. There is also a growing body of literature suggesting that improved self care can decrease hospitalization, cost and mortality – capturing the attention of health economists (Lucini et al. 2005, Malmstrom et al. 2008, Riegel et al. 2012).

As massage therapists (MTs), our role is to assist the client with functional recovery and his/her capacity to return to previous activities and support their ability to resume social responsibilities. These goals may not be achieved in the short term, necessitating a prolonged treatment and rehabilitation process (Diego et al. 2012). Additionally, this journey will necessitate ongoing client self-management, as interventions for client self-management support are critical to improving quality of care in the chronic care model (Holman & Lorig 2004).

Clinical Consideration

Clients can feel isolated in their 'bubble of trauma' (Gullick et al. 2014), learning to deal with their new body, caregivers after discharge and their new normal. Phenomenological research, of trauma suffered from a burn injury, from China, South Africa, Norway and America show the following results (Gullick et al. 2014):

- Patients perceive the event as a life crisis that shatters their understanding of the world and their place in it

- A reliable recall of events can be blocked by fragmented glimpses of disorganized memories, dreams, hallucinations and even delusions

- Recurring themes of social rejection for young burn survivors and reported experience of lingering feelings of anger and bitterness years after their burn injury.

According to a study from the *Journal of Trauma* (Holbrook et al. 1999), the magnitude of patient impact following major injury is often underestimated. Using the 12- and 18-month Quality of Wellbeing Scale (QWS; questionnaire) to measure outcome, the study concluded that seriousness of injury and intensive care unit days are significantly associated with patient post-injury depression and post-traumatic stress disorder.

Clinical Consideration

Trauma can be life-altering on many levels. Following significant trauma or injury, it is not unusual for a client to feel *betrayed* by their body. Movement and activity that previously were accomplished with ease can be experienced as arduous and painful and this can erode a person's sense of somatic trust, the confidence that our body will perform at the level we

Clinical Consideration (Cont.)

need it to. Eroded trust is generally accompanied by fear and anxiety, which can drive sympathetic nervous system (SNS) hyperactivity. When working with clients who have experienced significant trauma/injury, one important consideration is assisting the client with regaining their sense of confidence in their body's ability to function, and function as close to pain-free as possible. The authors have found this component of care to be integral to the client's recovery, sense of wellbeing and quality of life.

Clinical Consideration

Trauma can be life-altering on many levels. Following significant trauma or injury, it is not unusual for a client to feel betrayed by their body. Movement and activity that previously were accomplished with ease can be experienced as arduous and painful and this can erode a person's sense of somatic trust, the confidence that our body will perform at the level we need it to. Eroded trust is generally accompanied by fear and anxiety, which can drive sympathetic nervous system (SNS) hyperactivity. When working with clients who have experienced significant trauma/injury, one important consideration is assisting the client with regaining their sense of confidence in their body's ability to function, and function as close to pain-free as possible. The authors have found this component of care to be integral to the client's recovery, sense of wellbeing and quality of life.

Selfcare Maintenance, Monitoring and Management

Maintenance, monitoring and management are key concepts of self care (Riegel et al. 2012).

Maintenance

Selfcare maintenance is defined as those behaviors practiced by clients with chronic presentations to maintain physical and emotional stability. These behaviors may be entirely self-determined and directed and/or include recommendations that are mutually agreed on between client and healthcare provider. It is important for the healthcare provider to work collaboratively with the client and strategize how best to integrate as many of the advocated behaviors the patient can accept, with an emphasis on those measures rooted in evidence to support their value.

Monitoring

Selfcare monitoring comprises routine and vigilant body monitoring, surveillance, or *body listening* (Dickson et al. 2008). The goal of self-monitoring is recognition that a change has occurred.

Recognition of an emotional change is aided by personal insight and interpersonal awareness. Recognition of a physical change is facilitated by somatic awareness. As MT is a powerful tool for improving body awareness and literacy, we can see here the value of MT in improving client self-monitoring.

Clients who are skilled in self-monitoring are more adept at self care and can communicate information that will facilitate the healthcare provider's ability to deliver more effective treatment. Self-monitoring is the link between selfcare maintenance and selfcare management.

Management

Selfcare management is defined as the response to sensations and/or changes when they occur. As noted previously, awareness of, and changes in, emotional and physical state is facilitated by alertness to bodily sensations (somatic awareness).

An important component of self-management, facilitated by somatic awareness, is the client's ability to reliably determine how his/her sensations change in response to MT treatment and/or selfcare practices and activities.

Client-reported changes are an integral component in evaluating the effectiveness of implemented treatment and selfcare measures.

Healing and recovery following any trauma or injury extends beyond the treatment room. It is the massage therapist's role to assist the client with evaluating self-management options in order to determine a best course of action, as this will factor significantly into long-term outcomes for the client. The ultimate outcome of scar rehabilitation is for the client to be able to reintegrate into society and fully participate in life.

Clinical Consideration

According to Korn (2013), MT can assist the client with improving body awareness, sense of self and sense of connectedness/socialization and this seems to impact client selfcare and selfregulation behaviors.

Client and Therapist Partnership

To achieve the best possible outcomes, the client and healthcare provider must share complementary knowledge and authority in the healthcare process (Holman & Lorig 2004).

Effective care for chronic traumatic scars requires a partnership between the massage therapist (the MT) and client, working together to develop good strategies for management over time, as rehabilitation from a traumatic injury can be a lifelong process.

A collaborative process that supports the perspectives and experiences of the client, as the experts on their own lives and bodies and what they feel or experience, along with the therapist's knowledge

and expertise, will achieve the most effective and comprehensive outcomes. This is particularly evident when working with chronic presentations, as the client knows most about the consequences they are experiencing as a result of the traumatic event and subsequent traumatic scars. Client knowledge and input is a must for guiding sound management over time.

The client will be responsible for daily management, behavior changes, emotional adjustments and accurate reporting of changes, such as improvements or set-backs. In addition to the delivery of safe, effective and ethical care, the MT is responsible for providing encouragement, relevant information, meaningful activity or exercise recommendations and useful strategies for implementation.

When roles and responsibilities are properly executed, a true client-centered approach is created and more effective self care is achieved (Holman & Lorig 2004).

Client Engagement

All healthcare providers will attest that client compliance is essential for successful outcomes. All healthcare providers will also attest that generating client engagement is not always easy for a variety of reasons. Some aspects of engagement can be facilitated by the therapist and certain barriers diminished (see Box 10.1).

A growing body of literature illustrates the complexity that patients face when trying to incorporate advice from multiple healthcare providers. Misunderstandings, misconception and lack of knowledge all contribute to insufficient self care (Dickson et al. 2011, Riegel et al. 2012). It is therefore important to have full knowledge of what other care providers have recommended so as not to conflict or be redundant.

If the measure is too complex or lacks value in the eye of the client, the likelihood of compliance is impacted. The key is to keep any

Box 10.1

Factors affecting, effective selfcare engagement

Some of the major factors serving as barriers and facilitators to selfcare include (Reigel et al. 2012):

- **Clinician experience and skill**. As is the case with most things, the more experienced we are, the more skilled we become. Over time, the MT may devise more efficient and effective ways to instruct a selfcare measure or recognize what measure will achieve the best possible outcome for a given client. In addition to experience, collaborating or conferring with colleagues is another way to expand the therapist's client selfcare literacy and implementation strategies.

- **Client motivation**. The drive to achieve goals can be intrinsic or extrinsic. Intrinsic motivation is driven by an internal desire to perform a particular task because the individual, themselves, perceive the outcome as beneficial. Extrinsic motivation refers to changing a behavior because it leads to a specific predetermined outcome that is desirable and beneficial, such as to restore function following injury. Most trauma/injury-related selfcare behaviors are, initially, driven by extrinsic motivators. That is, the individual may not be internally motivated to perform a behavior, but the perception of the significance and importance, as conveyed by others, may motivate the client (Ajzen & Fishbein 2005) – motivation strategies with be covered in more detail further on in this chapter.

- **Cultural beliefs and values**. In cultures where independence is valued, selfcare behaviors might be seen as more important or desirable. In some instances, selfcare advice might contradict cultural beliefs, for example to promote rest during recovery, in contrast to activity (Davidson et al. 2007).

- **Habits/daily routines**. Some patients get used to performing certain selfcare behaviors and selfcare becomes part of their daily routine. Others, however, view self care as *work*. For them, the regimen might occur a continuous struggle. Typically, the clients who are the most successful in self care are those who adopt and perform recommended behaviors until the behaviors evolve into habits (Ekman et al. 2000, van der Wal et al. 2010). Here we can see the importance of assisting the client with finding selfcare measures that align with their preferences/values and ones they can more easily integrate into their lifestyle.

therapist directed measures straight-forward and meaningful. Additionally, any measure that can be incorporated into the client's lifestyle will likely be more consistently practiced and will therefore yield better outcomes.

Certain patient-related factors can adversely impair self care, including psychosocial status (e.g. depression, anxiety, less social support, lower self-efficacy, less formal education, socioeconomic status), having a higher number of symptoms, age-related changes (e.g. cognitive and sensory impairments, reduced functioning), lower health literacy and less health system experience (Ni et al. 1999, Morrow et al. 2005, Morrow 2007, Dunbar et al. 2008, Moser & Watkins 2008).

Those who are unable to make judicious decisions will have a more difficult time engaging in good selfcare practices. Focused attention and working memory capacity are required to perceive and process information prior to the selection and execution of a course of action. Individuals with limited attention and memory have diminished ability to understand and reflect and thus may struggle with, or be unable to perform, self care; for example, those with severe psychiatric illness may have difficulty performing independent self care (Riegel et al. 2012).

Likely more relevant to traumatic scar clients, situational influences on attention and memory such as certain medications, sleep deprivation or emotional stress can interfere with self care. In these situations, some degree of shared care, dependent care or community support may be needed (Lim & Dinges 2008, Naue 2008, Riegel et al. 2012).

In addition to support from family, friends, social and support groups, another consideration for improved client engagement in selfcare behaviors includes the use of mobile technology for access to information or to reinforce any self/homecare recommendations – technology considerations are covered in more detail later in this chapter (Bodenheimer 2003, Zwar et al. 2006, Kennedy et al. 2013).

Strategies to Facilitate Engagement

How can we present, phrase or demonstrate a selfcare measure in a way that the client will embrace it and engage, rather than view or interpret it as 'one more thing' to add to their already long list of instructions from their healthcare provider(s)? How can we inspire clients to invest, engage or *buy-in*? It has been the authors' experience that the therapist's level of commitment and interest in a client's wellbeing serves to inspire his/her own self-caring behaviors.

Communication: Encouragement and Empowerment

Encouragement, an effective extrinsic motivator, serves to inspire and bolster one's confidence and stimulate engagement. Encourage your clients to take responsibility – and credit – for what they feel, learn and apply as a result of their work with you. The old adage applies: *give someone a fish and they eat for a day, teach them to fish and they eat for a lifetime.*

Generating client interest in how their body works and how to best care for themselves can facilitate improved self-sufficiency. Self-sufficiency further bolsters confidence and a sense of empowerment, culminating in heightened engagement in selfcare behaviors.

In order to function well, ongoing care may be the reality for some traumatic scar clients. However, self-management, as much as possible, is the ultimate goal, and therefore it is important to establish the MT as facilitator not *fixer*. It serves no good purpose for any client to become dependent, as dependency erodes empowerment.

Although the healthcare provider is instrumental in identifying relevant selfcare measures, it is equally important to encourage clients to discover for themselves what they need to change or do to improve their situation.

In terms of client self/home care, as professional guide or facilitator, the therapist's responsibility is to provide information or guidance in an objective manner. It is the client's prerogative to make choices based on the information that has been provided – the very essence of informed choice.

As healthcare professionals, MTs are required to fully inform clients about proposed plans so the client can make an informed choice about the course of their care.

In addition to meeting professional requirements, information sharing with the client can serve to bolster their sense of empowerment, as information sharing provides the client with an opportunity to understand and weigh options and make choices.

Empowerment ensures the opportunity to act in accordance with one's values and interests, thereby supporting autonomy and a greater sense of feeling in control of matters pertaining to one's health and wellbeing. When one feels empowered, they are more likely to engage in a particular selfcare measure. **Empowerment drives change**.

Technology

No-one moves a muscle these days (pun intended) without consulting a device. Our device-driven world does have its benefits, and this is certainly true in healthcare.

There is a fundamental shift in healthcare systems around the world, facilitated by the emphasis placed on self-management and technological possibilities. Health and wellness information and measures can be accessed via the Internet and are often free, thereby reducing cost and increasing the availability to a larger population base (Bradway et al. 2015).

Various health apps, have taken significant strides in overcoming many of the barriers that patients have to self-management, including usability, relevance to the patient's lifestyle, compliance and understanding of their injury/impairment through readily available and recurrent viewing. Additionally, studies have shown that patients believe that this option is effective in increasing their sense of control over their situation and such tools help empower the patient and support their ability to enter into a more informed conversation with their healthcare provider. An informed client and collaborative care approach strengthens the therapeutic relationship (Tatara et al. 2013, Bradway et al. 2015).

Clinical Consideration

The authors utilize personal device technology to help reinforce or support the provision of client self or homecare instructions. Instead of providing verbal instructions at the end of a treatment session and/or static handouts with exercise illustrations, the client is encouraged to audio- or video-record any self/homecare measures so that they can review as often as needed. The authors have noticed a notable shift in compliance and/or engagement with clients who have video-taped 'how to', a homecare measure on their smartphone. The authors also admit to YouTube usage, as there are some great informative presentations and exercise, *how to*, clips available. Clients tend to welcome professionally scrutinized and useful links.

Relevancy

In addition to the judicious use of technology, the authors have found that it is helpful to get to know the client a bit before beginning the self/homecare information-sharing process to any great degree. Some clients may be eager for information and/or measures while others may require a more gradual or minimalistic introduction or approach.

The authors suggest refraining from providing extensive client self/homecare measures after the initial treatment, with the exception of basic measures to facilitate the treatment or minimize the possibility of post-treatment soreness.

Getting to know the client a bit better will provide valuable insight as to how best to communicate or present selfcare measures. Recall as students, some of us show a preference for visual, auditory, kinesthetic or tactile learning; this applies to clients as well.

Research may support that a particular measure derives the best outcome; however, if the client views the measure as irrelevant or unrealistic, the likelihood of engagement is highly … unlikely. Simply telling the client that a particular measure is supported by research or will be helpful for them may not work for every client. This calls upon the therapist to be creative.

Discover your client's interests and utilize your own creativity to present the information in a manner that somehow relates to the client's interests or to a relevant meme. Or devise a compelling analogy, for example: a car engine requires oil to lubricate moving parts in order to reduce friction – our bodies require proper hydration to serve the same purpose.

Providing information in a manner that is interesting, understandable and meaningful (i.e. seems to make sense to the client) will nurture client self-interest and stimulate a change in behavior. Change begins with awareness.

Also, as noted, it is always best to keep client self- and homecare measures uncomplicated and easy to integrate into daily life.

Client Self/Home Care

The usual spectrum of self/homecare measures apply to traumatic scar clients. Each individual will require individual consideration and recommendations. Basic protocol guidelines include:

- Identify the client's needs and goals and what might facilitate the MT treatments

- Prioritize: generally begin with, or provide measures for, what the client identifies as the most troublesome; or begin with a measure that is sure to derive a benefit as this can serve to inspire the client

- Keep it simple, address each issue individually.

Client self care to be administered at home may include injury and care education, various exercises, and other measures taken following treatment to facilitate the work or reduce the incidence of post-treatment discomfort (e.g. heat or cold applications and adequate hydration). No specific measure, other than general post-treatment care and relaxation measures, will be covered in depth in this book as each could justify a book of its own.

The techniques, as described in this book, do not have to be painful to be productive – this includes both during and post-treatment. However, it is not unusual for a bit of tenderness or mild post-treatment soreness to occur in some instances. Make your clients aware of this. And, if they experience atypical soreness (e.g. moderate to intense pain), ask them to call and let you know so you can document it in their file and figure out why an atypical response occurred. And, so that you can suggest appropriate client selfcare measures to address the atypical soreness (e.g. heat or cold application, client-directed pain management options).

Thermal and Cryotherapy

It is suggested that the therapist adhere to MT competency standards and common protocol for hot/cold applications. And be mindful of any client specific precautions or contraindications (CIs) to hot or cold applications.

As discussed in Chapter 9, following the skin/CT and myofascial techniques covered in this book, the client will generally benefit from heat application in the therapeutic range. Readily available, cold application is an effective and cost-effective analgesic, with virtually no side-effects when administered properly, and no CIs to cold exist.

Relaxation Measures

Various relaxation measures are commonly employed during treatment and can be utilized as a form of client self/home care. These include:

- Heat application

- Deep/relaxed breathing

- Muscle relaxation techniques.

Clinical Consideration

The authors suggest a certain amount of caution with using the phrases *relax, just relax, I need you to relax*, or any derivative. *Telling* a client to relax may only serve to increase any feelings of anxiety or cause the client to feel like they are doing something wrong. A more productive approach may be to gently touch or hold where the therapist can see that the client is tensioning; for example, when working around a client's neck you may observe them bring his/her shoulder(s) forward/elevate the shoulder off the table if they are supine. By gently placing one hand on an elevated shoulder, more often than not, the client will register the somatic information and self-adjust.

Deep/Relaxed Breathing

Vital to life and a cornerstone of most MT practices are relaxed breathing techniques.

Deep or relaxed breathing is known by several different names such as diaphragmatic breathing, abdominal breathing, belly breathing and paced respiration (Harvard Health Publications 2015).

When you breathe deeply, the air coming in through your nose fully fills your lungs and the lower belly rises. Deep breathing may seem abnormal to some, leading to *chest breathing* – shallow breathing from the chest which increases tension and anxiety (Harvard Health Publications 2015).

Shallow breathing restricts the diaphragm's range of motion. The deepest part of the lungs do not receive a full share of oxygenated air, which can make the client feel short of breath and anxious.

Deep abdominal breathing encourages full oxygen exchange which, in turn, helps to slow the heartbeat and lower or stabilize blood pressure (Harvard Health Publications 2015).

At this juncture, careful consideration should be given to what is within our scope of practice, such as relaxation breathing methods and simple exercises. Also within our scope is encouragement, demonstrating measurable positive outcomes and staying current with research on scar management.

Muscle Relaxation Techniques

Muscle relaxation techniques can be incorporated into a treatment session or can be recommended as client self/homecare and generally relaxed breathing is performed simultaneously.

Progressive muscle relaxation (PMR), developed by Jacobson, involves the sequential tensing and releasing of major skeletal muscle groups with the aim of inducing relaxation by promoting awareness of tension in skeletal muscles

(Jacobson 1938, Cooke 2013). Bernstein and Borkovec (Bernstein et al. 2000) developed a shortened, modified and most commonly used form of PMR.

Simple tense/release involves one muscle or muscle group.

It is thought that mind–body therapies, such as PMR, induce a relaxation response by altering SNS activity, which in turn results in a decrease in pulse rate, blood pressure and musculoskeletal tone, and altered neuroendocrine function. It has been suggested that deep somatic restfulness and muscular relaxation reduces anxiety and physical arousal (Campos de Carvalho et al. 2007, Payne & Donaghy 2010, Cooke 2013).

Nutrition and other wound care considerations

Nutritional counselling or guidance is not typically within the MT scope of practice. The information provided is simply meant to inform the MT about the role of certain macronutrients (proteins, fat and carbohydrates) and micronutrients (vitamins, minerals and trace elements) in wound healing and inflammation and pain management.

Nutrition is known to significantly influence successful wound healing outcomes. The exuberant cellular and biochemical events that constitute the wound-healing cascade require energy, amino acids, oxygen, metals, trace minerals and vitamins for successful completion. Certain nutritional deficiencies can impact wound healing by impeding fibroblast proliferation, collagen synthesis, and epithelialization (Blass et al. 2012).

During wound healing, adequate protein intake supports the healthy formation of tissue fibers (e.g. collagen and elastin). Adequate intake of healthy carbohydrates provides the body with the energy needed to facilitate processes, and healthy fatty acids enable the formation of prostaglandins, which mediate physiological inflammation in the early stages and help control inflammation later on. Various vitamins, trace minerals and elements are also essential for new formation of stable new tissue (Geiersperger 2009, Van den Berg 2010). Van den Berg (2012) notes that acidic pH retards fibroblast function, which in turn can reduce healing efficiency.

According to Blass and colleagues, the supplementation of antioxidant micronutrients and glutamine is associated with accelerated wound closure (Blass et al. 2012).

As noted in Chapter 2, Vitamin C has been identified as an import component in the formation of healthy cross-links, therefore adequate intake during tissue remodeling following exercise and trauma is an important consideration (Boyera et al. 1998).

Capsaicin, found in hot peppers, is well-known and widely used in pain management.

Essential fatty acids, and certain culinary spices and herbs, fruits and vegetables and beverages have been shown to contain anti-inflammatory properties. Whereas foods containing arachidonic acid (e.g. dairy and meat fats) stimulate inflammation (Hankenson & Hankenson, 2012).

Other Wound care Considerations

Although these are not part of MT care, they are commonly used in wound care and therefore warrant mention for information purposes.

Silicone gel and silicone sheeting

Silicone gel and sheeting are commonly used in wound dressing as a means to improve the appearance and texture and/or feel of scars.

Although the exact mechanism of the action of silicone is not known, proposed mechanisms include increases in temperature and collagenase activity, increased hydration, and polarization of the scar tissue leading to scar shrinkage. Other proposed benefits include a reduction in the production of pro-inflammatory agents, such as

TGF-β2, redness, pain and itching, and improved scar elasticity (Berman et al. 2007, Janis & Harrison 2014).

Topical onion extract

Onion extract is a common ingredient in some over-the-counter scar management products – demonstrating improved dermal collagen organization, but no reduction in scar hypertrophy or scar elevation. When compared with a petrolatum-based ointment there was no difference in scar erythema, hypertrophy, or overall cosmetic appearance (Saulis et al. 2002, Chung et al. 2006).

Medicinal honey

The use of honey for medicinal purposes dates back to the ancient Greeks and Egyptians.

Honey offers an affordable, effective topical treatment for wounds, shown to facilitate healing and suppress microbial proliferation. Honey's antibacterial effects are attributed to its acidity, hydrogen peroxide content and high osmolality. Multiple studies have reported on its infection-fighting effectiveness, citing complete resolution of methicillin-resistant *Staphylococcus aureus* with its use.

Meta-analysis supports the greater efficacy of honey compared with alternative dressings. The exact amount of honey needed for antibiosis and wound healing is unknown and the composition and geographical origin of the honey may influence its medicinal value (Blaser et al. 2007, Gethin & Cowman 2008, Mandal & Mandal 2011, Hanazaki et al. 2009, Wijesinghe et al. 2009, Al-Waili et al. 2011, Lee et al. 2011, Janis & Harrison 2014).

Therapist Self Care

Simply put, practice what we advocate: make wise nutritional choices, adequately hydrate, engage in regular exercise, get adequate rest and apply the rule of *moderation*.

As noted in the opening of this chapter, both the physicality of the work and empathetic demands can take a toll if not well managed. Sadly, attrition is high in our profession and so good body mechanics and sound selfcare measures, out of the gate, are essential to career longevity.

Wise Use of Your Body

It is not essential to be muscularly strong to do this work. Proper body mechanics factor into technique effectiveness and will minimize potential strain and over-use injury.

Appropriate positioning of the therapist's and the client's body, use of gravity, control of the therapist's body and body weight can all be used to apply pressure rather than being reliant on hand and upper body strength.

In addition to potential injury, if your own body is distressed chances are so is your mind and you will have greater difficulty being 'in the present' to what you are palpating/feeling and delivering in the form of treatment. As noted in Chapter 9, if during treatment you cannot seem to find a position that feels comfortable to your body, pause and change your position – or you may need to ask the client to change position. Be ever mindful of your positioning and at no time compromise your own comfort or wellbeing.

Myofascial techniques require the use of your hands and body in ways that differ from some of the other techniques (e.g. lymphatic, nerve sedating and fluid movement). Much like a graded exercise program, it will reduce the incidence of injury; the same applies for new or different techniques. If new to you, it is prudent to gradually introduce the myofascial techniques into your treatments.

Train yourself to use your left and right hands/ arms as equally as possible. Use various points of contact (i.e. various aspects of your body to make contact with your clients) throughout the treatment. Change your point of contact often (e.g. fingers, knuckles, base of palm, thenar, hypothenar eminence, forearm, elbow etc.).

Box 10.2

Tips for reducing work related injury and burnout

- Develop the habit of checking in with your own body during treatment, be mindful of your alignment (feet, back, shoulders, arms/hands and neck) and breathing

- Pace yourself: be mindful of your energy output during each treatment and establish a daily/ weekly treatment schedule that you can maintain with relative ease over the lifespan of your practice

- Take periodic breaks during the treatment (change positioning and how you are using your hands, fingers etc., take a sip of water)

- Allow for some rest time between appointments

- Receive MT treatment on a regular basis

- Regularly engage in restorative, supportive, bio-mechanically enhancing forms of activity or exercise, something that helps to balance the demands associated with this profession

- Learn and utilize more than one approach or technique style, this helps reduce the risk of over-use injury and burnout

- Be a lifelong learner, be intrigued and energized by what you learn

- Keep the work meaningful and inspiring!

Be flexible in your approach as it may take some adjusting to figure out the positioning that will be the most effective for you and your client.

Empathy Strain and Burnout

Empathy, an appreciation for the feelings and emotions of others, involves a certain amount of cognitive and emotional effort. Empathy strain refers to a healthcare provider's overextension of psychological resources, contributing to burnout and, for some, even causing emotional pain (Weiner & Auster 2007).

Burnout describes the physical and emotional exhaustion that MTs can experience when they have low job satisfaction or feel overwhelmed by their work or workload.

There are a few guiding principles to gauge empathy strain and investigate if you are feeling burnout (Khalsa 2008):

- Are you a caregiver or caretaker? Caregiving (what is provided by a healthcare professional) is the giving of treatment and aid to a client with no obligation to produce certain results. Caretaking (or taking over care of a person who cannot provide for himself or herself) often derives from the therapist's need to be needed and is a fast road to burnout.

- Changes in eating or sleeping patterns (over- or undereating, difficulty sleeping, over sleeping or no motivation to get up in the morning)

- Feelings of depression and helplessness

- Ongoing and persistent fatigue

- Withdrawal from social contacts or activities (e.g. regular exercise).

If you recognize any of the above symptoms, take action to get your life back on the path to balance. Find the one thing you enjoyed doing and begin again. Build the time into your schedule for you. And when necessary, seek professional assistance. There is no shame in asking for help; our profession asks much of us.

Just Say NO

Providing care for our clients is an important responsibility; however, when your appointment book is filled with the maximum amount of clients you can physically and mentally handle, trying to squeeze in one more may tip the balance.

Saying no for some may not be easy but *sometimes No is the best/healthier answer, to support stress relief and life balance.* Being overloaded is individual. Just because other MTs can juggle more doesn't mean you should be able to or have to. Only you can know what is too much for you.

Box 10.3

A reflection on reasons for saying no (Mayo, 2013)

- **Saying no isn't selfish**. Saying no to a new commitment is honoring your existing obligations and can make certain that you can devote high quality time to them. Quality of life is as important to the therapist's wellbeing as it is to the client.

- **Always saying yes isn't healthy**. When you are overcommitted and under a lot of stress, you may feel run-down which can contribute to getting sick.

- **Saying yes can cut others out**. By saying no, you give the opportunity to other therapists or care providers. This can build your and your client's interprofessional network.

Learning to say *no* appropriately is an important part of managing professional boundaries and managing your stress-load. Take into account the following guidelines when deciding what is best for you (Mayo Clinic 2013):

- Weigh your obligations and priorities before making any new commitments. If the new client will benefit from your work, and your schedule will allow, then schedule them in. If not, refer out.

- Weigh time commitment demands. Is the new client a short- or long-term commitment? For example, if the healthcare team feels therapeutic scar management is needed for 6 weeks, can you accommodate the client weekly for that amount of time? If the client is long term – 6 months or more – can you make arrangements for the amount of time to properly care for the client's needs? This includes any paperwork involved in the patient's care. Don't say yes if it will mean months of burdensome stress. Your burnout serves no good purpose.

- Guilt should not be part of the equation. Don't agree to a take on a new client out of guilt or obligation. Agreeing will likely lead to additional stress and resentment every time you see the client on your schedule.

- Sleep on it. If you have a compressed schedule, take a day to think about the request and how it fits in with your current commitments before you respond to the client. If you can't sleep on it, at least take the time to think the request through before answering.

- Just say no, when no is the right answer. Provide a brief, professional, explanation when stating your reason for declining to take someone on as a client or when requested to overextend your regular appointment schedule. Do not offer complex and lengthy justifications or explanations. Provide a referral to another care provider if you can.

- Be honest. The truth is always best. Your integrity should maintain intact when saying no.

- Be ready to repeat. You may need to refuse a request several times before your *no*, is accepted. If that happens, calmly and professionally repeat your no, with or without your original rationale, as needed.

Clinical Consideration

In the authors' experience, a powerful clinical experience is making physical contact with someone's pain for an hour or more. As MTs we make the somatic

Clinical Consideration (Cont.)

connection with our hands on the very spot that hurts – and we receive feedback immediately as we watch our client's face change in that instant.

Such validation and acknowledgment is immeasurably significant to our clients. The experience that someone else feels *it*, not in the same way they do, but a validation none the less. In the authors' experience it is a profound moment when a client has the realization that the therapist acknowledges, 'Yes, I can feel that, too.'

Our ability to physically touch and feel, and our empathy, are powerful elements that contribute to the overall effectiveness of MT.

The work of providing care requires MTs to open their hearts and minds to their clients – unfortunately, this very process of empathy is what can render us vulnerable to being profoundly affected, sometimes negatively, by our work. As noted in Chapter 8, vulnerability is both a powerful part of healing and is potentially risky for client and care provider.

Compassion Fatigue and Indirect Trauma

Fatigue

Compassion fatigue, the *cost of caring for others*, refers to the profound emotional and physical exhaustion that helping professionals and caregivers can develop over the course of their career. The inability to refuel and regenerate can lead to a gradual erosion of all the things that keep us connected to others: our empathy, our hope, and of course our compassion – not only for others but also for ourselves (Figley 1982, Mathieu 2012).

The biggest contributors to compassion fatigue are where you work, your workload, your working conditions and the amount of high quality training you have received in trauma-related care (Mathieu 2012).

When overtaxed by the nature of our work we may begin to show symptoms that are similar to our traumatized clients: difficulty concentrating, intrusive imagery, feeling discouraged about the world, hopelessness, exhaustion, irritability, high attrition and negative outcomes (dispiritedness, cynical outlook, boundary violations) (Mathieu 2012).

Indirect Trauma

Every scar has a story and there is a high likelihood of massage therapists bearing witness to a client's story. Their stories can be horrific and the recounting of them may have lasting impact on both the client and therapist.

Indirect trauma is the cumulative response to working with many trauma survivors over time. The indicators for indirect trauma resemble those of direct trauma (e.g. intrusive imagery, SNS stimulation, anxiety and feeling overwhelmed) and can impact the therapist's personal and professional relationships (ISTSS 2015).

As is the case with trauma survivors, indirect trauma will look and feel different for each person. Some of the characteristics that may contribute to indirect trauma are the therapist's personal history, usual ways of coping with challenge and distress, and current life circumstances (e.g., other stressors, lack of support network) (ISTSS 2015).

Prevention

Ways of coping and current life circumstances can contribute to a greater likelihood of compassion fatigue and indirect trauma. So it goes without saying that taking measures to minimize stressors, develop effective stress coping skills and build solid, personal and professional, support networks are important preventative measures.

The therapist's way of working with survivors may contribute to or diminish the incidence of compassion fatigue and indirect trauma. For example, managing boundaries effectively can help protect the therapist from compassion fatigue indirect trauma. The importance of professional boundaries for the sake of client safety and therapist wellbeing cannot be emphasized enough.

Care for the care provider

It is important to be able to recognize indicators of compassion fatigue indirect trauma, as awareness is the first step toward change.

Any professional working with trauma survivors can benefit from identifying specific difficulties, assessing the contributing factors, targeting specific steps to take, and getting support from friends or colleagues in taking those steps (ISTSS 2015).

Compassion fatigue and indirect trauma can be addressed by attending to basic self care: work-life balance, ensuring quality time for play and rest. Healthy nutritional practices and regular exercise are also essential.

Additionally, massage therapists can benefit from appropriate professional training, connection with their colleagues, ongoing consultation for their work, and a place to talk about their experience of indirect trauma and, when necessary, professional assistance.

Finally, it is essential to embrace or restore meaning and hope. Each individual must find ways to connect with whatever in life is meaningful and gives purpose for that person (ISTSS 2015).

References

Ajzen I, Fishbein M (2005) The influence of attitudes on behavior. In: Albarracin D, Johnson BT, Zanna MP, eds. The handbook of attitudes. Hillsdale NJ: Lawrence Erlbaum Associates.

Al-Waili NS, Salom K, Butler G, Al Ghamdi AA (2011) Honey and microbial infections: a review supporting the use of honey for microbial control. Journal of Medicinal Food 14: 1079–1096.

Berman B, Perez OA, Konda S et al (2007) A review of the biologic effects, clinical efficacy, and safety of silicone elastomer sheeting for hypertrophic and keloid scar treatment and management. Dermatologic Surgery 33: 1291–1302; discussion 1302.

Bernstein DA, Borkovec TD, Hazlett-Stevens H (2000) New directions in progressive relaxation training: a guidebook for helping professionals. Westport CT: Praeger.

Blaser G, Santos K, Bode U et al (2007) Effect of medical honey on wounds colonised or infected with MRSA. Journal of Wound Care 16: 325–328.

Blass SC, Goost H, Tolba RH et al (2012) Time to wound closure in trauma patients with disorders in wound healing is shortened by supplements containing antioxidant micronutrients and glutamine: a PRCT. Clinical Nutrition 31(4): 469–475.

Bodenheimer T (2003) Interventions to improve chronic illness care: evaluating their effectiveness. Disease management 6: 63–71.

Boyera N, Galey I, Bernard B (1998) Effect of vitamin C and its derivatives on collagen synthesis and cross-linking by normal human fibroblasts. International Journal of Cosmetic Science 20(3): 151-158. Available from: MEDLINE with Full Text, Ipswich, MA. [Accessed 4 November 2014].

Bradway M, Årsand E, Grøttland A (2015) Mobile health: empowering patients and driving change. Trends in Endocrinology and Metabolism 26(3): 114–117.

Campos de Carvalho E, Martins FT, dos Santos CB (2007) A pilot study of a relaxation technique for management of nausea and vomiting in patients receiving cancer chemotherapy. Cancer Nursing. 2007; 30(2): 163–167.

Chung VQ, Kelley L, Marra D, Jiang SB (2006) Onion extract gel versus petrolatum emollient on new surgical scars: Prospective double-blinded study. Dermatologic Surgery 32: 193–197.

Cooke H (2013) CAM-Cancer Consortium. Progressive muscle relaxation [online document]. Available at: http://www.cam-cancer.org/CAM-Summaries/Mind-body-interventions/Progressive-Muscle-Relaxation. December 17 [Accessed 8 March 2015].

Dahl O, Wickman M, Wengström Y (2012) Adapting to life after burn injury – reflections on care. Journal of Burn Care and Research 33(5): 595–605.

Davidson PM, Macdonald P, Moser DK et al (2007) Cultural diversity in heart failure management: findings from the DISCOVER study (Part 2). Contemporary nurse: a journal for the Australian nursing profession. May–Jun 25(1-2): 50–61.

Dickson VV, Deatrick JA, Riegel B (2008) A typology of heart failure self-care management in non-elders. European Journal of Cardiovascular Nursing 7(3): 171–181.

Dickson VV, Buck H, Riegel B (2011) A qualitative meta-analysis of heart failure self-care practices among individuals with multiple comorbid conditions. Journal of Cardiac Failure. May 17(5): 413–419.

Diego AM, Serghiou M, Padmanabha A et al (2012) Exercise training after burn injury: a survey of practice. Journal of Burn Care and Research, 34(6), e311-7.

Dunbar SB, Clark PC, Quinn C et al (2008) Family influences on heart failure self-care and outcomes. Journal of Cardiovascular Nursing 23: 258–265.

Ekman I, Ehnfors M, Norberg A (2000) The meaning of living with severe chronic heart failure as narrated by elderly people. Scandinavian Journal of Caring Sciences 14(2): 130–136.

Figley CR (1982) Traumatization and comfort: close relationships may be hazardous to your health. Keynote presentation at conference, 'Families and close relationships: individuals in social interaction'. Lubbock, TX: Texas Tech University.

Geiersperger K (2009) Wundheilung und Ernahrung. Master Theisis fur der Universitatslehrgang fur sports physiotherapy. Paris Lodron Universitat – Abteilung Sportwissenschaften.

Gethin G, Cowman S (2008) Bacteriological changes in sloughy venous leg ulcers treated with manuka honey or hydrogel: an RCT. J Wound Care 17: 241–244, 246.

Gullick JG, Taggart SB, Johnston RA, Ko N (2014) The trauma bubble: patient and family experience of serious burn injury. Journal of Burn Care and Research 35(6): e413–e427.

Hanazaki K, Maeda H, Okabayashi T (2009) Relationship between perioperative glycemic control and postoperative infections. World Journal of Gastroenterology 15: 4122–4125.

Hankenson, Hankenson (2012) Nutrition model to reduce inflammation in musculoskeletal and joint diseases. In: Schleip R, Findley T, Chaitow L, Huijing P (eds) Fascia: the tensional network of the human body. Edinburgh: Churchill Livingstone Elsevier, Ch. 7.23, pp 457–464.

Harvard Health Publications (2015) Relaxation techniques: Breath control helps quell errant stress response. Available at: http://www.health.harvard.edu/mind-and-mood/relaxation-techniques-breath-control-helps-quell-errant-stress-response. [Accessed 2 June 2015].

Holbrook TL, Anderson JP, Sieber WJ et al (1999) Outcome after major trauma:12-month and 18-month follow-up results from the Trauma Recovery Project. Journal of Trauma and Acute Care Surgery 46(5): 765–773.

Holman H, Lorig K (2004) Patient self-management: a key to effectiveness and efficiency in care of chronic disease. Public Health Reports 119(3): 239.

ISTSS (2015) International Society for Traumatic Stress Studies. Available at: http://www.istss.org/

SelfCareForProviders/5189.htm [Accessed 10 February 2015].

Jacobson E (1938) Progressive relaxation. Chicago: University of Chicago Press.

Janis J, Harrison B (2014) Wound healing: part II. Clinical applications. Plastic and Reconstructive Surgery 133(3): 383e–392e.

Kennedy A, Bower P, Reeves D et al (2013) Implementation of self-management support for long term conditions in routine primary care settings: cluster randomised controlled trial. British Medical Journal 346, f2882.

Khalsa KPS (2008) Taking care of yourself. Available at: http://www.massagetherapy.com/articles/index.php/article_id/1589/Taking-Care-of-Yourself.

Korn L (2013) Keynote: Somatic empathy - restoring community health with massage. Lecture notes from the International Massage Therapy Research Conference. Boston, MA, April 25–27.

Lee DS, Sinno S, Khachemoune A (2011) Honey and wound healing: an overview. American Journal of Clinical Dermatology 12: 181–190.

Lim J, Dinges DF (2008) Sleep deprivation and vigilant attention. Annals of the New York Academy of Sciences 1129: 305–322.

Lucini D, Di Fede G, Parati G, Pagani M (2005) Impact of chronic psychosocial stress on autonomic cardiovascular regulation in otherwise healthy subjects. Hypertension 46(5): 1201–1206.

Malmstrom RK, Roine RP, Heikkila A et al (2008) Cost analysis and health-related quality of life of home and self-care satellite haemodialysis. Nephrology, dialysis, transplantation: official publication of the European Dialysis and Transplant Association - European Renal Association. Jun 23(6): 1990–1996.

Mandal MD and Mandal S (2011) Honey: its medicinal property and antibacterial activity. Asian Pacific Journal of Tropical Biomedicine 1(2): 154–160.

Mathieu F (2012) The compassion fatigue workbook: creative tools for transforming compassion fatigue and vicarious traumatization. New York: Routledge.

Morrow DG, Weiner M, Young J et al (2005) Improving medication knowledge among older adults with heart failure: a patient-centered approach to instruction design. The Gerontologist 45: 545–552.

Morrow DG (2007) Patients' health literacy and experience with instructions: Influence preferences for heart failure medication instructions. Journal of Aging and Health 19: 575–593.

Moser DK, Watkins JF (2008) Conceptualizing self-care in heart failure: a life course model of patient characteristics. The Journal of Cardiovascular Nursing 23:205.

Mayo Clinic (2013) Stress management. Available at: http://www.mayoclinic.org/healthy-living/stress-management/in-depth/stress-relief/art-20044494 [Accessed 2 June 2015].

Naue U (2008) 'Self-care without a self': Alzheimer's disease and the concept of personal responsibility for health. Medicine, Health Care and Philosophy 11(3): 315–324.

Ni H, Nauman D, Burgess D et al (1999) Factors influencing knowledge of and adherence to self-care among patients with heart failure. Archives of Internal Medicine 159: 1613–1619.

Orem D (2001) Nursing concepts of practice. Philadelphia: Mosby, Elsevier.

Payne R, Donaghy M (2010) Payne's Handbook of relaxation techniques: a practical guide for the health care professional, 4th edn. London: Churchill Livingstone Elsevier.

Riegel B, Jaarsma T, Strömberg A (2012) A middle-range theory of self-care of chronic illness. Advances in Nursing Science 35(3): 194–204.

Saulis AS, Mogford JH, Mustoe TA (2002) Effect of Mederma on hypertrophic scarring in the rabbit ear model. Plastic and Reconstructive Surgery 110: 177–183; discussion 184–186.

Tatara N, Årsand E, Stein Olav Skrøvseth SO, Hartvigsen G (2013) Long-term engagement with a mobile self-management system for people with type 2 diabetes. JMIR Mhealth Uhealth 1, e1.

Van den Berg F (2010) Angewandte physiologie – Band 1: Das bindegewebe des bewegunfsapparates; verstehen und beeinflussen [Applied Physiology – vol. 1; The connective tissue of the locomotor apparatus; understanding and influencing]. Stuttgart: Thieme Verlag.

Van den Berg F (2012) In: Schleip R, Findley T, Chaitow L, Huijing P (eds) Fascia: the tensional network of the human body. Edinburgh: Churchill Livingstone Elsevier, pp 149–155.

Van der Wal MH, Jaarsma T, Moser DK et al (2010) Qualitative examination of compliance in heart failure patients in The Netherlands. Heart Lung 39(2): 121–130.

Weiner SJ, Auster S (2007) From empathy to caring: defining the ideal approach to a healing relationship. Yale Journal of Biology and Medicine 80: 123–130.

Wijesinghe M, Weatherall M, Perrin K, Beasley R (2009) Honey in the treatment of burns: a systematic review and meta-analysis of its efficacy. New Zealand Medical Journal 122:47–60.

Zwar N, Harris M, Griffiths R et al (2006) A systematic review of chronic disease management. Canberra: Australian Primary Health Care Research Institute.

Resources and further reading
Scar patient support networks/organizations

American Burn Association: www.ameriburn.org

Spiegel Burn Foundation: www.spiegelburnfoundation.com

Phoenix Society for Burn Survivors: www.phoenix-society.org

National Lymphatic Network: www.lymphnet.org

For the therapist

AMTA Selfcare Tips: http://www.amtamassage.org/career_guidance/type/7?utm_source=%2fselfcaretips&utm_medium=web&utm_campaign=redirect

Body Mechanics for the Massage Therapist: http://www.amtamassage.org/courses/detail.html?CourseId=36

Salvo SG (2015) Body mechanics, client positioning, and draping. In: Salvo S (ed) Massage Therapy: Principles and Practice, 5th edn. St Louis: Elsevier, pp 112.

Appendix Massage therapy research resources

Research databases and repositories

The following resources provide massage therapy research or are research informed:

BioMed Central – peer-reviewed journals: http://www.biomedcentral.com/browse/journals

CaseRe3: Case Report Research Repository: http://www.casere3.org/about-casere3/

Cochrane Collaboration: http://www.cochrane.org/

Evidence Informed Massage Therapy Facebook page: https://www.facebook.com/massage.evidence

IN-CAM Health Outcomes Database: http://www.incamresearch.ca/content/welcome-cam-health-outcomes-database

Massage Net – online research network: http://www.massagenet.org

Massage Therapy Foundation (MTF): http://www.massagetherapyfoundation.org/research-agenda

National Center for Complementary and Alternative Medicine (NCCAM):

http://www.nccam.nih.gov

PedCAM: http://www.pedcam.ca

PubMed: http://www.ncbi.nlm.nih.gov/pubmed/

Touch Research Institute: http://www6.miami.edu/touch-research/TRIP database: www.tripdatabase.com

It is important to note that many of the more robust professional MT associations provide access to large online research databases as part of the membership benefit (e.g. PubMed, MerckMedicus, Biomed Central, Medscape and the Cochrane Collaboration).

Massage therapy (and related) research organizations

Massage Therapy Foundation: http://www.massagetherapyfoundation.org/

IN-CAM Research Network: http://www.incamresearch.ca

International Society for Complementary Medicine Research (ISCMR): http://www.iscmr.org/

Fascia Research Society: https://fasciaresearchsociety.org/fascia-research-congress

National Center for Complementary and Alternative Medicine: (NCCAM): https://nccih.nih.gov/health/massage

Conferences

Massage Therapy Research Conferences

International Massage Therapy Research Conference: http://www.massagetherapyfoundation.org/research-conference

MTAS Interdisciplinary Research Symposium (held annually): http://www.saskmassagetherapy.com/index.php

Conferences which include massage therapy research

IN-CAM Research Symposium http://www.incamresearch.ca/

International Congress on Complementary Medicine: http://www.iccmr2015.org/

International Fascia Research Congress: http://www.fasciacongress.org/2015/

International Research Congress on Complementary and Integrative Health: http://www.icimh.org/

Funding for massage therapy research

Massage Therapy Foundation Grants: http://www.massagetherapyfoundation.org/grants-and-contests/

Massage Therapy Research Fund: http://www.incamresearch.ca/content/massage-therapy-research-fund-mtrf

Additionally, some professional MT associations provide research grants available to their members.

Books

Menard MB (2009) Making sense of research. Toronto: Curties-Overzet Publications

Dryden T, Moyer C (2012) Massage therapy: integrating research and practice. Champaign, IL: Human Kinetics

Andrade CK (2013) Outcome-based massage: putting evidence into practice. Baltimore: Lippincott Williams & Wilkins

Journals and magazines

International Journal of Therapeutic Massage and Bodywork: http://www.ijtmb.org/index.php/ijtmb/issue/archive

Journal of Bodywork and Movement Therapies: http://www.journals.elsevier.com/journal-of-bodywork-and-movement-therapies/

Journal of Burn Care and Research: http://journals.lww.com/burncareresearch/pages/default.aspx

Journal of Wound Care: http://info.journalofwoundcare.com/

Massage and Bodywork: http://www.massageandbodywork.com/

Massage Therapy Canada Magazine: http://www.massagetherapycanada.com

Massage Therapy Journal: http://www.amtamassage.org/articles/3/mtj/index.html

Massage Today: http://www.massagetoday.com

Research literacy courses

It is imperative that massage therapists are research literate. Many (entry to practice) MT training and education programs do not include research literacy in the entrance requirements and so this is an important continuing education consideration. Here are a couple of excellent online courses:

Massage Therapy Foundation – the basics of research literacy: http://www.massagetherapyfoundation.org/research-literacy-courses/

University of California – Understanding Research, An Overview for Health Professionals: https://www.coursera.org/course/researchforhealth

INDEX